Knapsacks and Roses

Knapsacks and Roses

Montana's Women Veterans of World War I

EDWARD E. SAUNDERS

Copyright and Library of Congress Information

Knapsacks and Roses

© 2018 Edward E. Saunders, all rights reserved
Published by Edward E. Saunders; Laurel, Yellowstone County, Montana, 59044

No part of this book may be reproduced in any written, electronic, recording, or photocopying form without written permission of the author, Edward E. Saunders.

Emily Dickinson quote from "Collected Poems of Emily Dickinson," first published as "Poems," 1890.

Paperbound ISBN: 978-0-9973265-1-2
Interior and cover design by the publisher

First edition
First paperbound printing, 2018
Printed and bound in the USA

1. Montana. 2. World War I. 3. Women veterans. 4. Veterans affairs.
5. Nurses. 6. Nursing. 7. History.

Type setting in Adobe Garamond Pro. Robert Slimbach designed Garmond Pro for Adobe Systems. Font released in 1989.

*To America's women
veterans, who served well
the cause of freedom.*

"*We never know how high we are
Till we are called to rise;
And then, if we are true to plan,
Our statures touch the skies.*"

- Emily Dickinson

CONTENTS

ILLUSTRATIONS viii

FOREWORD ix

ACKNOWLEDGMENTS xii

INTRODUCTION xiv

1. A TRAIN CAME TO GLASGOW: "The Hope and Promise" 1

2. LUCY'S TICKET: "No parades for them" 12

3. THE DRAFT: "I enlisted, I wasn't drafted" 28

4: FRONTIER NURSING: "Angels under the big sky" 41

5: THE PROFESSION OF CARE: "Calamities and war" 56

6. THE YEOMANETTES: "The keys of victory" 70

7. THE CALL: "Clouds of war reach Montana" 87

8. A TELEGRAM FROM MARGARET: "Help that wouldn't come" 102

9. THE GREAT FALLS SIX: "Thick or thin, hell or high water" 121

10. GOING ACROSS: "The only cowards were..." 140

11. OVER THERE: "War becomes real" 166

12. UNDER FIRE: "Into the cauldron" 185

13. GOING HOME: "A veiled pride" 221

EPILOGUE: "Forgotten no more" 237

APPENDIX A: Biographical summary of the women 240

APPENDIX B: Montana towns where the women enrolled 248

APPENDIX C: Alphabetical list of the women WWI veterans 254

NOTES 260

SELECTED BIBLIOGRAPHY 283

INDEX 289

ABOUT THE AUTHOR 297

ILLUSTRATIONS

Cover	Florence Biddles Myers, nurse, Army Nurse Corps, WWI
26.	Glasgow, MT, 5th Street, year 1913
27.	Lucy Walters, nurse, Army Nurse Corps, WWI
27.	Malta, MT, hospital, ca. year 1920
55.	Signatures of nurses of Montana Board of Nursing
86.	Navy yeomen (F), San Francisco, CA
129.	Six graduate nurses, Great Falls, MT
139.	Recruit tents, Fort Riley, KS
139.	Camp Funston, KS, influenza ward
165.	Virginia Flanagan, graduation photograph
165.	Army nurses, gas mask training
215.	Alice H. Ralston, nurse, Army Nurse Corps, WWI
215.	Base Hospital 10, Le Treport, France
216.	Harriet O'Day, nurse, Army Nurse Corps, WWI
216.	Elizabeth Sandelius, nurse, Army Nurse Corps, WWI
217.	Elizabeth Sandelius, War Dept ID
217.	Elizabeth Sandelius, WWI "dog tags"
218.	FT Riley, WWI nurses
218.	U.S. Army horse-drawn ambulance
219.	Field Hospital 112, Cohan, France
219.	Nurses at Field Hospital 112, Cohan, France
220.	Telephone operators, Army Signal Corps
220.	Merle Egan, Army Signal Corps, WWI
234.	Eula B. Butzerin, nurse, Army Nurse Corps, WWI
234.	Frank and Susie Welborn (siblings)
234.	Susie Welborn's AEF ID document
235.	Base Hospital 53, Langres, France
235.	Chateau-Thierry American Cemetery
236.	Eagle Circle Veterans Wall of Remembrance
236.	Regina McIntyre-Early engraved name
239.	Headstone of Florence Ames

FOREWORD

Diane Carlson Evans served as a combat nurse, Army Nurse Corps, Republic of Vietnam, 1968/69. She is co-founder of the Vietnam Women's Memorial Project, and initiated and led the effort to successfully add the Vietnam Women's Memorial to the Vietnam Veterans Memorial in Washington D.C. She has been honored by many national organizations and institutions for her steadfast work.

THE GUNS OF WORLD WAR I RAINED DEATH IN EUROPE one hundred years ago. Alongside America's doughboys, brave women from America volunteered to serve in that frightful conflagration. In history, America has never drafted women to serve in the Armed Forces, they have all volunteered: many knowingly went into harm's way. As an Army nurse, I witnessed and endured a terrible war in Vietnam. Wars differ; I cannot speak of the heartrending destruction in World War I that America's women of the Great War witnessed, nor of the emotional wounds they suffered. But a common thread weaves across history to the war I endured and saw firsthand: especially with the role of women in war.

Ed Saunders' scrupulously researched book tells those differences in vivid detail and with powerful accounts of the sacrificial work of military nurses and other women on America's home front and in the European theater in World War I. This powerful narrative presents the priceless contributions of America's women and those with ties to Montana who, during World War I, volunteered to go where they were desperately needed. They were courageous forerunners of the modern calling of women in the human experience.

Their courage while nursing in disease-infested military hospital wards in America and while facing enemy fire in rudimentary field hospitals on war-torn battle lines in France, showed their fierce dedication to duty wherever found. These women also labored under the mundane chores of important military paperwork, their weapons were typewriters. Their technical skills in war zones ensured telephone calls and messages went through: desperate calls in battle for help and life-saving support.

Knapsacks and Roses reveals triumphs over adversity and lessons that must never fade from America's core. Saunders' book forever preserves the visceral recollection of these gallant women and their untold stories.

I rightfully earned and proudly wear the title, "Army Nurse." *Knapsacks and Roses* adds to the rich legacy of army nurses. Women who served with America's military a century ago were not accorded equality in pay, status, and honor, as with the male soldiers. These women worked under hostile conditions and experienced bloody, wretched circumstances challenging them physically and emotionally. You will learn their names, where they came from, and why they entered military service for the most dangerous and frightening duty on earth. When victory came, these women returned home, mostly alone, from distant war. America rarely shared honors with them. The women faded into history.

America's women in uniform shared agonies in World War I. Saunders gives a voice to the women who left incomparable and compelling stories of service in war. He also helps us understand the spirit in which these women bore their burdens. America no longer has living veterans of World War I. Saunders' exceptional and diligent work found the records of these women, uncovered their past, and provided a galvanizing record of heroines who provided hope where there was little. He tells of women who sacrificed their health and security to save the lives of those who fought for freedom so far from home.

Knapsacks and Roses illustrates the influence of horrific worldwide events upon the personal destinies of Montana women: including the worldwide influenza epidemic of 1918. Saunders gives us a comprehensive history of the times while interweaving the lives of women he determined should never be forgotten.

Saunders, a war veteran himself, has previously said of those in uniform, "Our standard is not in numbers, but in the nobility and human spirit in uniform, which never forgets the price we pay for a free America." This filled my heart. Years ago, in my effort for a memorial to honor America's women military veterans of Vietnam, I was told that a Vietnam Women's Memorial in our nation's capital was irrelevant as "so few of us" served during the Vietnam era. I testified before Congress that this was not about "numbers" but about the immeasurable contribution, the courage, devotion, and tenacity of America's women who served in support of the Armed Forces: many of them saving thousands of lives of America's servicemen and —women in Vietnam and worldwide.

Our numbers in service do not diminish the value of one of the most important contingents in war and in the human endeavor—women.

From the light of the past, and through the eyes and experiences of the women in this book, I believe our next generations, so distant from World War I, will understand the futility and anguish of that terrible war that made the heavens weep sorrowful tears.

These women veterans of World War I represent and personify thousands of other women throughout America who also volunteered to serve. Through Saunders' work, the story of these women is now in the annals of history and is a shining beacon for young women and men everywhere. We owe America's women who walked the path of honor before us, that we will never forget them, their calling, and their devotion to a better world for all. This book helps fulfill that promise.

Diane Carlson Evans
Helena, Montana

ACKNOWLEDGMENTS

DEDICATED MONTANANS WITH PASSION AND FORESIGHT preserve Montana's rich heritage, history, and culture. These people helped immeasurably with this book. Traveling Montana's vast mountains and prairies to visit many county museums and historical societies brought these Montana World War I women veterans to life. Montana's enthusiastic local and state historians have many records, photographs, letters, and artifacts that helped my research.

This book could not have happened without the Montana State Library's Montana Memory Project (MMP), Jennifer Birnel, director. MMP has much publicly available print material, Montana newspapers, photographs, resources, and other contributions. My thanks to the staff at the Montana State Library, Helena, Montana, who helped greatly with my many queries and diligently helped find records and files supporting my research.

I owe much to these Montana county historical societies and museums: Valley County Museum in Glasgow; Phillips County Museum in Malta; Yellowstone Gateway Museum, and Livingston-Park County Library in Livingston; Range Riders Museum, and Miles City Library in Miles City; The History Museum in Great Falls; the Yellowstone County Museum and the LDS Bi-Stake Family History Center, in Billings. To the Billings City Library and the Butte-Silver Bow Library in Butte. To the St. Vincent's Hospital Foundation in Billings for allowing me access to their historical archives. To the Confederated Salish-Kootenai Tribes, Pablo, Montana, whose invaluable assistance helped me identify and prove the first known female WWI veteran from a Montana American Indian tribe.

I found many people still have remarkable artifacts, letters, diaries, and photographs in dusty boxes on closet shelves from their ancestor's service in World War I, and are eagerly willing to share these treasures. My sincere thanks to the people who eagerly shared stories, photos, and information.

Nationally my thanks to the Office of the Historian, U.S. Army Medical Command, Fort Sam Houston, Texas, for their support and quick answers to my many questions about the Army Nurse Corps. To the United States World War One Centennial Commission, Kansas City, Missouri, for their continued help and dedication in preserving the history of America's involvement in a terrible war. To the Wisconsin Veterans Museum, Madison, Wisconsin, for their information and photographs on Clara C. Peterson, who entered World War I service from Billings, Montana. To the U.S. Library of Congress and the National Endowment for the Humanities for their "Chronicling America": digitized newspapers from America's history. This is an invaluable resource in reading newspapers of World War I.

A thanks to the staff and executive leadership of Hathi Trust Digital Library and to Google. Their foresight in putting online digitized historical reports, free-of-charge electronic books, and other voluminous print materials made my research much easier and rewarding. To the U.S. National Archives and Records Administration and to the National Library of Medicine for putting many digital photographs online for public use.

A special thanks to Alan S. Miller and Tracy L. Livingston, of Sheridan, Wyoming, for their invaluable review, critique, and constructive criticism of the draft manuscript of this book.

To Diane Carlson Evans, nurse, Army Nurse Corps, Republic of Vietnam, who wrote the foreword to this book; I am honored she did.

Last, I sincerely thank and respectfully honor Montana's and America's women veterans of World War I for their commitment and courage. A century ago they walked a road few dared. May these remarkable women rest in peace clothed in the honor they richly deserved but rarely received.

Ed Saunders
Laurel, Montana

INTRODUCTION

THIS BOOK TELLS TRUE STORIES OF MONTANA WOMEN who volunteered for war in World War I. Regardless of where they were born, lived, or died, almost all these women entered military service from Montana. The women in this book are real, I did not invent any woman or create a composite one to represent many. The dialog quoted came directly from the women, their letters, or written records in newspapers and magazines when the women lived.

When World War I began, Montana had slightly less than 700 registered nurses; the U.S. Army Nurse Corps [ANC] could muster only 400 nurses. In time the Army estimated it would need almost 40 percent of all America's graduate nurses to support the war. It would get less than a third of that number. A nurse from Glasgow, Montana, Lucy Walters, when writing home from war, quietly pleaded for more nurses to help.

Official records read over 200 women entered the U.S. military from Montana in World War I: most were nurses in the ANC, ten were in the U.S. Navy Nurse Corps. Of the women veterans of World War I who entered military service from Montana, eighty-nine volunteered for overseas duty: a remarkable 42 percent.[1] At least five Montana women served in World War I with the Women's Telephone Unit of the American Signal Corps (WTU): the "hello girls" who operated military switchboards in France.

Public Law 95-202, signed by President Jimmy Carter, November 23, 1977, and amended, gives veteran status to now sixty-four categories of American civilians who served in active military service. This law included the ANC, Navy Nurse Corps, and the WTU.[2] Based on this public law, Alice Hough Ralston, from Butte, is Montana's earliest officially recognized female military veteran. Ralston entered the Navy Nurse Corps in 1914. She resigned and then later entered the ANC in 1917. At least seventeen Montana women became yeomen [Female] in administrative support for the Navy.[3] Sadly, many of these Montana women veterans of World War I faded into history, what became of them isn't widely known.

Collectively America knows little about its women World War I veterans. The last U.S. male veteran of World War I, Frank Buckles, died in 2011; the last female U.S. female World War I veteran, Charlotte Louise Berry Winters, yeoman [Female], U.S. Navy, died in 2007. America no longer has living eyewitnesses to World War I, but we have the written record. Personal accounts are rare. During World War I the Army prohibited soldiers from keeping war diaries and journals. The Army censored war letters and didn't allow soldiers and nurses to have cameras for photographs. Looking at the written record through the lens of its day requires great discipline, openness of mind, and perhaps healthy skepticism as to who wrote the record and why. A century after World War I, we are familiar with, as far as written records allow, the many aspects of that terrible chapter in American and world history. In history some conclusions based on the written record are self-evident, others more fleeting.

No story told secondhand accurately reflects the emotion, the resolve, the fear, and the motive of the person who walked the road before us, and about whose story we write. Judgment of men and women who walked the path we didn't, and with whose priorities we may disagree, is a sirens' song writers, researchers, and historians take great risk in doing. The women World War I veterans who went to France crossed an ocean infested with enemy submarines. On ship they slept in street clothes with life belts around their waists. They waited and wondered about their fate. In France these women nurses served in some of the worst winter conditions in modern times. Mud, rain, and cold were also enemies.

These women faced danger in other ways: physical and emotional exhaustion, accidents of war, disease, and the terrible influenza epidemic of 1918. These women saved lives and gave hope to common soldiers, America's doughboys, in a conflagration of carnage not yet seen or imagined in the annals of mankind. These women served an indifferent federal government that denied them equality in status, recognition, and benefits as the men. The women would struggle for decades for their rightfully earned place in America. These military women from Montana and America began a storied roll-of-honor in service, commitment, and courage that continues to this day.

The Montana women in this book were born in eight countries and one United States territory. In America these women were born in twenty-eight states, fifty were born under Montana's big sky. Those born elsewhere soon made their way to Montana, few said why. They settled in fifty-six Montana towns, cities, river crossings, forgotten mining camps, and one lonesome windswept railroad siding named "siding 45": soon named "Glasgow."[4] Few people accurately remember how the names came to many of these remote places where sky, horizon, and relentless Montana winds were the settlers' daily companions: places like Ollie, Belmont, Alton, Box Elder, Casady, Comet, Cokedale, and Grace. History challenges historians to find these forgotten stops in Montana where settlers held hard, fast, and dear to hope.

Montana grew from a person's hope, however misguided, fleeting, or foolish, for a better life. Adult single women had few opportunities in Montana at the turn of the twentieth century, opportunities that made money and a good living. Opportunities that created independence and a future: a future unshackled to a hardscrabble ranch or scrubbing floors in a white-washed unadorned building having a sign reading "boarding house." A future better than being a bucket girl making lunches for the bucket pails of miners working in the dangerous and dark depths of Montana's mines. Opportunities that lifted a woman beyond the common and created a sense of worth, value, honor, and pride in accomplishment. Being a trained, certified, and licensed registered nurse gave Montana women a chance few had then.

Death made everyone equal in Montana in the early 1900s. The copper mines of Butte brought mineral wealth, but with a heavy price of crushed skulls and backs from rock falls deep underground where a miner died almost every day. Toxic smelter fumes at Anaconda destroyed lungs. Railroads brought prosperity to Montana, but railroads brought crushed hands, broken limbs, and death from derailments. Falling timber killed many a lumberjack in Montana's vast western forests. Montana had its share of back alley fights with fists, knives, or any piece of metal an angry man grabbed to settle a score. Montana brought death in other ways: hypothermia in fierce winters, complications in child birth, and always the invisible killer of disease: diseases with names few could pronounce or could treat. Getting the injured, wounded, sick, or women due in childbirth, to anyone with more than a layman's knowledge of first aid, became an instant desperate priority. If a doctor was a hundred miles distant, maybe–just maybe–a trained and experienced nurse was closer and could save a life.

Swords of war also made people equal. America entered World War I, the "Great War," on April 6, 1917. Historians still debate the reasons for the outbreak of general war in Europe. America initially struggled to stay out of the war in Europe. America thought it another war among perpetually squabbling people: unstable people in garishly plumed military garb with peacock-strutting egos and toxic national pride, who held to centuries old antagonisms and bad blood. Where points-of-honor and self-respect transcended reason. Where agreements made in secret bound countries to act with violence, ignoring any chance for peaceful settlements. Where countries played a deadly international chess game revolving around complex webs of alliances designed for survival and domination. Countries smiled and politely bowed in public, but behind closed doors continually suspected neighbors of treachery and perfidiousness. Nations resolved to die before their honor allowed them to tip over their king in resignation of the deadly game. Isolation meant death; agreeing to friendships, however fleeting and shallow, ensured survival. Countries clenched their collective fists of nationalism and settled disagreements, not with diplomacy but with guns: the heavier caliber the better. On April 7, 1917, the day after America's entry into war, the editorial of the Missoula, Montana, newspaper, the *Daily Missoulian*, read, "The lusts of power and the pomp and circumstances of kingly power," were responsible for the war.

Despite President Woodrow Wilson's high-minded neutrality stance, others in America saw the need to prepare for war. Innovation looked at organizing military hospitals with medical staff and equipping the hospitals in ready-to-deploy configurations. Beginning late spring 1917, America needed war nurses from anywhere—even Montana.

The nurses came mostly from the American Red Cross [ARC]. Nurses like Cora Viola Craig, a shy introverted woman born in Ohio and trained a nurse in Kansas City. She homesteaded alone three miles from her nearest neighbor, and fifteen miles from the nearest town on the vast plains and prairies in northeast Montana. Cora wasn't ruggedly handsome or even pretty, her short unadorned hair didn't cover a plain and ordinary face. No man's ring ever graced her left hand, and no child ever came forth from her womb. She wanted to be a missionary, but she would be honored by an earthly king.[5] Louise LaFournaise, a mixed blood Canadian metis from Glasgow, Montana, became a war nurse. On her official war department photograph, her piercing eyes, unkept hair, and determined countenance showed a resolute woman. In time she would survive spinal meningitis: one of the first known to do that.[6] Elizabeth "Sandy" Sandelius, a daughter of Swedish immigrants, was born and reared in Cokedale, Montana: a small mining camp choked by over one hundred smoldering coke ovens in a narrow valley beneath timber-covered mountains near the Yellowstone River. She hid a deep secret from the Army to enter the war. The Army would cite her for heroism under fire at a desperate field hospital on the battle lines of France.[7] Harriet O'Day, from Billings, Montana, had weary eyes in a photograph as she wore a smartly attired Army nurses' uniform.[8] She would be cited for heroism under fire at a forward evacuation hospital: a cluster of Army tents near the human cauldron of Verdun in the war's final days.[9] After the war, and in her photo in a college annual as a faculty member, O'Day's easy closed-mouth smile and full face, all under a stylish flapper hat, maybe hid what she saw in war.[10] Regina McIntyre-Early, whose Canadian father married an American Indian in the late nineteenth century, would be the first known and proven female World War I veteran of a Montana American Indian tribe. McIntyre-Early was Salish-Kootenai through her mother. In July 2017 her name was inscribed in Pablo, Montana, on the Salish-Kootenai's ornate and majestic *Eagle Circle Veterans Wall of Remembrance.* Honored forever with Native American song and ceremony.[11] Lucy Walters was sailing to France for war service, while underway, she almost went to her death during a German submarine attack.[12]

The nurses held to each other. When war came, the "Great Falls Six," six young women training as nurses at the Columbus Hospital in Great Falls, Montana, agreed to stay together as friends, colleagues, nurses, and women. They decided to go to war together—and they did. The decision almost caused the death of one of them.[13] One of the six, Mina Andy Aasen, became one of three Montana WWI nurses to make the Army a career.[14] A veteran of two world wars she served in uniform for almost thirty years. History would honor Captain Aasen, ANC, as one of the sixty-six Army "Angels of Bataan": American Army nurses in World War II held as prisoners-of-war of the Japanese in the Philippines.[15] Butte, the gritty hard rock mining town filled with immigrants and miners, sent thirty-seven women to war. Seven of the thirty-seven, like the "Great Falls Six," would stay together throughout.[16] No Montana World War I nurse died in war, but Marcia Lange, an Army nurse from Havre, Montana, who served in France, almost died from influenza. She wrote: "Of the nineteen nurses I knew who went [to France] seventeen came back as invalids."[17]

The great influenza epidemic struck Montana in 1918. The few qualified nurses remaining in Montana faced a terrible decision: help America's military wounded, sick and dying in the war effort, or stay in Montana to care for family, friends, and citizens dying too. Newspaper editorials demanded that nurses staying in the civilian sector, become public health nurses to serve everyone and not become private nurses for affluent families. The slashing derogatory term "slacker nurse," grew in intensity.[18]

Missoula, Montana, a scenic city in the western part of the state, lies where several mountain valleys come together. The Clark Fork River flows nearby. Missoula would give much in World War I, eighteen daughters of Missoula would enter the ANC and go to war.[19] Eula Butzerin, graduated with honors from Missoula High School, became a nurse, and served in war-torn France in an Army hospital. Her father served as state senator from Missoula, her mother a suffragette. Her two brothers served in the Army. One brother was killed-in-action. After the war she struggled to find her brother's grave: marked with his dog tags on a stick. Eula went on to become a woman of letters as a professor of nursing training on university faculties.[20]

These women came home from war largely by themselves. The military usually discharged them when they returned from war and disembarked at New York City. The military gave them a one-way railway ticket back to where they came. When the women returned to Montana, few parades and victory celebrations waited for them. In Great Falls during a victory celebration, the nurses were asked to march in the parade, but march behind the victorious Montana doughboys.[21]

As time passed, the women began dying: many too young. Few Montana women WWI veterans have veteran headstones showing their service. Eighteen are known buried in U.S. national cemeteries: three of the eighteen in Arlington National Cemetery.[22] One Army nurse, Anne Samson, died after the war at age twenty-four in Billings, Montana, from complications in childbirth. She lay in an unmarked grave for over ninety years. She was finally found and honored.[23] Susie Welborn McCrumb, a life-long nurse in peace and war is buried across the street from Anne. McCrumb served in France in World War I. Her brother, Frank Welborn, a Montana infantryman, was killed-in-action there. At her death in 1996 in Billings at age 103, Susie was thought the last surviving nurse of the ANC of World War I. Shortly before her death, the diminutive and quiet Susie, still proudly wore her World War I victory medal and ARC nurse lapel insignia.[24]

When war came, Montana and America weren't prepared, but both knew what was coming. On Sunday, August 2, 1914, the month World War I began in Europe, you could buy the Sunday edition of the *Daily Missoulian* for five cents. Your five cents bought the *Daily Missoulian*'s bold and troubling headline: "Sunday's Sun Rises on a Grim Scene This Morning." A large macabre cartoon was underneath the headline with a mocking caption, "Three Cheers for War." The cartoon showed three nightmarish skeletons covered in coarse garb. Each haunting skeleton carried an emblem of what the skeleton-of-war represented: the left-hand skeleton, titled "death," waved a large cutlass sword; the middle skeleton, titled "debt," poured money into a burning cauldron; the right-hand skeleton, titled "devastation," waved a burning torch. Readers of the *Daily Missoulian* that day could also find a portion of Theodore O'Hara's haunting poem, "The Bivouac of the Dead."

> The muffled drum's sad roll has beat
> The soldier's last tatoo;
> No more on life's parade shall meet
> That brave and fallen few.
> On fame's eternal camping-ground
> Their silent tents are spread,
> And glory guards, with solemn round,
> The bivouac of the dead.

The next day, Monday August 3, the *Daily Missoulian* printed a small graphic in the newspaper's upper right corner of the front-page reading, "War is Hell at any time and this one seems due to set a new infernal record." The large morning cartoon graphic read a cryptic "War," and showed two older men, with bowed and dropped heads, watching the setting sun. One man prays. America, Montana, and Montana's women would need a lot of prayers and soon; the sun wouldn't shine again for a long, long time.

Chapter 1
A TRAIN CAME TO GLASGOW

"The hope and promise"

ON FRIDAY, NOVEMBER 2, 1917, SETTLERS, CITIZENS, young and old, with growing patriotic fervor, gathered at the Valley County courthouse, Glasgow, Montana. Businesses and local schools had closed that day allowing everyone to attend a planned celebration at the courthouse.[25] Fierce Montana winters with punishing winds and temperatures well below zero hadn't arrived yet, but they would and soon. The Canadian border was three good days horseback ride north. Winds would soon come from the sprawling Saskatchewan prairies: hard winds vexing a settler's soul and causing the most ardent of Christian to vigorously blaspheme his luck and curse his decision to move to Montana. In the vast prairies and rolling hills in northeast Montana, no mountains, forests, or great divides blocked the weather from west or north. Few trees grow there, except in thickets along the Milk River flowing west-to-east on Glasgow's south side, and along the Missouri River farther south. The meandering and sluggish Milk River flooded twice a year during early spring rains and summer snow melt. These floods continually plagued Glasgow. In 1928 Valley County built a levee around Glasgow's south side protecting the town from annual floods.[26] What remained of autumn in 1917 was kind to Glasgow that Friday. No snow was on the ground or forecasted. At sunrise the thermometer read eighteen degrees; sunshine would warm the day to a pleasant sixty-seven degrees, winds thankfully calm.[27]

The Montana legislature created Valley County in 1890 with county seat at Glasgow. Valley County needed a courthouse, a good solidly built and noble looking courthouse. Completed in 1893 at the south end of 5th Street in Glasgow, the two-story brick courthouse building wasn't elaborate, but it had enough dignity to stand ninety years for the county.[28] It also served as a makeshift gallows in June 1903 when Valley County vigilantes hung John "Jack" Brown from a second-floor window. Brown, a burglar and petty thief who had recently stolen a coat in Glasgow, made the mistake of joining a jail break on June 6 with convicted killer, William Hardee.

This was Brown's second jail break and locals were getting riled.

A year before, Hardee was sentenced to be hanged for murdering Charles Snearly near Culbertson, Montana: east of Glasgow. This would be the first legal hanging in Valley County. But Hardee wasn't born to be hanged. He and others dug a hole through the jail's brick wall and escaped at night.[29] In the jailbreak another prisoner, George Pierce, grabbed a Winchester rifle and shot and killed Valley County deputy sheriff Jack Williams. Pierce and the others escaped into the night. Valley County formed a posse; the chase began. On June 10 the posse found Brown, who didn't put up a fight, and took him back to the Glasgow jail. Hardee, a cold-blooded killer with nothing to lose except his neck on the gallows, headed south. Hardee crossed the Missouri River on a stolen raft, the posse in pursuit. On June 17 the fifty-member posse found Hardee seventy-five miles southwest of Glasgow. While beating the bushes for Hardee, a shot rang out killing posse member Charles R. Hill. Hill had been Hardee's boyhood schoolmate in Buffalo, Wyoming. Having had enough of Hardee, the posse opened fire and riddled Hardee with lead. The posse then unceremoniously buried Hardee where he fell.[30] History doesn't say if any words were said, either Christian or coarse, over Hardee's now forgotten grave somewhere in the rugged country south of the Missouri River on the windswept and treeless Montana plains.

That night, seeking Montana justice of sorts and revenge for Hardee's killing of Charles Hill, vigilantes formed in Glasgow. Hardee was dead, but Brown, the luckless coat thief recaptured days before, would do in Hardee's place. Hanging trees of the tall strong variety are hard to find in the vast treeless plains of Valley County. The courthouse, a supposed hall of justice standing next to the jail, would do in a pinch for nefarious purposes. Dragging Brown from jail and up the courthouse stairs to the second floor, vigilantes tied a rope around the hapless Brown's neck and tossed him out the window: ironically the county attorney's window.[31] How long Brown hung alongside the courthouse wall [and who hung him] no one ever said. The *Billings* [MT] *Gazette*, June 23, 1903, condemned Brown's lynching in the harshest terms saying it was revenge pure and simple, and reflected poorly on the entire state. The *Gazette* said it was mob law and all efforts in that direction should be condemned in unmeasured terms. A bit late for Brown. The first legal hanging in Valley County, Montana, would have to wait.

When craftsman and workers built the Valley County courthouse, architects added a pillared vertical extension on the front of the main roof directly over the courthouse front door. The extension had its own pointed roof sloping on four sides. The side of the extension facing the street had space for a large clock. Citizens could check their watches with the courthouse clock, especially when a train was due at the railroad station two blocks north.[32] The clock, it appears, was never installed.

That same November day in 1917, an unscheduled passenger train was coming to Glasgow: due before noon. The train would ride the northern transcontinental railway built decades before. The railway would cross hundreds of miles of vast Montana prairie and mountain foothills heading west. It would strain heavily up the Rocky Mountains, then down into the Columbia River Valley of Washington. The train would go through the Cascade Mountains and then south along the coast of Puget Sound to a growing Army training base south of Seattle. The train on the Great Northern transcontinental railway that day wasn't carrying passengers for pleasure, the train was carrying Montana men to war—a far distant war.

James J. Hill had a vision, a vision for a transcontinental railroad across the northern plains of America, then through the Rocky Mountains and into the Puget Sound of Washington. Born 1838 in Canada, Hill grew up in Minnesota. With a reputation as a pleasant, capable, and straightforward man with boundless energy, he soon learned the railroad and river shipping business. He started a successful shipping agency and commission business in St. Paul, Minnesota, to carry freight on Minnesota's railroads and river traffic.[33]

In 1869 the Central Pacific and the Union Pacific railroads met at Promontory, Utah, and completed America's first transcontinental railroad. Serious discussion began among private investors and businessmen about building a second transcontinental railroad from Lake Superior to the Puget Sound region of the Pacific coast. The line would parallel the original transcontinental railroad, but farther north somewhere near the Canadian border. The challenges many, investors few, and optimism low.

By the 1870s gold mining slowed in Montana. Populations dropped. What major settlements remained were near army forts and Indian reservations. Montana offered little except challenges, hardships, cold weather, and always the wind. In the early 1880s prospectors in Montana discovered coal, silver, and copper: copper in abundance at Butte. Business interests looked to Montana again. Two prominent Montana men, Paris Gibson, an entrepreneur and future U.S. senator from Montana, and Martin McGinnis, a newspaper man, business man, and member of the U.S. House of Representatives from Montana from 1873 to 1885, began convincing Hill to invest in Montana. The region between the Great Falls of the Missouri and Butte had extensive mineral wealth. When Hill and his business partners took control of the St. Paul, Minneapolis & Manitoba Railway Co., Gibson and McGinnis continued lobbying Hill for a railroad to Montana's mineral areas. The Northern Pacific Railway was Hill's major competitor and rival. Chartered in 1864, the federally subsidized Northern Pacific had already built a line extending through southern North Dakota, into southern Montana, and extending west to Helena.[34][35] Hill wasn't keen on investing heavily in another long distance and expensive east-west railroad line into Montana when his competitor was already there. Hill also knew large Indian reservations existed in Montana, and the federal government hadn't granted railroad rights-of-way through the Indian lands.

The area beckoned around the Great Falls of the Missouri. Coal deposits and opportunities for hydro-electric power existed at the town of Great Falls. Missouri riverboat traffic also terminated at Fort Benton, north of Great Falls. The Missouri River had been a water highway since the Lewis and Clark expedition of 1804/06. The earliest successful voyage of a steamboat to Fort Benton was July 2, 1860, when steamers *Chippewa* and *Key West* reached the fort. Steam boats would travel the Missouri for the next thirty years. The overall decline of steam boating began in the 1880s. After 1879 no record exists of a steam boat built exclusively for sailing the Upper Missouri River.[36] From 1886 to 1890 heavy riverboat traffic to Fort Benton carried needed railroad construction material for James J. Hill's strategic railway plan.

By 1890 Missouri riverboat traffic decreased on the upper Missouri River as shallow bottomed side-wheel boats could not carry enough freight to compete with railroads.[37] The shallow draft steamers *Far West* and *Josephine* carried about 200 tons of freight each when the Missouri River became shallow in late summer.[38] By 1890 the steamboat *F. Y. Batchelor* carried the last appreciable commercial cargo to Fort Benton. After that, Fort Benton no longer saw river boats on the Missouri docking at Fort Benton's riverside wharfs. Missouri River steamboats never had the size and opulence of those grand and glorious rear-wheeled palaces gracing the Mississippi River. Passengers who once rode the smaller Missouri River steam boats, no longer had a reason to do so.[39] People began riding trains and not river boats. Gone forever was the chance to disembark from the river boats at Fort Benton and walk the short distance on the riverside path to Fort Benton's three-story ornate and brick Grand Union Hotel: thought the finest accommodations between Chicago and Seattle.[40]

In 1884 Hill visited Montana and saw firsthand the opportunities for a new westward bound railway. Hill's political connections in Washington D.C. would resolve in Hill's favor the matter of rights-of-way through Indian reservations. Hill knew if he didn't first get a railroad into Montana's rich mineral regions first, the Northern Pacific would. The Northern Pacific said central Montana belonged to the Northern Pacific, everyone else stay out. The political and monetary wars between Hill and the Northern Pacific would wage for years. Hill created three major business in Montana: Great Falls Water Power and Light Company, the Red Mountain Coal Mining Company, and the Montana Central Railway. The Montana Central Railway would connect Helena and Butte. Although Hill had no readily apparent business relationship with the Montana Central Railway, few ignored Hill's involvement.[41]

Hill's grand scheme was to build an east-west railway paralleling the Northern Pacific Railway, but hundreds of miles farther north. Hill began informally calling this route, the "high line": the high-line being a railway connecting the west terminus of the St. Paul, Minneapolis & Manitoba Railway near Devil's Lake, Dakota Territory [present North Dakota] to Great Falls, Montana. A planned rail link to the Montana Central Railway would follow. All this was a serious gamble. Hill was putting it all on the table to get a railway across northern Montana, then across the Rocky Mountains, across the Cascades in Washington, and to the Puget Sound: win or lose, succeed or bust. This was all in a day's work in Montana, the land of grand opportunity or disastrous failure: little room in between. As future mayor of Glasgow, Montana, Dr. Mark Hoyt, MD, said in 1937, "We are a community of optimists. An optimist, you know, is one who sees the flame in the candle where there is no candle, and a pessimist is a damned fool who comes along and tries to blow it out."[42]

At the end of harvest season, 1886, Hill freed his existing locomotives and trains for the big push across Montana and into Helena. During summer 1887, workers laid 643 miles of track for Hill's St. Paul, Minneapolis & Manitoba Railway between Minot, Dakota Territory, and Helena. At the eastern Montana border, the Great Northern descended into Montana's Milk River Valley. The Milk River did not begin in the mountains and followed a meandering path with an erratic, uncertain flow. The railway would twice cross the river on the railway's westward path. The line would continue up the Missouri River plateau and into the farthest north regions of the Great Plains. Railroads hadn't conquered the Rocky Mountains that far north. As he built the railway, Hill began informally referring to it as the "Great Northern route," or the "Great Northern Railway." The name stuck. Hill, in time, officially changed the business name of the St. Paul, Minneapolis & Manitoba Railway to the "Great Northern Railway."[43]

The line would go west to Fort Assiniboine, southwest of present Havre, Montana, then southwest past Fort Benton. Passing Fort Benton, the rail line would go to Great Falls, arriving there October 16, 1887, then later to Butte that year. At Butte the Great Northern connected to a Union Pacific spur line south to Utah, and then via the Central Pacific/Southern Pacific, to California. All by-passing the rival Northern Pacific Railway.[44]

By 1889 Hill debated his next move with his Great Northern Railway to the Pacific Coast. He considered buying out the Northern Pacific, but the Northern Pacific wasn't strong financially and Hill would have to contend with the U.S. government and the government's subsidies of the Northern Pacific.[45] Hill decided to press on with building the Great Northern across the Rocky Mountains in northwest Montana. Hill knew he had to find the easiest practical route for construction: if that was even possible in the high mountains near present Glacier National Park west of Browning. Hill had on his payroll John F. Stevens: a young college-trained engineer and rugged outdoorsman. Stevens took on the challenge to find a route through the mountains. A route through the mountains had been rumored, but no one had precisely found the pass. In early 1889 Stevens set out westward from Fort Assiniboine.

Using a reluctant Blackfoot Indian guide, Stevens trudged through the snow along the Marias River headwaters. On December 11 Stevens realized he was at a low point on a ridgeline, and that low point was the ideal route for the Great Northern Railway over the northern Rocky Mountains. Given the challenges of gradient, less curves around high peaks, and other construction criteria, Stevens reported this route was the most efficient to the west coast. He had discovered Marias Pass. Great Northern Railway followed this northern route through the Rocky Mountains.[46][47]

During the 1890/91 construction season, the Great Northern Railway extended west across Marias Pass and into the sprawling valley north of Flathead Lake. In 1892 the railway was approaching Spokane, Washington, with its flat plain, large population and hydroelectric possibilities. Continuing west across into the Cascade Mountains, Hill drove the last spike on January 6, 1893, completing his dream a northern transcontinental railroad. He owned the railway from Minneapolis-St. Paul, across North Dakota, into Montana, and west across northern Idaho, Washington, and to the Puget Sound. Twenty-five years later, the railway would help carry America to war.

Steam locomotives don't run on dreams, locomotives need water and fuel: tons of coal and ample water. Surveyors on the Great Northern Railway planned rail sidings about every sixty miles along the Great Northern Railway as the railway traversed northern Montana. Sixty miles was about as far a locomotive of the late 1880s could go without refueling and taking on water.[48] In July 1887 surveyors plotted sidings along the route of the future Great Northern Railway. On the map one site was named "siding 45" and had a large coaling and water station.[49] Siding 45 was seventeen miles north of the Missouri River where the Lewis and Clark expedition traveled and later where steamboats steamed up and down. "Siding 45" would become Glasgow, Montana. The change in northern Montana began in earnest, largely due to the Great Northern Railway.

Railroads make money hauling freight—not passengers. Getting greater railroad traffic and hauling greater freight loads, meant attracting users to the railroad. That meant attracting settlers to land near the railroad. People were drawn to rail sidings where trains stopped and refueled. Railroad men gathered at the stops to maintain the trains, and get something to eat, drink, rest, and relax a bit. For something to drink, railroad men didn't always prefer water. In 1888 Glasgow had one street: the street facing the railway. Saloons along this street outnumbered all other commercial businesses.⁵⁰ For relaxing, madams arrived, and not the cultured and genteel kind.

At rail sidings along Montana's high line, railroad men named the rail sidings at sixty-mile intervals after European towns: maybe a try at making Montana sound genteel and a bit more refined and proper. Rail stops or sidings in northern Montana had names like Shelby, Dunkirk, Devon, Inverness, Gildford, Havre, Zurich, Harlem, Glasgow, and Malta. Glasgow was sixty miles east of Malta, and named after the Scottish city.⁵¹ Tents and squatters set up in Glasgow after the Great Northern Railway came through in 1887.

In 1887 Glasgow was in Dawson County with county seat at Glendive, 150 miles south. The county sheriff was in Glendive, a long way from Glasgow. In Glasgow railroad men, cowboys, drovers, and settlers settled things with fists and guns. If Glasgow was to survive and prosper—and if the Great Northern was to make money in the area—permanent settlers had to come and create a community for families and their children, with law and order and available medical care with doctors and nurses.⁵² The final plat for Glasgow was finished and approved in 1897. Glasgow would be a typical Montana railway town with a T-plot layout. The top of the T was Front Street paralleling the east-west railway. Fifth Street was the leg of the T going south two blocks and ending at the courthouse.⁵³

Hill needed settlers to come to northern Montana. He had to convince them these lands were productive and promising. Hill supported the Newlands Act of 1902. This federal law began the modern U.S. Bureau of Reclamation. This act covered fourteen western states that have arid or semi-arid land.⁵⁴ Montana was among these states. These lands needed water from damming existing rivers and providing irrigation. Hill eyed the Milk River in Montana for a large-scale irrigation project.⁵⁵ Hill also began advocating dryland farming and an enlarged Homestead Act creating homesteads of 320 acres rather than the previous 160 acres allotted in the Homestead Act of 1862. To get immigrants to North Dakota and Montana, Hill even offered immigrants the chance to rent all or part of a railroad box car as an immediate home for $22.50 to $50.⁵⁶ Hill made traveling promotional rail car exhibits showing abundant sheaves of wheat and other crops of agricultural plenty to show people willing to believe him.[57]

Hill's competitor, the Northern Pacific, also began extensive advertising enticing settlers to the upper Great Plains and Montana. The Northern Pacific's year 1889 promotional brochure told settlers Montana has "remarkable irrigated wheat regions yielding from thirty to fifty bushels an acre."[58] For cattlemen the brochure continued, "All of Montana…is essentially a grazing country and is occupied by large herds of cattle and flocks of sheep. …This grass is the most nutritious known have properties of hay and grain. Cattle fatten on it more rapidly than on the blue grass of Kentucky or the buffalo grass of Nebraska and Colorado."[59] Even after the disastrous winter of 1886/87 when millions of livestock lay dead in Montana from starvation due to heavy snows, and domestic cattle largely wiped out, the Northern Pacific's brochure ignored stark reality when it read: "Range cattle are not sheltered or looked after in winter. They run over the open country, and pick up their living on the dried, standing grass. The raising of horses is also a growing and profitable industry. No winter care is given them, and when rounded up in the spring they are found to be as fat as if they had been stabled and well fed all winter."[60]

Both Hill and the Northern Railroad knew northern Montana brought hostile conditions with vast distances and isolation for anyone willing to come. Daytime temperatures ranged from one hundred degrees to minus twenty-five. As late as 1917, Janet M. Geister, federal advisor for child welfare of the Department of Interior's Children's Bureau, and later director of the American Nursing Association, wrote of northern Montana when she visited:

> Ninety-eight miles from the nearest 'phone, railroad, or telegraph wire. The work is fascinating. I never have met such splendid people as these ranchers, nor any in greater need of public health work. You have no idea of the isolation of these people. We drive miles and miles over dim trails, across the hills and buttes before we find the tiny little one-room shacks that folks live in. We can't possibly get back to the little communities every night, we carry tarpaulins and sleep in haystacks. …We leave in five minutes for some of the most beautiful country in the west, the

Brakes [sic] up by the Missouri River. We will travel by auto, afoot, and horseback. I wear a khaki-colored flannel riding suit, mountain boots and no [sic] much else. When we go to bed we undress by taking off our hats and putting on heavy coats.[61]

Wide-open land and plenty of it, beckoned intrepid and adventurous people to Montana. With railroads crossing Montana, and agricultural and mining opportunities growing, settlers saw opportunities and hope for a better life. The land rush began. By 1886 Indian tribes in the Great Plains and Montana began giving up their treaty rights and lessening the size of their reservations. By 1888 the Milk River Valley was open to settlement.[62] In 1908 Montana senator Paris Gibson wrote: "[Montana] is a state of unbounded natural possibilities and gilt-edge opportunities, and the world is finding it out and immigration is coming our way."[63] Congress passed legislation in 1909 increasing homestead acreages from 160 acres to 320 acres.[64] Restrictions applied: Among them homesteaders couldn't mine for minerals on their homestead land. Settlers also had to continuously cultivate at least one-eighth of the land after the first year of settlement.[65] Women could apply for homesteads.

By 1913, except where the Northern Pacific Railway entered Montana at the North Dakota border and turned south along the Yellowstone River, Hill's Great Northern Railway was the only railway north of the forty-seven north latitude line in Montana. The forty-seven north latitude line cuts Montana largely in half north and south.[66] In 1913 President Wilson opened over 1.3 million acres of land for homesteading in America. In northeast Montana the government opened forty thousand acres for homesteading on the Fort Peck Indian reservation.[67] The U.S. Department of the Interior began extensive preparations for a land lottery. This meant opening lottery offices in Montana cities of Glasgow, Havre, and Great Falls. The 8,400, 160-acre land parcels from the Fort Peck reservation would be chosen by lottery. If you registered and your name drawn first, you had first choice; if picked last, good luck. Interested people could register at land offices in those three Montana cities from September 1 to September 20, 1913.[68]

Montana newspapers reported people from all over America came to register. Special trains and extra coaches on regular trains brought thousands to Montana for the land lottery. The *Great Falls* [MT] *Tribune* reported on September 19, 1913, that one Burlington train brought 442 people from Missouri, Kansas, Oklahoma, Iowa, Illinois, and Nebraska. Promptly at one-minute past noon, September 1, 1913, the Glasgow land office opened for registering. The Glasgow land office could process about seventy-five applicants per hour. The first person to register in Glasgow was Mable Sims: the deputy county superintendent of schools in Glasgow.

Glasgow and the Great Northern Railroad had made ample preparations to accommodate the thousands of people expected to come.[69] On September 18 over two thousand land seekers registered at the Glasgow land office.[70] Hoke Smith, the Great Northern Railway's publicity agent said optimistically of people, "They want to live in Montana and while only a limited number of them can hope to get land in the drawing, many of them will see the opportunities that the state offers and will return later and buy land."[71] Over forty thousand hopefuls eventually registered for the land drawing. Fourteen thousand people registered at Great Falls.[72]

The golden lottery was held September 23 at Glasgow: watched by Judge James W. Witten and Clay Tallman, commissioner of the general land office in Washington D.C. The drawing was planned outside, but bad weather forced the event indoors to the chagrin of many waiting outside to watch the grand event. Zita Friedl, the young daughter of Glasgow mayor R. H. Friedl, drew the first name of Samuel A. Crow of Hammond, Indiana. A Hoosier won the lottery. The fifteenth name drawn in the lottery was Hazel Richardson from Great Falls: the first woman drawn. Richardson, a stenographer in Great Falls, said she saw no reason why a girl shouldn't be able manage a ranch, and while she has not had any experience on a farm she felt certain could do it. [73] [74] Other women agreed. Lucy Walters, Cora Craig, and Ann Dobias, all lived in Glasgow. They had much in common: they were single, would file for homesteads near Glasgow, and they were nurses. Soon to be war nurses.

Chapter 2
LUCY'S TICKET

"No parades for them"

THAT FRIDAY MORNING, NOVEMBER 2, 1917, Lucy Walters, with her luggage, was at the Glasgow, Montana, train station. The westbound Oriental Limited, the Great Northern Railway's elegant flagship passenger train, was due at 9:30 a.m. Lucy had to be on it. The train had a remarkable on-time record, but people in their quiet nervousness kept checking their time pieces: either pocket watches or lapel pendants. Looking east and west along the rails, people silently strolled up and down the platform with quiet but uneasy thoughts. Would the train be on time? Did it derail? Where was it?

Lucy dressed warm as the day began cold.[75] Passengers kept their tickets ready. Lucy didn't get a ticket, she got an official notification and transportation order from the War Department directing her to proceed without delay and assigning Lucy "to active service in the military establishment." The notification told her to report to a specific military base. The War Department also sent her an unsigned printed oath of office. She was instructed to take the oath on the morning of a specified day before a notary public or other official authorized to administer oaths. Lucy would sign the statement confirming she took the oath and send the signed statement in a provided envelope to the War Department. Lucy and other Montana nurses had to first take the oath of office before making travel arrangements.[76]

The War Department transportation order was the same as a train ticket. Lucy would board the train and travel west to America Lake, Washington: beyond the Rockies and along the Puget Sound south of Seattle. She was going to Camp Lewis: named for Meriwether Lewis of the Lewis and Clark expedition. Camp Lewis, a large Army training base for World War I military recruits, had a growing hospital that needed doctors and nurses. That November day in Glasgow, Lucy took the required loyalty oath to America and became Nurse Walters, ANC. At the Glasgow train station, Lucy, age thirty-nine, wasn't going on holiday, she was going to war.

Another train was coming to Glasgow that morning, an hour after

Lucy and the Oriental Limited were to depart. Forty-one men from Glasgow, Valley County, Montana, would board a special west-bound troop train at 10:30 a.m. America drafted the men to fight in the Great War. Based on Montana's population, the federal government said Montana's total draft quota in 1917 was 6,350 men.[77] Valley County had to fill its military draft quota. Forty-nine men from Sheridan County, east of Glasgow, were already on the train. Assembled citizens at the Glasgow train station cheered these forty-nine men. The *Glasgow* [MT] *Courier* reported the men seemed happy: happy to go see the Kaiser [Kaiser Wilhelm or "Kaiser Bill"] with his funny-looking pointed helmet, and "get his goat."[78] The men boarding at Glasgow that Friday would be the fourth draft quota sent from Valley County, and the last for a while. The third quota departed Glasgow a month before on October 3.

On October 5 the *Glasgow Courier* reported thousands of people gave the soldier boys a rousing farewell, and ensured the recruits had every comfort before they departed. The manager of Glasgow's Orpheum Theater gave the men, free-of-charge, a special movie show the day before. Glasgow held a free dance benefit Tuesday night. Early Wednesday morning, the day the men were to depart, the Glasgow band began playing patriotic music at the courthouse. County attorney Carl D. Barton and the Reverend Stone gave patriotic speeches. The Glasgow Red Cross Society served the men a fried chicken dinner at noon. After the dinner a grand parade escorted the men to the Glasgow train station.[79] The Glasgow fire department led the parade followed by Civil War and Spanish-American war veterans. School children followed carrying American flags. Citizens gave the men an abundance of cigars, tobacco, candies, and fruits. The men boarded the troop train and filled three Pullman passenger cars: each with upholstered seats and a few fold-down bunks. A large banner, reaching from one end of the three cars to the other, read: "112 Men from Glasgow, Montana."[80]

Other Montana cities and towns held grand departure ceremonies for local boys going to war. On September 23, 1917, seventy-nine recruits departed from Missoula. Missoula held a large parade led by a local band and drum and bugle corps. Citizens draped a large banner on the troop train showing the recruits were from Missoula, Montana. On September 6 the first twenty-eight recruits from Great Falls, Montana, had their picture taken in pressed suits and ties for the *Great Falls*

Tribune. They departed Great Falls at 2:25 p.m. on Great Northern train 43. For a month Great Falls had been planning the departure ceremony for these men. The ceremony had marching bands and other activities unlike anything the city had seen. It was the first occasion of its kind in the city's history. All businesses and schools closed that day.[81] The town held a special luncheon at the Hotel Rainbow, with a concert by the Black Eagle band. The parade to the train station formed at 1:00 p.m. at the Masonic temple. All Great Falls citizens were invited to join the parade. Local officials gave short farewell speeches at the train station. The recruits departed with fanfare, music, waving crowds, cheers and tears.[82]

On September 5 from six to seven thousand people gathered at the Custer County courthouse in the eastern Montana prairie city of Miles City. They were sending off the town's first ten draftees. The gathering was thought the largest in Miles City's history. At least eight local organizations formed a parade. Patriotic ceremonies were held with music, singing, and rousing cheers. Speeches were given to honor the recruits. At the conclusion of his speech to the departing men, the honorable Judge D. L. O'Hern said: "There is only one other piece of advice I want to leave with you, and it's the most important of all. If the Kaiser ever should…get near one of your trenches…remember, Montana is shouting to you, 'Boy, hold steady, and shoot straight,' and if you get him the war will be over."[83]

When war began, the Second Infantry Regiment of the Montana National Guard, headquartered at Fort William Henry Harrison, Helena, Montana, became the 163rd Infantry Regiment. The regiment was preparing to go to war, and the citizens of Helena, Montana's state capital, raised $3,000 dollars to buy tobacco, fruit, and other trimmings to stock the departing train for the soldiers. Helena invited all Montana to come for the send-off. The Great Northern and Northern Pacific railroads even reduced train fare to Helena for Montana citizens to attend.[84]

Montana citizens wanted their recruits to keep high personal standards to reflect upon the hometown. Running a bayonet through "Kaiser Bill" and his pointy-helmeted troops was acceptable, encouraged, and even expected, but not while you're drunk. Killing the Hun would give a man a first-class ticket to heaven amid angelic cheers of welcome at the pearly gates. Drinking demon liquor would send you straight to hell on a one-way ticket to eternal damnation, along with the damnable Huns you killed. Montana newspapers editorialized about liquor being furnished to recruits as the recruits traveled across Montana to military training camps farther west.

Phillips County, Montana, borders the Canadian province of Saskatchewan. Malta is the county seat sixty miles west of Glasgow on the Great Northern railway. When a troop train arrived in Malta on September 23, county sheriff Rolla Crabb, also chairman of the Phillips County draft board, appealed to the ninety-six Montana recruits boarding at Malta to be good citizens of America and abstain from liquor. No liquor was to be on troop trains carrying Montana boys to war. Crabb, who would later move to Maryland after being voted out of office for beating a Montana sheep herder half to death, said at the Malta train station, "I know each of you boys, and I don't want it ever said of our county that we sent a bunch of boozers to fight in war."[85] The Malta ladies' relief committee had pinned a red ribbon on the Phillips County boys going to war. The red ribbon alerted others too. Malta saloons refused to serve the departing boys if the boys were wearing the red ribbon. When the ninety-six Phillips County draftees boarded the train at Malta, the *Great Falls Tribune* reported not a drop of liquor was found on the train.[86]

Temperance wasn't a Montana priority when troop trains carrying new recruits departed many Montana towns. Word reached the Spokane County sheriff, Spokane, Washington, that a troop train from Butte, Montana, would be passing through Spokane and full of liquor. Butte, a gritty western Montana mining town full of immigrants, always had its own way of doing things. Good luck finding a man with soft hands in Butte. Callused hands and strong arms from swinging pick axes and working shovels in Butte's deep and dangerous copper mines, backed up whatever a man from Butte felt and said about things: especially about having a shot of whiskey or pint or two of ale after his dirty, dangerous, and debilitating shift a thousand feet underground.

To save Butte's military recruits from demon rum, the Silver Bow County Ministerial Association, the Women's Christian Temperance Union, and other kindred organizations, intended to push through a municipal ordinance requiring city and county authorities to close city saloons ten hours before the departure of any contingent of troops from Butte. These temperance organizations passed a resolution having three "Whereas's" and one "Resolution." The first "Whereas" read the departure of the first contingents of recruits was attended by deplorable scenes due to the intoxication of large number of the men. The second "Whereas" read riotous outbreaks on the troop train and twenty-five gallons of liquor were reported to have been seized in Spokane, Washington. The third "Whereas" read local authorities encouraged the free use of liquor and did nothing to discourage drinking on the train before the recruits departed the Butte train station. The "Resolution" read that citizens of Butte, in mass meeting assembled, petitioned the law and governor of the state to take steps to ensure these deplorable conditions cease when the next contingent of men going to war departs from Butte. It is not known if Silver Bow County sheriff, John K. O'Rourke, a determined Irishman among many determined Irishman in Butte, ever heeded the resolution.[87]

Butte men didn't deserve all the suspicion for being 90-proof ruffians bent on sending the Huns to hell. A few weeks before at the Washington state border, Sheriff Reid from Spokane had seized a shipment of whiskey from Missoula. Clever men heading toward Seattle hid the shipment in unmarked glass bottles. Reid said if the federal government would permit him, he would arrest all men found to be violating Washington state liquor laws: even men from Montana on the troop trains.[88] History doesn't say if Sheriff Reid inspected the train from Butte for illicit liquor. Maybe better heads prevailed that day. Good luck, Sheriff Reid, in trying to arrest a train load of Montana men from Butte heading to war.

The mayor of Missoula, H. T. Wilkinson, perhaps concerned about upholding the image of the scenic western Montana university city as being more refined, educated, and proper, approved an order of the Missoula city council. The order read that for the best interests of good order in handling drafted men leaving Missoula, the sale of liquor is prohibited when the men departed. To do this, the mayor and the city council ordered all saloons and places where intoxicants were sold retail or wholesale, be closed and sales of liquor be prohibited from midnight of the day the troop train departs until the train leaves Missoula.[89]

Even Montana's Cascade County sheriff, L. H. Kommers, had his fill of drunk recruits. Kommers said he would search the train for liquor before the train departed Great Falls. Kommers heard the last train taking Cascade County men to war had three barrels of beer and a large amount of liquor. Montana men going to war were not to have a last drink. The pulpit of sobriety standing resolutely before the pearly gates forbade it. The draftees bought booze before departure, and probably drank it abundantly. Kommers said if he found any intoxicants on the train or in the luggage of the men, Kommers would arrest the offender and turn him over to the federal department of justice.[90]

The last quota of Valley County draftees gathered November 2 at the Glasgow courthouse. The troop train taking them to war would arrive at 10:30 a.m.: an hour after the fast and elegant passenger train, the Oriental Limited, had departed. Another patriotic and grand send-off ceremony was planned on the courthouse lawn for this last group of draftees. Glasgow mayor Matt Murray gave a speech, the Reverend Brickert said the county would back the boys to the last dollar, the last man, and to the last breath—a breath free of alcohol that is. A choir having two men and two women from each church in Glasgow sang songs; cheers rang; flags waived; mothers and fathers, wives and sisters, showed pride. Everyone waved farewells. There were few dry eyes at the station. Men boarded the train: men like John Vatne from North Dakota; Billy Evashenko, a Russian; Knute Soreng and John Hovland, both Norwegians; Olaf Olson a Swede, and Joseph DeFao, an Italian. Few men that day were Montana born and reared. Most were immigrants following a dream to the promised land of northeast Montana: land that James J. Hill, the great railroad "Empire Builder" said would be ideal for homesteading.[91] Hill never said anything about riding his train to war.

Fred Louis Truscott, twenty-six years old, was a promising hometown boy born and reared in Glasgow. A handsome clean-shaven bachelor he had smooth features and pleasant eyes not covered by spectacles. Truscott had a stylish contemporary haircut and wore a smartly tailored suit over a white shirt with starched high collar. He boarded the westbound troop train with the others. He was in charge of all the Valley County men that day going to Army basic training.[92] A Notre Dame graduate, class of 1913, with an electrical engineering degree, Truscott was on the Glasgow chamber of commerce board of directors. A recognized leader, he served on the Liberty Loan committee and organized the ARC drive in Glasgow. Truscott was also a lieutenant in the Glasgow Home Guards: a paramilitary organization in Montana with questionable authority to do anything other than carry the American flag and ensure others followed.[93]

Truscott, along with the others, was going to war. Traveling the northern tier of Montana along the "high-line," the train started from Plentywood near the North Dakota border, and headed west. The train carried fifty-six men from Sheridan County, forty-six men from Valley County, twenty-five men at Malta from Phillips County, and twenty-six men at Chinook from Blaine County. Fifty men from Fort Benton, Choteau County, would meet the train at Havre.[94] Before leaving Havre, the county seat of Hill County, the Hill County boys were guests of the people of Havre for most of the day with entertainment and dinner at the Methodist church. The farewell program included speeches and music. The boys received comfort kits of tobacco, candies, tooth brushes, shaving powder, pencils and paper to write home with, and other things before the boys departed. Ten recruits from Harlem, in Blaine County, were given a rousing send-off at a dance and reception at Harlem. The Women's Study Club of Harlem gave comfort kits to the ten recruits. Automobiles took the ten to Chinook to meet the westbound troop train.[95]

History doesn't say if Truscott waved goodbye to Glasgow, his hometown. Soldiers and those entering the armed forces of the United States, especially those going to war, do look back: not in regret, but with one last look to that where they grew, the life they knew, the people they loved. A last glance for support and courage, and to convince themselves their decision to enlist had merit. A last glance to reaffirm a value system ingrained in them from birth. A last glance to say to their family or to themselves, "I'm a man now," and to view the home they knew that in the deep recesses of their minds and hearts they may never see again. The romance of war lingers in the minds of young men, a certain psychology that tends to overpower personal identities and fears a person has made for themselves. All armies in the world, that have ever been and ever will be, have exploited and manipulated the veiled and hidden warrior ethic that is ingrained in the human male.[96]

American Civil War veterans living in Valley County marched in the send-off parade that day to the Glasgow train station. In 1917 the youngest Civil War veterans were in their late 60s and early 70s. They had seen hard war in bloody battles at Shiloh, Gettysburg, Cold Harbor, and the trenches of Petersburg. These veterans knew the young men leaving that day at Glasgow would in time "see the elephant":

meaning seeing the huge animal of war charging them headlong.[97] Montana's Gertrude Zerr would later ride the same railroad west to serve America. Zerr would become one of two Montana chief yeomen (Female) in the U.S. Navy of World War I. She would write for *Harper's Magazine*: "...Youth is daring, and when it has a reckless leader then there are no boundaries to its adventuring."

At the Glasgow station when the last recruit boarded, the train engineer blew the whistle twice in quick succession, signaling he was ready to ease forward the train's throttle and pull the troop train west. The special train wasn't heavy that day, it was carrying men and their baggage. The engineer released steam slowly but resolutely into the large driving pistons, relief valves blasting steam exhaust, and the smoke stack belching acrid coal smoke. The engine came to life carrying men with their hopes, dreams, and veiled fears. A skilled and inventive engineer could make a train's steam whistle sing a guttural opera, whistle, and spit. You could generally tell what engineer was at the throttle based on the whistle he composed. On November 2 at Glasgow, Montana, the engineer that day and the whistle he played, isn't remembered.

As the train whistle faded west, and crowds at the Glasgow train station dispersed and walked away, a serious matter loomed: Fred Truscott wasn't physically strong. If he knew, Truscott didn't say, and he didn't write it down. Draftees filled out World War I draft registration cards. The cards asked basic questions of name, family, citizenship, marital status, who the draftee financially supported, employer, any previous military service, and if the draftee claimed an exemption.[98] If the draftee was an American of African descent the draft registrar would cut or tear away the lower left corner of the completed registration card: a quick look indicator that the draftee was "colored."[99]

Truscott had passed the local draft physical. Doctor Alfred N. Smith, MD, a Glasgow doctor, was the Valley County draft board's physician.[100] Smith had to examine hundreds of county men for military service. Smith didn't have time to give comprehensive physicals to each. He apparently didn't catch what was wrong with Truscott, or Truscott didn't tell him. The draft registrar's report listed the draftee's height, physical build, color of eyes and hair, or baldness, and if the person had lost a limb or was blind. Nothing more. The examining physician asked basic questions and performed a simple examination.

The physician checked if the draftee had teeth, could the draftee see and hear, could he breathe, did he have venereal disease, was he mentally sound or an idiot, and did he have all his limbs, fingers and toes. That was largely it. The draftee passed or failed. If he failed, he was given a written reason why. Next in line, please.

Patriotic intentions can take a military recruit so far, then and now. At military basic training bases hard realities instantly arrive. Recruits face a regimented life few can explain. Green recruits quickly learn about marching with heavy loads having pack straps cutting your shoulders, marching in poorly fitting uniforms and new unbroken-in poorly-fitting boots. Recruits soon learned of carrying rifles that grew heavier each marching mile. All this soon erased hometown cheers and music at Glasgow's and thousands of America's train stations in World War I: stations where fledgling dough boys departed to test and prove their manhood in the great adventure of a distant war.

Truscott returned to Glasgow from Camp Lewis a month later, he never completed Army basic training.[101] An unknown disability sent him home. Truscott, an educated and disciplined man, didn't give up; he kept trying. In July 1918 the Army, needing more recruits, accepted Fred again. This time he wouldn't return to his home, family, and friends. A week after arriving at the basic training camp at Jefferson Barracks, St. Louis, Missouri, Truscott caught influenza. Pneumonia, the flu's lethal companion, battered Truscott's lungs. The Army notified his father, J. L. Truscott, that Fred was dying. J. L. Truscott, a prominent mercantile owner in eastern Montana, hurriedly went from Montana to Missouri to be with Fred but arrived too late. Fred Truscott died at Jefferson Barracks, St. Louis, Missouri, October 17, 1918, less than a month before the war ended. A youthful, educated, promising leader, Fred went to fight the Kaiser, but never got farther east than Missouri. The flu killed Truscott as sure as a Kaiser's bullet.

Truscott's friends and family grieved greatly. They brought him home to Montana and buried him in Resurrection Cemetery in Helena, next to his sister, Florence, who died years before.[102] The *Glasgow Courier* on October 25, 1918, read Fred Truscott "died in the service of his country." He never saw the Kaiser or the Kaiser's funny helmet. Fred never heard the train whistle at Glasgow again.

In early October 1917, Lucy Walters received her notification to go to Camp Lewis. On Wednesday, October 10, the Valley County

Nurses Association honored Lucy with a farewell dinner at the Glasgow nurses home: a two-story, nicely constructed apartment house for nurses across the street west from the Glasgow hospital. At the close of the dinner, the association presented Lucy with a Bible wrapped in a beautiful silk American flag. All nurses present joined in wishing her God-speed in the work she chose for the war effort. Her friends regretted her leaving.[103]

Walking the streets, the Glasgow train station was about a half-mile north of the nurses' home: a good distance on cold Montana mornings if you carry luggage. Maybe someone helped Lucy to the train station, maybe not. She would be traveling alone, no colleagues, friends, or family would go with her. When the fast-moving Oriental arrived around 9:30 a.m., she would have to be ready. She would have five minutes to board the train along with everything she brought. The Oriental wouldn't wait. The Army provided Lucy a first-class Pullman car ticket and would pay her up to $4.50 per day food and expense allowance to Camp Lewis.[104] In the new lightweight steel Pullman sleeper cars, she got a lower berth. Lower berthed passengers faced forward. Before evening when the Pullman car attendant folded the seat flat as a bed, she could sit and look out the window. She wouldn't have to clamber up to the top bunk.[105] The Army authorized her one hundred pounds of excess baggage to bring. What few photos exist of her in history show she dressed appropriately, but not flamboyantly. She was a professional woman and her attire showed it.

No bands, cheers, speeches, or patriotic banners met Lucy when she arrived at the train station along Front Street. No dance was held in her honor the night before, no bands played for her, and no parades marched with her to the station. Grateful patriotic clubs in Glasgow didn't give her a comfort kit. The single-story, stylish, Glasgow train station bordered the rails away from the city activity and patriotic crowds gathering a few blocks south at the courthouse. The farewell ceremony for the men would begin in an hour, but not for Lucy; she would be gone by then. Gone with her thoughts, eagerness, and trepidations. If she waved goodbye to anyone at the station, or if she shed farewell tears, she took that with her and left no record.

The westbound Great Northern train 1, the Oriental Limited, began at St. Paul, Minnesota, and came across vast prairies and rivers of the northern plains. Three hundred miles west of Glasgow, at

Browning, Montana, the Oriental would begin the steady climb up the Rocky Mountains. The Oriental was coming fast, it was built for speed. In 1909 the Great Northern boasted it could run the Oriental from Tacoma, Washington, to Chicago, via the Burlington road, a distance of 2,217 miles, in seventy-two hours.[106] It didn't carry livestock, lumber, grain, or coal; it carried passengers, and carried them in comfort. The train was dependable and on time.

The Great Northern Railroad used a new, modern-for-its-day, steam locomotive: the Baldwin class K-1 Atlantic locomotive. Classified as a 4-4-2 locomotive, it had four leading wheels, four driving wheels, and finally two trailing wheels under the cab.[107] The locomotive carried eight thousand gallons of water and held thirteen tons of coal. It would drink Niagara Falls amounts of water and burn coal like it fueled an immense mythical fire-breathing dragon. Fuel, flame, and water create steam, lots of steam for the new fast locomotive: 200 pounds-per-square-inch pressure of saturated steam driving fifteen-inch diameter pressure cylinders connected to drive wheels over six feet tall.[108] On north-central Montana's flat and level railroad grades, the Oriental could run fast with speeds over eighty miles-per-hour.[109]

The Oriental had to stay ahead of the troop trains going west. The Oriental's passengers paid good money to ride in comfort and safety. They expected the Oriental to be on time, every time. In 1915 the Great Northern Railway reported its crack train, the Oriental Limited, was late only fourteen times on its run to the coast and was on time every day from April 14 to July 19, 1914.[110] [111] Construction caused what delays held up the Oriental. Danger lurked. On June 3, 1916, the eastbound Oriental Limited struck a rock slide near Katka, in northwest Montana. The engine plunged into the Kootenay River. The engineer and fireman went missing and presumed drowned. No passengers were injured, but two cars derailed.[112] Winter snow slides also blocked the rails.

The new Oriental Limited began May 23, 1909. The Oriental had custom built ornate steel rail cars for better safety. The cars had fine colorful trim and richly upholstered seats. The Oriental had electric lights and carried the finest equipment in the service, compartment observation cars, standard and tourist sleeping cars, dining cars and day coaches. The train even had a vacuum cleaner. For women the Oriental Limited train directory read, "A women's lounge room with shower bath in connection and a maid who is also a manicure, expert hair dresser and masseuse, in attendance." A manicure, facial massage, hairdressing, and shampoo, each cost seventy-five cents. Shower bath cost fifty cents. You could even make a telephone call from the train when the train was stopped at terminals in Chicago, St. Paul, Seattle, and Tacoma. The directory read the train was "As wonderful as the country it serves."[113] Each sleeper car was named after oriental ports such as Yokohama, and Manila.[114] For seventy-five cents passengers could get lunch and dinner on the train.[115] A summertime coast-to-coast round-trip ticket from Portland, Oregon, to New York City, was $118.20.[116]

Winter comes early to northern Montana and stays long; cold winds blow. The Oriental would cross the high Marias Pass a few hundred miles west of Glasgow. Marias Pass in November had cold, snow, and sometimes avalanche danger. In December 1917 a snow slide near Essex, Montana, blocked both eastbound and westbound Oriental Limited trains.[117] In Montana, Lucy Walters was far from the dry arid and warmer land where she was born and knew as a girl.

The Sacramento Mountains of southern New Mexico give birth to the Rio Peñasco, or the Peñasco River. The Peñasco River on a wet year might flow to the junction of the Pecos River farther east near present Artesia, New Mexico. Lucy was born July 24, 1878, on the Lower Peñasco River where her father, Jim, got ranch land in New Mexico Territory on the pastures and flatter land there.[118] The Spanish word "peñasco" means "rocky." Glasgow, Montana, was far from being aggressive rocky land. In Montana the Milk River flows south and east of Glasgow until it meets the Missouri River. The Peñasco River was but a spit compared to the upper Missouri River. Generally the Milk and the Missouri rivers were easy-going shallow rivers, but they could get angry in spring, terribly angry.

James Volney Walters, born in Kentucky, 1827, made his way to California and lived there in the 1850s. In California, September 1861, Jim and other men joined the Union Army during the Civil War. They marched as part of the "California column" to the New Mexico Territory that included present Arizona. These Union soldiers saw no combat in the territory but patrolled the region. Jim was mustered out of service, November 1864, in New Mexico Territory. In 1869 James married Frances Gonzales-Baca in Tularosa, New Mexico Territory.

History reads Frances was a midwife and a "practical nurse."

Twelve children were born to them: three sons, nine daughters.[119] Lucy was one of the nine daughters.[120] As she matured, Lucy wasn't svelte or rotund, but short and solid. Her face wasn't harsh, but full and with smooth gentle curves. She had her mother's Spanish eyes: dark, engaging, and romantic. Lucy's eyes also had a positive look of purpose, resolve, and courage. No man's ring would ever adorn her hand, and she never bore a child. Being a nurse with credentials gave her freedom: employment freedom, economic freedom, travel freedom, and freedom over her womb. She was her own woman, free to come, free to go, and she did.

By 1906 Lucy was working as a trained nurse at the German Hospital, Kansas City, Missouri.[121] German immigrants founded the hospital in 1884, and it became a place of quality health care. The hospital established a nursing school in 1905.[122] By 1918, owing to the war effort and not wanting to appear supporting the Kaiser, directors of the German Hospital changed the hospital name to "The Research Hospital."[123]

On October 5, 1906, Lucy was placed in charge of the German Hospital medical tent at the Salvation Army encampment on the 1300-acre Swope Park in Kansas City. Several women had left the encampment to take a walk. At the Blue River, Nellie Akers, age 15, and Mrs. A. W. Howard, decided to wade in the river. They both slipped into a deep pool in the river and went under. Lucy was standing on the river bank. She had learned to swim on her father's ranch. Seeing the two women going under, Lucy wearing long flowing nurses' garb, plunged into the river and swam first to Akers. Lucy pulled Akers to shallow water and then swam to Howard, who had gone under a second time. Lucy, after a hard struggle, pulled the unconscious Howard to safety. Both Akers and Howard were unconscious for several hours but were revived and lived. The *Kansas City Star* reported all who saw the accident said Lucy's displayed remarkable coolness and bravery.[124]

Lucy, like many Montana women who would go to war, didn't leave a diary. In World War I Army security rules prohibited soldiers from writing in small books, kept in breast pockets next to their hearts, their thoughts, experiences, observations and fears. Few of Lucy's letters survive. She never recorded when, how, and, most importantly, why, she came to Glasgow, Montana. Glasgow was a distant and, some would say, remote place far from Kansas City, and the New Mexico Territory where Lucy was born. Whether she followed the great land rush to northeast Montana, believed James J. Hill's promotional brochure for immigrants, or simply followed wanderlust and adventure, is lost to history. Lucy never said if she followed a nurse's altruism to help, or if her decision was a business one: multitudes of people, regardless of where they congregate, need medical care and will pay good money for it.

At Glasgow before the war, Lucy worked for Dr. Smith. He was affiliated with Glasgow's Francis Hoyt Mahon Memorial Hospital. The hospital opened November 21, 1911. A. W. Mahon had donated an entire city block for the new hospital. Workers built a pleasant-looking and comfortable two-story nurse's residence or dormitory, called the Nurses Home, across the street from the hospital.[125] Dr. Mark Hoyt, MD, came to Glasgow in 1891. A contract surgeon for the Great Northern Railway, the Great Northern hired Hoyt to convert three boxcars into a medical clinic at Glasgow and try doing something about the many deaths in the area.[126] The boxcars were arranged in a letter H configuration. One car was the office and sleeping room, the second a combined surgical and supply room, and the third was the recovery ward. There were no nurses; patients were attended by family, friends or volunteers.[127]

Hoyt developed a large local practice in Valley County. He later became a World War I Army physician and eventually Glasgow mayor.[128] Smith and Hoyt partnered in Glasgow. The Army would call Smith to active duty months later. Hoyt would also be called to active duty at Base Hospital 38 formed at Philadelphia. History doesn't record what duties Lucy did while working with Smith. Since Smith did all the World War I draft physicals for the Valley County men, Lucy probably helped: especially with recording the paperwork. Lucy never said or wrote when she decided to join the ANC.

A very capable woman, Lucy, before her fortieth birthday, would travel the length and breadth of America: from the Mexican border to the Canadian province of Saskatchewan, and from the Pacific Ocean to the Atlantic. She would crisscross the Atlantic Ocean. Born sixty miles north of the Mexican border, at Glasgow she lived sixty miles south of the Canadian border. In less than a year she would see the large troop hospital in Camp Lewis, Washington, and then cross to the other side of the planet to the distant and romanticized land of France where war had become terribly real.

In time more Glasgow women joined the World War I U.S. military. Along with Lucy, Cora Viola Craig, Ann Dobias, Bertha Becker, and Florence Ford, would become nurses in the ANC. Ethel Lezie Brown, a young Glasgow hometown girl, would be one of the few Montana women to join the Navy as a yeoman (Female). Throughout Montana women going to war went largely as Lucy did: individually or in small groups. Only two Montana nurses, Eula B. Butzerin, from Missoula; and Alice Ralston, from Butte, would go to war as members of a complete military unit.[129] Regardless of their individual circumstances, for Lucy and over 200 women from Montana, the Great War had begun.

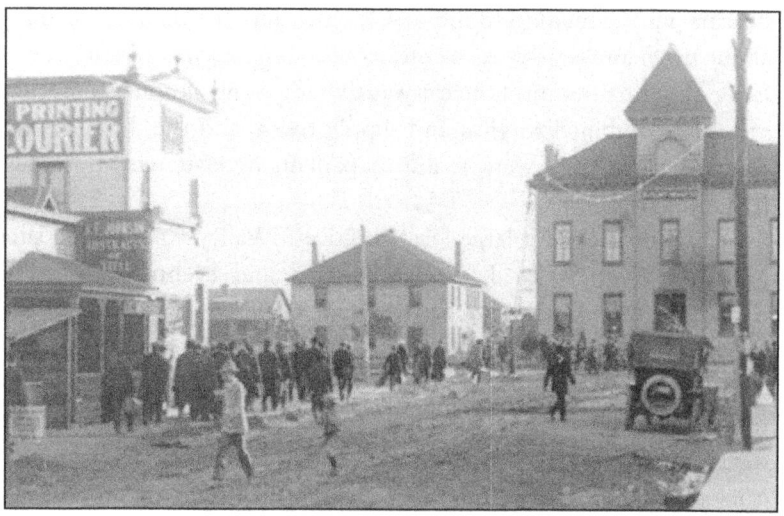

Glasgow, Montana, 1913. Registering for the Fort Peck land lottery.
Valley County courthouse at right, with county jail in middle.
Courtesy Valley County museum.

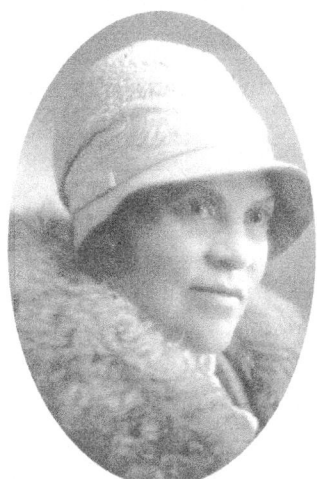

Lucy Walters
Courtesy Kathy Goins

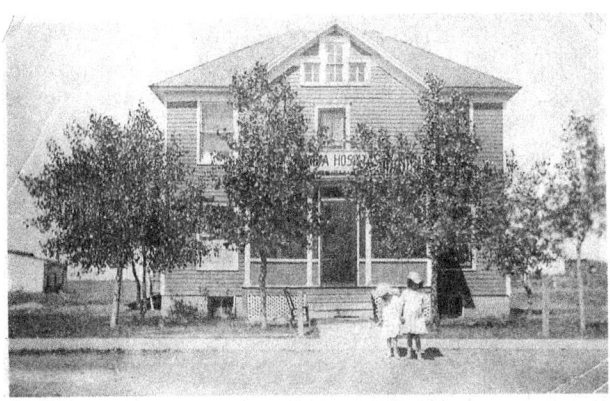

Malta, Montana, hospital, ca 1920. Lucy Walters owned and operated the hospital after WWI. Ann Dobias, WWI nurse, helped Walters at the hospital. As of 2017 the building still stands as a private residence in Malta.
Courtesy Kathy Goins.

Chapter 3
THE DRAFT

"I enlisted, I wasn't drafted"

HUNDREDS OF HONORABLY SERVED VETERANS ARE BURIED in the 31-acre Eastern Montana State Veterans Cemetery at Miles City, Montana. The cemetery is about a mile or two south of town: a town named after General Nelson Appleton Miles, the famous Indian fighter of the American west in the late nineteenth century. Prairie winds blow here. The popping of flags in the wind is heard many times at the quiet and reverent cemetery on the Montana plains. A Word War II veteran wanted history to know his intention, resolve, and perhaps unbridled patriotism in going to war. The cryptic phrase "I enlisted, I wasn't drafted" is engraved at the base of his upright white marble veteran headstone. He volunteered for war and forever wanted people to know.[130]

In America's history the federal government has never required or drafted women to serve in the military. To date, women serving in the United States armed forces have all volunteered. Beginning with the American Civil War, the federal government has drafted men to serve in the military: millions of American men. The prosecution of hard war and bloody combat was seen as men's business. Starting a century ago, the federal government had to enroll, in some manner, women to serve: not because the military wanted women but needed women. This was true when the military needed skills, which society, culture, and provenance of the day, relegated to women.

"Conscription," "selective service," and "the draft," are terms in history naming the process America uses to require men, under penalty of law, to enter the United States military. Congress can do this when Congress deems opposing military forces threaten the safety and security of America. Congress then passes legislation, subject to presidential review, to implement conscription.

In history America ideally wanted volunteers to enter the military. Volunteers were thought more motivated, patriotic, and more willing to serve. Usually not enough men volunteered. The federal government first used conscription to fill the need for soldiers in the Union Army in the American Civil War. President Lincoln's call for volunteers fell woefully short of the millions of soldiers needed to fight the Confederacy. The respective states in the Union, not the federal government, had the responsibility to raise volunteer regiments. In 1861 at Lincoln's first call for volunteers to serve in the Union Army, men enlisted for patriotic reasons, adventure, or peer-group pressure. By 1863 these soldiers were already in the Army—or dead. Grim realities of war made less motived man think again about wearing the uniform of the North. War makes good business. Jobs were plentiful in the north in war industries, why fight in uniform when there's money to be made in business? Congress decided the federal government needed conscription, or the draft, to fill needed military ranks. Congress now said conscription would be a national process and not left to the states.[131]

To fill needed military ranks, Congress passed a conscription act on March 3, 1863. It was "an act for enrolling and calling out the national forces and for other purposes."[132] Lincoln would issue four separate calls for new troops under the conscription act. The act required men in the Union, ages twenty to forty-five, and immigrants who filed for citizenship, to register for a three-year tour-of-duty in the Union army. The act did not allow many exemptions to conscription. The draft had two classes of draftees: class 1 had all single and married men aged twenty to thirty-five, and class 2 had married men over thirty-five. Men from class 2 would not be drafted until all those in class 1 went first. This basically meant married men over thirty-five would not be drafted. The conscription act authorized the Provost Marshalls Bureau of the War Department to enforce conscription.

The Army would administer the draft. The first task was to count the eligible men in each northern congressional district. The War Department assigned a quota for each district based on the number of eligible men in that district and the proportional allocation of soldiers Lincoln called for. If the district didn't raise enough volunteers, a conscription draft would be held in that district to fill the remaining required number of men. This was all a very intricate and complicated process done nationally above the Mason-Dixon Line with paper and pencil.[133]

The conscription act was flawed from the start and was one of the poorest managed laws of that time. The act allowed for men to buy their way out of a draft call by paying a $300 fee: largely an unreachable sum for a poor man. Men could also hire substitutes to take their place for a privately negotiated sum. Fraud began in earnest. Inaccurate counts, bribes to those doing the counting, and bribes to doctors doing physicals made the Civil War draft almost unworkable. Draft evasion became a problem with men disappearing into the vast interior of America, escaping across the border into Canada, or simply not showing when their name was called. "Bounty jumping" became an art form of clever men. Some places paid cash bounties or cash bonuses to men who enlisted: sort of a monetary inducement to serve your country. A man would enlist under an assumed name, pocket the enlistment bonus, and vanish. The same fellow would take another false name, enlist elsewhere, collect bonuses, and vanish again.

Conscription had another less visible purpose: bolster the number of volunteers by implying a volunteer was a better citizen, a more courageous man and a man to be honored. A volunteer could receive state and federal enlistment bonuses, join the regiment of his choosing, and proudly escape the stigma of the draft by saying he was a better man than those being led by the dog's leash of conscription.[134] In short, the boast, "I enlisted, I wasn't drafted."

In time draftees accounted for a low 8 percent of the Union army.[135] Regardless of the low number of draftees, frustration and anger boiled over the inequities of the conscription law of that time. The deadliest civil riot in American history began in New York City, July 1863, because of the Civil War draft. Public and political sentiment began calling the draft "rich man's war—poor man's fight" and viewed it as class struggle rather than a need for national survival in war. Economically poor white men, especially Irish immigrants, had few alternatives in the draft. They could not afford the $300 draft buy-out fee, had no job due to discrimination, and had no money to hire substitutes. If they left their families to enlist in the military and were killed-in-action or disabled, their families would suffer greatly in the densely packed, disease-infested immigrant ghettos of New York City.

The smoldering volcano blew. On Saturday, July 11, New York City conscription officials drew the first names of the draft. In lower Manhattan, groups of men drank themselves into violent courage. They resolved to correct the matter, perceived or actual, with their fists. Taking to the streets the next day, angry men didn't see Sunday as a day of physical and spiritual rest, but as a day of cleansing the sins of the draft by fists and blood. Wholesale mob violence began. Draft offices and draft officials were the first targets of smoldering rage. Mobs then turned their violence upon blacks, who the mob saw as taking jobs from them. Lynchings happened and rioters burned an orphanage for black children. Newspaper offices were destroyed and editors threatened. Homes of the wealthy and Protestant churches were also burned. Determined to restore order, the federal government sent regular Army troops into Manhattan. Many of the troops had just returned from fighting in the terrible battle of Gettysburg two weeks before. By Wednesday and Thursday military troops and New York policemen had restored order. The rioting lasted four days and killed an estimated 105 people.[136] The struggle with conscription for military service would vex America for the next one hundred years.

Citizens challenged the Civil War draft in court. Did the federal government have the authority to force a man [women weren't drafted] to leave his home, family, and job to fight in a war the man may not agree with or didn't want to fight? Did conscription violate individual liberties and the reserved rights of the states? The first challenges in court began in Pennsylvania.[137] The Pennsylvania Supreme Court said the Draft Act of March 3, 1863, was not an invasion of the rights of the several states and of the nation's citizens. Justices said the law was a valid exercise of power constitutionally conferred upon the United States by the people. The ultimate ruling in America was the Draft Act of March 3, 1863, was valid and constitutional.

Woodrow Wilson, a Democrat and former president of Princeton University, was elected president of the United States in 1912. When war began in Europe, he pledged American neutrality and offered to broker a peace settlement in Europe. These were lofty goals consistent with Wilson's high-minded and uncompromising ideals on the human experience, bordering on self-righteous. The Navy Bill of 1916 specifically stated Wilson's policy; the bill read: "It is hereby declared to be the policy of the United States to adjust and settle its international disputes through mediation or arbitration to end that war may be honorably avoided."[138] This was not workable in early twentieth century Europe where competing and conflicting ideals of nationalism had reached a level where vengeance and punishment eclipsed compromise. America could not dismiss the escalating war in Europe.

The war began affecting America physically and psychologically.

Germany's unrestricted submarine warfare was sinking commercial ships. Americans were dying on the high seas. Over one thousand men, women, and children died in the German sinking of the British-flagged liner the *Lusitania*, May 7, 1915. One hundred twenty-eight Americans on the *Lusitania* went into the water off the Old Head of Kinsale on Ireland's southern coast and drowned.[139] In January 1917 America learned of Germany's top-secret efforts to get Mexico into the war on Germany's side. Germany had promised Mexico full recovery of Mexican territory lost to America in the Mexican War of 1845.[140] America finally had enough. Senator Frederick Hale from Maine said, "How is it that any nation could put up with the affronts we have."[141] Even Wilson concluded in the spring of 1917 that war was inevitable. He changed his mind on America's neutrality and sought congressional approval of a resolution for war.

On April 4, 1917, the U.S. Senate passed a resolution for war. On April 6 the U.S. House of Representatives met to debate and vote for the same resolution. Two amendments to the resolution failed: that Congress had to approve transporting troops to Europe, and only troops who volunteered for duty in Europe could go to Europe.[142] Shortly after 3:00 p.m. Washington D.C. time, the House voted 373 to 50 to approve the resolution of war. Montana's Jeanette Rankin, born near Missoula, a graduate of the University of Montana and life-long pacifist, sat with her head bowed through the first roll call vote: failing to answer when twice her name was called for "yay" or "nay" on the resolution. On the second roll call vote she rose despairingly in the House chamber and supported herself against a desk. Wearied by the hours of protracted debate on the resolution, cries of "vote, vote," came from members of the House. Rankin said in a sobbing voice, "I want to stand by my country, but I cannot vote for war." She slumped back in her chair and apparently whispered "no." Chief clerk of the House, Jerry South, went to Rankin's seat to confirm her vote of "no" against the war resolution.[143] [In 1941 Rankin would vote "no" against declaring war on Japan in World War II: the only person in Congress to vote against war with Japan.]

From August 1914 to April 1917, when America entered World War I, efforts bordering on a crusade began in America by powerful organizations and political men: former president of the United States, Theodore Roosevelt, and the National Security League among

The Draft   33

them. They advocated a "preparedness" movement to ready America for an inevitable involvement in the European war. Wilson initially didn't support preparedness, as he saw it a violation of his neutrality policy. Public sentiment and the reality of war were against Wilson.[144] Preparedness for America's entry in war began in earnest with Congress passing on June 18, 1916, the National Defense Act of 1916. This broad scale and comprehensive legislation reorganized America's military and greatly increased the overall military structure and strength.

America had to decide if it needed the draft. Wilson first advocated an all-volunteer force for largely the same reasons dating to the American Civil War: volunteers would be more beneficial and expedient than conscripts. An unwilling conscript was thought mediocre soldier material. A national draft would also signal to foreign countries that America was preparing for war, and this would be inconsistent with Wilson's neutrality stance. Roosevelt, Wilson's long-time political adversary, wanted to show Roosevelt's continuing leadership and swagger against Wilson's aversion for war: the rough-rider cowboy and war veteran, against the liberal intellectual.

Born 1858, by age fifty-one, when Roosevelt had finished his second term as president, his personal and political accomplishments were many and distinguished: Harvard and Columbia university graduate, Dakota cowboy, New York assemblyman, assistant secretary of the Navy, governor of New York, Spanish-American war troop commander and combat veteran, Nobel Laureate, noted author, vice-president, and president of the United States. [In 2001, Roosevelt would be awarded the Medal of Honor for his courage under fire while leading troops up San Juan Hill in Cuba. The only president thus far so honored.[145]] A genuine non-stop engine of energy and activity, the many times bombastic Roosevelt was dissatisfied with the political direction of America after he had left the White House. Roosevelt had been to the mountain top and liked the view on high; he showed no inclination of coming down. He ran for a third term as president in 1912 on his newly founded Progressive "Bull Moose" Party.[146] He lost convincingly to Wilson. Even with losing the presidential election, Roosevelt still had a national political base and wasn't backing down to stay out of the national and international political arena—especially to Wilson.

Beginning with the Civil War, America had a regular army and a volunteer army. The U.S. Constitution (art.1, §8, cl.12) reads in part, Congress has the power to raise and support armies. This is the regular army, or America's full-time professional standing army whose job is the profession-of-arms. To augment the regular army, the president as commander-in-chief, could call for volunteers. The regular army would then train the volunteers. In 1898 during the Spanish-American War, federal law and Army general orders allowed volunteer units to be raised and formed locally. The federal government would fund the units and then integrated them into the regular army.[147]

Given this law as precedent, Roosevelt wanted to raise, command, and take to war in Europe, a volunteer force like his Rough-Riders of the Spanish-American War. Eight years after Roosevelt's presidency, he went to the White House and personally lobbied Wilson for the right to raise a volunteer army and go to war. Roosevelt was challenging Wilson's leadership and Wilson knew it.[148] Realizing volunteers could not fill the need for millions of soldiers for war, Wilson wanted new laws to abolish the old volunteer system and institute national conscription. He also wanted to block Roosevelt. Part of the law would read only volunteers would be allowed in the regular Army and the newly created National Guard.[149] This was to prevent Roosevelt from raising Roosevelt's personal volunteer army.

America officially was at war in April 1917. Congress began debating how to raise the needed troops for war. America's choices were relying on volunteers or begin conscription. Mindful of serious problems with the draft during the Civil War, and fundamental questions of the draft versus personal liberties, strong opposition of the draft existed in Congress. Missouri's senator James A. Reed said, "The nation will be better defended by men whose heart and soul are freely given for it. There is a difference in going to war with his mother's blessing and a brute with a bayonet dragging him out from her arms."[150] Conversely others felt national conscription would be more democratic, and the less motivated [so-called "slackers"] would "no longer be able to evade their duties and seek security at the expense of their loyal and courageous fellows. Its rank injustice is the fatal weakness of the volunteer system."[151]

Many congressmen still believed volunteers could fill the ranks. Wilson disagreed. Secretary of War Newton Baker reiterated the volunteer system could not raise sufficient troops, and as an added psychological effect, the draft would show America's resolve and earnestness to Germany.[152] Roosevelt supported what he called "universal obligatory military service" [he was careful not to say "draft" or "conscription"]. He continued advocating for a volunteer force to augment the draft. Roosevelt said in a letter April 12, 1917, to the chairmen of both the Senate and House Military Committees that he could raise and train a volunteer force. Then in four months take them to Europe to meet the immediate war need. Roosevelt wrote, "There are many hundreds of thousands of men in this country who are first-rate fighting material and available for service within a short time, who would eagerly volunteer for immediate service at the front."[153] [The thought of the aging rough-rider Roosevelt and his quickly trained volunteers charging headlong into entrenched defensive positions manned by the Kaiser's battle-hardened troops, expert with machine guns and artillery, is too terrible to imagine. The French learned tragically at Verdun, and the British at the Somme.]

Members of the House Military Committee first wanted to try raising an army of 500,000 men through the old volunteer system. The Army said this wasn't possible. The supporters of the volunteer plan to raise half a million men wanted to try the plan for thirty days. If the plan didn't work, they would be willing to vote for compulsory service. The Army's position was the volunteer system, ineffective and undemocratic, would not raise sufficient men needed in the present national emergency. The Army also said if the volunteer system failed, as the Army predicted it would, then foreign nations would conclude America was against the war and not willing to support it.[154] Opposed to the war and conscription, Wisconsin representative William J. Cary, introduced a resolution. It read in raising an army by selective conscription, the first selection should be made from "such male citizens of proper military age as are officers or members of the New York Stock Exchange, or any other similar body, or officials in banks, lawyers, magazine editors and other citizens engaged in non-productive pursuits." Whether this also meant congressmen, Cary didn't elaborate. The resolution failed.[155]

The matter of conscription and the draft reached Montana. John Morgan Evans, a Montana representative in the U.S. House during World War I, sent word to Montana that he wanted Montana's views on the conscription bill before Congress. Evans favored the volunteer plan but the Missoula Chamber of Congress, and the Missoula Women's Club that also received Evans' telegram about the conscription bill, overwhelmingly rejected the volunteer plan. Both organizations also sent word to Jeanette Rankin, Montana's other congressional representative, about their rejection of the volunteer plan. Missoula's Chamber of Commerce unanimously passed a resolution, without dissent, and with a standing ovation and cheers, reading:

> Resolved that we express to our senators and representatives in congress that we favor the policy of selective conscription for active military service, rather than the undemocratic volunteer policy under which one patriot shoulders the shirked military duties and dangers of other citizens who are less patriotic.[156]

Montana cities of Butte and Hamilton also wired Rankin telling her to "stand alone" if she had to in support of Wilson's conscription bill.[157] Rankin's votes on the subject confused Montana. The *Daily Missoulian*, April 29, 1917, read Rankin voted for the volunteer plan and opposed the War Department and Wilson's selective conscription. However, the *Daily Missoulian* the next day said Rankin opposed conscription but in the final vote supported conscription. Rankin would later miss a vote to recommit the Army bill as she missed her name in a roll call vote.[158]

Great Falls favored conscription. The *Great Falls Tribune* in its April 8, 1917, editorial, "The Conscription Idea," wrote:

> The secretary of war and the army officers are all thoroughly committed to the desirability of conscription as a principle in raising the new army planned for, but we have yet to see how congress [sic] and the country will take to it. ...The United States is conservative...when any change comes that seems copied from military nations and infringes on personal liberties. However, the Tribune is agreed with the general staff of the army and the administration officials in regarding the conscription principle as the best when it comes to raising an army.
>
> ...Conscription is not only the fairest way to

raise an army, but it is best for the country and best for the men conscripted. ...Even the man who thinks it is his duty to volunteer is going to be told by wife or children or mother or loved ones in his family that he is mistaken as to the call of duty. That his first duty is toward them. Or they will tell him that it is too soon, and that some other fellow should go first. ... But if the same man is conscripted there is no doubt or argument left about his patriotic duty left. ...He is saved much inward debate and mental struggle, and so are his kinsmen and women folk. ...He must answer the call of his country in any event...

...That is why we present the argument in favor of conscription here. For our part we like it better than the volunteer system, with its implication of cowardice cast upon those who do not respond by enlisting, though they may have very good and sufficient private reasons why they do not enlist that the public knows nothing about.

On April 18 Wilson went to Capitol Hill to lobby the Senate for passage of the compulsory military service bill. The strongest dissent for conscription came from the South and the Midwest where agriculture was strong. Southern senate opponents to the draft argued the draft would take men needed for farming. Despite continuing opposition, Wilson's compulsory military service bill passed the Senate Military Affairs Committee 10 to 7.[159] Future president of the United States, Warren G. Harding, then a U.S. senator, added an amendment to the conscription bill [the so-called Roosevelt amendment] to authorize four volunteer divisions. The amendment, however, did not direct the president to accept the volunteer divisions.[160] The legislation did not mention Roosevelt by name, but Congress knew the amendment meant Roosevelt.[161] Senator William J. Stone, D-Missouri, had vigorously opposed the Roosevelt amendment saying Roosevelt had a political agenda and not much more. Stone also implied Roosevelt was too old to command troops in the field and wouldn't take military orders from anyone senior to him in rank.[162] Stone was correct. The old rough-rider would never lead troops again. Roosevelt, age sixty, died less than two years later, January 9, 1919, at his New York home.

The House had previously passed the draft bill, and on May 18 the Senate passed the bill 65 to 8. The major provisions of the bill, after compromises between the House and Senate versions were: Drafting with certain exceptions, 500,000 men between ages twenty-one and thirty; federalizing all National Guard units; and increasing military pay. Another provision, surely not to be received cheerfully and with vigor by all draftees, was liquor could not be served at or near any Army training camp "to protect the morals of the soldiers." The World War I draft bill ensured all evils of the Civil War draft were corrected: draftees couldn't buy their way out of the draft or hire substitutes. The bill included the Roosevelt amendment that Wilson never enacted. Immediately after Wilson signed the bill, he declared a national holiday allowing all draft eligible men time to sign up.[163] Montana soon confirmed the ineffectiveness of the volunteer system versus the draft. The *Daily Missoulian*, May 9, 1917, read:

> No better argument for conscription can be found than one right at our door. In April, 109 men were enlisted at the recruiting station in Missoula. For the same period there were 165 enlistments in Spokane, which boasts of a population of 120,000, six times larger than that of Missoula. There is no need for argument now for the conscription bill is a law. These figures merely show the injustice of the volunteer system.

In World War I the draft was challenged in the U.S. Supreme Court. In 1918 the Court in unanimous opinion in Selective Draft Law Cases, 245 U.S. 366, said the Selective Service Act was constitutional. The Court examined and rejected all of the challenges against the World War I draft act.[164] The court also said "Congress may conscript for military duty in a foreign country, and the militia clause [of the Constitution] is not a limit upon the war power."[165]

Army brigadier general Enoch H. Crowder and his assistant, Army major Hugh Johnson, created the system to manage the draft in America. Crowder looked to decentralize the day-to-day draft procedures down to local levels. The governors of each state would manage the apportionment down to the local level, then tell each draft board [normally the county boards] their quota of men to be furnished.[166] In time over four thousand local draft boards across America, composed of civilian members of the community, decided on the induction, rejection, or deferments on local eligible men.[167] Draft quotas were based on total population, not on how many men registered for the draft. In Montana this caused problems. Congressman Evans criticized the system as being unfair to Montana. He said:

> The quota as finally arranged is not based on the number of men registered but is based on the estimated population of the several states. ...Montana is given a million people and must furnish 10,000 men. Nearly 3,000 of these men have already volunteered, leaving about 7,500 to be drafted.
>
> We who are familiar with the state know that this is about 25 percent too high. This estimate makes Montana furnish more men than Colorado, which has four congressmen; more than Washington, which has five congressmen and more than North Dakota which has three congressmen.[168]

The U.S. government federalized Montana's National Guard on July 25, 1917. The guard reported to Camp America, Washington, [present Fort Lewis, Washington] to begin extensive training. While the guard reported for duty, Montana men began registering for the draft. The first draft call wouldn't be until September 1917. Montana men had to complete a questionnaire at the local draft board. The draft had five basic categories of enlistees with thirty subcategories; draft boards had to determine which of the categories and subcategories each man fell under.[169] Not an easy task. This included determining conscientious objector status. Federal draft law allowed long-established religious pacifists such as Quakers and Mennonites to serve in noncombatant roles in the military. The *Great Falls Tribune* was critical of this narrowly focused exemption to traditional religious groups. The *Tribune*, July 10, 1917, read: "It [the law] makes no provisions for those who may hold similar views if they do not belong to such recognized religious groups. Even in that case the law does not excuse the drafted conscientious objector from service to his country, though it does excuse him from service on the fighting line."

The *Tribune* was skeptical about men who suddenly found religion when war trumpets sounded. The *Tribune* offered if a man says he was a conscientious objector to war and not a Quaker or Mennonite, then put the man to work in a proposed agricultural branch of the Army. The man would be a farm laborer and required to grow food for the war effort. In short, fight for America or grow food for America.[170]

It is also amazing how cupid's arrows affect a man's heart when draft boards come calling. Men knew that being married might affect their draft status: meaning they wouldn't have to go. The marriage business got good. Preachers were suddenly busy at the altar. Read the fine print fellows. For the draft the War Department said any man who married after the declaration of war on Germany would be treated the same as a single man. The War Department said "slackers," thinking they can get out of military service by marrying, had better think again.[171]

The local draft board received the list of names drawn by lottery. The number of men needed for the first draft call would be notified to report for a medical physical. The men also had seven days to apply for a draft exemption from the date they were notified to report for a physical. If they failed the physical, the local draft board would give them a written reason.[172] Automatic exemptions included, ordained ministers; members of religious sects forbidding its members to go to war; German citizens; state legislators and governors; county and municipal officers; mailmen, pilots, and not surprisingly, United States congressmen. Many exemptions existed for various family situations involving marriage, children, and dependents.[173] For an exemption to the draft, babies began arriving miraculously fast. The *Ronan* [MT] *Pioneer* reported August 31, 1917, that seven different couples in Butte had used the same baby to claim dependent status. A Butte woman had also acted as wife to two separate men for the men to claim marriage.[174]

But Montana's men rose to be counted and mostly complied with draft requirements. By population, Butte was required to provide the most men in Montana: 791; Broadwater County, the fewest at thirty-one.[175] Montana men began gathering, waiting, and wondering. Wondering when the call would come for them to go to war and wondering if they would ever see their families or Montana again.

Chapter 4
FRONTIER NURSING

"Angels under the big sky"

THE EASTERN PART OF THE CEMETERY IN BILLINGS, MONTANA, is over a century old with tipping and broken granite, marble, and stone grave markers. Wrought iron fences, once decorative and ornate, now rust and fall around several graves. Large expanses of grass along a narrow lane have no grave markers. Many unknowns, paupers, or human remains lost to disease a century ago, are thought buried there. The old part of the cemetery struggles for any remaining nobility and reverence. Few people visit the old cemetery: except local history tours and those interested in genealogy or the macabre. The interred there are forgotten ancestors, or simply forgotten. Workers maintain this part of the large cemetery as best municipal budgets allow. However, workers can't do much other than mow uneven ground, or gather broken limbs and leaves when wind storms come, and wind comes often and hard.

Her headstone faces east on a hill in the old cemetery. Large tall trees, pine and leaf, a hundred years old or more, surround her grave and others nearby. The path to her grave goes steadily uphill. A person's legs pay a small price in muscle to get to the destination: an upright, white marble headstone on the south side of the path at the crest of the hill. During midday the trees shelter hers and other graves from heat, weather, and Montana's fierce persistent winds. Her white marble headstone, forty-two inches long, thirteen inches wide, and four inches thick, with a slight uniform curve at the top, weighs about 250 pounds. Workers set the stone sixteen inches into the ground making the crest of the curved top between twenty-four and twenty-six inches high. The modest headstone stands among many more decorative grave markers when size and ornateness of carved granite ensured the living knew the deceased person's stature in service, earthly wealth, or love by family. In time people who visit cemeteries recognize these modest and unadorned upright white marble headstones mark the grave of an honorably served U.S. military veteran.

The captivating headstone on the hill reads: "Florence Ames, Montana, Nurse, Army Nurse Corps, World War I." At the base of her headstone, someone, probably her older sister, Emma, buried next to Florence, ensured the lyrics to the bugle tune "Taps" were engraved to honor Florence. In the one lithograph known, taken when Florence was in her mid-30s and probably while sitting, shows her plain, long, narrow, and unadorned face. She had short hair and may have been tall. She wore a simple, long, almost fragile necklace, and a modest dress.[176] Florence never walked down the aisle of marriage, and never suckled a baby at her breast. In the lithograph her eyes seem tired, perhaps because Florence traveled the world serving in peace and war. In life Florence fought wars against two deadly enemies: bullets and bombs from Kaiser Wilhelm's battle-hardened World War I troops in France, and a more ancient foe of mankind, a microscopic organism called mycobacterium tuberculosis, or simply TB.

William Ransom Ames, born 1830 in Tioga County, Pennsylvania, traveled widely before settling in Nebraska City, Nebraska, near the Missouri River. He married Louisa Balfour, together they had nine children. Florence, born February 12, 1882, was the second youngest.[177] Ames began farming on the south branch of the Weeping Water Creek in southeast Nebraska. A highly respected man of publicly noted integrity, he was elected as a Democrat to the Nebraska state legislature in 1890. Ames died at his home in Nebraska, 1903, of what was then called "Bright's Disease": a summation of many chronic kidney diseases. At his death, two of Ames' children, Roy and Florence, still lived in Nebraska City.[178]

Little is known of Florence's upbringing, her education, her ambitions, her dreams and future hopes. With her father's excellent reputation and work ethic, Florence probably had a good upbringing. Her father's lingering death from painful kidney disease may have influenced her to nursing. The same year of her father's death, Florence went to Chicago, Illinois, and entered the Illinois Training School for Nurses [now Cook County School of Nursing]. Founded 1881 the school, with a board of directors numbering twenty-five women and fifty men, was an adjunct to the Cook County hospital and the first school in the Midwest to follow the Florence Nightingale training curricula and methods begun in London, England.[179] The school advertised in newspapers and national magazine about its three-year comprehensive nursing program and opportunities. With strict entry requirements, pupils had to sign a contract agreeing they would adhere to the school rules and courses of study. Student nurses would also live in a nurses' dormitory.[180] The school proudly wrote a summary of the course of instruction:

> They [students] will also be given instruction in the best practical methods of supplying fresh air, warming and ventilating sick-rooms in a proper manner, and are taught to take care of rooms and wards, in keeping all utensils perfectly clean and disinfected, to make accurate observations and reports to the physician of the state of secretions, expectoration, skin, pulse, appetite, temperature of the body, intelligence as delirium or stupor, breathing, sleep, conditions of wounds, eruptions, formation of matter, effect of diet, or of stimulants or of medicines and to learn the management of convalescents.[181]

Not forgetting bedside manner, the school expected their nurses visiting patients in private service, to have an appropriate bedside manner: "A nurse shall never, under any circumstances, relate to her patient sad or exciting experiences with other patients; she shall maintain a dignified reticence in regard to the diseases, their treatment or the methods of other physicians." The school also ensured nurses knew who was boss and said: "Nurses are to take the whole charge of the sick-room, doing everything that is requisite in it, when called upon to do so, obeying implicitly the orders of the physician in attendance without note or comment."[182]

Florence graduated with thirty-one other women in the Illinois Training School for Nurses, class of 1906.[183] By then her brother, Roy, and widowed mother, had moved to the Yellowstone River Valley near Billings to be near other Ames family members who had begun sheep ranching. Florence followed her family.[184] Florence was a "graduate nurse." At the turn of the twentieth century, a graduate nurse was someone [mostly women] who had successfully completed a two or three-year comprehensive course-of-study at an established nursing school having faculty with credentials. A graduate nurse was the highest level of nursing qualification then.

Definition of "nurse" varies greatly in history to the early twentieth century. Formal nursing training, with uniform standards and curriculum, didn't begin until Florence Nightingale showed the need and benefits of trained people with standards of care for the military wounded during the Crimean War of 1854/56. She revolutionized inadequate British army medical services to cope with deplorable squalor and disease conditions facing British troops in the Crimea. She also began the world's first school of nursing at St. Thomas' Hospital in London. At this school Nightingale created the first uniform standards of medical care for nursing, and also began dignifying the profession of nursing.[185] In time American hospitals began Nightingale's principles of patient care. Using Nightingale's methods and standards, American women began volunteering their expertise and willingness to help America's sick and wounded during the American Civil War.

When the Civil War began, the federal government was ill-prepared for casualties on Civil War battlefields. Private relief organizations helped. In 1849 Dr. Elizabeth Blackwell, MD, was the first American woman to earn a medical degree. She began organizing three thousand women in New York to coordinate the work of smaller relief agencies. Her efforts formed the nucleus of the Women's Central Association for Relief, or the WCAR. The WCAR created a training program for nurses. The WCAR soon became the core of the United States Sanitary Commission. The Sanitary Commission was a civilian organization that supported the government. Many in government did not want civilians on battlefields. The Army Medical Bureau, headed by an aged fellow known as a "bigoted blockhead," didn't want upstart civilian busybodies in his business. He also didn't want women nurses mucking around men. In time the Sanitary Commission and its nurses showed skill in saving lives on battlefields and in troop hospitals. President Lincoln initially didn't support the Sanitary Commission. He didn't want to grant them a charter. Eventually he changed his mind. On June 13, 1861, Lincoln signed the order creating a charter for the Sanitary Commission.

The Sanitary Commission's demonstrated excellence in organization, efficiency, and soldier care soon impressed the surgeon general of the Army Medical Bureau, William Hammond. The newly appointed, younger, and effective Hammond ordered one-third of Army nurses in general hospitals be women. By war's end three thousand northern women had served as paid Army nurses. These women, however, did not work *in* the Army but rather *with* the Army [italics added]. Several thousand women continued as volunteers and salaried staff of the Sanitary Commission. The Civil War brought nursing to a higher level than before. Dorothea Dix and Clara Barton rose to high levels of national influence on nursing and nursing care based on their wartime Civil War experiences. Barton lobbied for America to become associated with the International Red Cross.[186] The ability, courage, and persistence showed by America's women during the American Civil War, began uplifting the profession of nursing in America. The profession would need another fifty years to fully mature.

Among the earliest nurses in Montana may have been Mrs. Katherine Babbage. She arrived on a Missouri River steamboat at Fort Benton in 1874. Trained in a maternity hospital in Washington D.C., Babbage started her practice as a nurse midwife. At the urging of Jesuit Father Pierre DeSmet, who founded St. Mary's Mission at Stevensville, Montana, the Sisters of Charity of Leavenworth, Kansas, in 1870 began Montana's first true hospital: St. John's Hospital in Helena. By 1890 other hospitals operated by the Sisters of Charity opened in Montana towns of Deer Lodge, Virginia City, Butte, Anaconda, Missoula, Fort Benton, and Billings. More followed.[187] Nurses began trickling into Montana.

The challenge for nursing in Montana and America at the turn of the twentieth century, was lack of standards prescribed in law. Most anyone, even those with dubious credentials, experience, and training, could say they were a "nurse." If you could bandage a bleeding body, set a broken limb, [horse or human] and give a shot of whiskey to deaden the pain, you could call yourself a nurse. The *Montana Standard* in Butte, printed a story in January 1910 about false nurses with disreputable agendas: "There have been many cases of demented invalids, particularly aged men, who have fallen victims to designing nurses and instances are constantly being exposed where these women have secured the license and made all the arrangements for marrying in cases where the patients had money." Instances of falsified nursing diplomas from "diploma factories" were reported in northern Wyoming not far from Billings. Officials found the chief nurse at the Sheridan branch of the Wyoming State Hospital in Sheridan, Wyoming, had false nursing credentials.[188] In 1903 New York State began an effort, soon to go national, to pass laws defining standards for nurses and requiring nurses to register with the state and pass an examination. North Carolina, New Jersey, and Illinois soon passed registration and examination laws. The law in New York had strong support in the state legislature. New York newspapers read:

> When a citizen employs for his family a nurse and pays the standard price for the trained service he wants to know that he is getting trained service. As the law stands now there are many incompetents practicing nursing who have had no training at all. Yet they demand and get as good pay as the conscientious young woman who has given two or three years of the best years of her life to the study and practice of nursing.

New York wanted to ensure the public knew the difference between a thoroughly trained hospital nurse and one partially qualified. The state wanted to assure the public and doctors that someone calling themselves a nurse was fully trained. New York also wanted to protect a fully qualified nurse from unjust competition with someone with lower standards of training; and protect young women from wasting their time and money by going to a so-called nursing school with suspect credentials.[189]

The laws included establishing state boards of nursing. In 1905 the Montana Deaconess Hospital in Great Falls graduated the first class of the hospital's nursing school. The class had two graduates: Harriet Fritschie from Pennsylvania, and Susie Kent from Bozeman, Montana. But Montana still had no laws governing nursing standards. Graduate nurses in Montana had created an organization called the Montana Association of Graduate Nurses. Using New York as an example, the Association of Graduate Nurses began lobbying the Montana state legislature for laws creating nursing standards and registration. In 1909 the first try at requiring the registration and examination of qualifications of trained nurses, Montana House bill No. 179, died in committee.[190] It failed largely due because so-called "practical nurses," or "trained nurses," were making their living by hiring out their abilities of questionable merit: skilled or not.

The trained nurse and practical nurse of that day learned their craft largely by on-the-job training and not through successful completion of a comprehensive course of study and training. If Montana required registration and passing of examinations, then the less qualified or frauds, might be out of a job. In 1908 private duty nurses in Montana, meaning those hired for specific families or cases, received $25.00 a week plus board. The private duty nurse was expected to work a twenty-hour shift. She would have to bathe, and feed the patient, give medications and clean the patient's room. She slept in the patient's room and was expected to include time for meals in her four hours off each day. [By 1935 in Montana nurses' work hours finally decreased to an eight-hour shift.] In 1908 nurses carried their own thermometers, syringes, and even narcotics until the passage of the Harrison Narcotic Act of 1914. The Act began a national effort to regulate opium, cocaine, and their derivatives.[191]

Mrs. Catherine Flynn, a 1911 graduate of St. Patrick's School of Nursing in Missoula, Montana, wrote of the challenges of nursing in turn-of-the-century Montana:

> Most of the private duty nursing in the early years (1908-1914) was done in the homes. Since there were no special extras, such as oxygen, intravenous injections and blood transfusions used at that time, there wasn't much advantage to hospitalization. Hence, the nurse went to the home if the doctor thought it necessary.
>
> ...Her work was very hard and tedious. She had 24-hour care of the patient in addition to maintaining relations with the family and hired help. Most of the homes had no modern conveniences such as plumbing and electricity. There was no doctor to come immediately for the simple reason that there was no telephone. Someone had to be sent with a message. The nurse had to meet each emergency with her own resources, and as was the case before modern medicines, severe illnesses ran their complete course with nursing care as the only treatment. ...Most of the nurses who went into homes were young girls just out of training and with little experience in this field.

> Communicable diseases were the greatest trial. There were so many and isolation was a real problem. It was hard to keep the patient isolated from the family and to get the necessary equipment to care for the patient …
>
> Maternity work was another problem. Nurses were engaged for the estimated date of delivery. They couldn't work on any other case from the one, and then the patient usually fought paying them for those days they waited for delivery. It was hard on both sides as the nurse couldn't afford to be off without pay and the family couldn't afford the cost of paying a nurse for waiting as much as two weeks…
>
> One great factor in home nursing was the policy of the doctor on the case. Some demanded their nurses have every accommodation and protection possible and backed her decisions at all times. Others were very indifferent and allowed people to take advantage of these young girls and left the responsibility of the patient on the nurse's shoulders.[192]

Montana's Graduate Nurses Association kept trying to have Montana pass laws requiring standards of nursing training and registration. The graduate nurses said they were not asking that untrained or unskilled nurses be barred from helping family, friends, or when asked in largely rural Montana. The graduate nurses wanted to protect the word "nurse" and make it apply exclusively to those who had shown proper preparation in caring for the sick. The graduate nurses wanted educational standards for nursing be written into law, and that the public still would have a choice in the publics' medical care.[193] In 1911 Montana state senator James M. Burlingame, from Great Falls, introduced senate bill 53. The bill set nursing standards, examinations, and registration procedures for trained nurses in Montana. The bill would make registration of nurses compulsory, with trained and untrained nurses distinguishable. With this bill, the trained graduate and registered nurses could sign their name with an "RN."

The bill included establishing a state board of nursing and qualifications for registered nurses in Montana. The bill read that medical doctors would comprise the board: not nurses. Montana graduate nurses opposed this. The law was changed to read trained nurses would make up the board.[194] Part of the proposed law established a state board of nursing examiners in Montana. The law read the board shall consist of five members of the Nurses Association of Montana, and who have been actively engaged in nursing for at least five years prior to the appointment. Two of the board members shall have at least two years' experience as nursing instructors. The president of the board shall act as inspector of all Montana training schools for nurses. Burlingame ensured the law didn't give nurses license to practice medicine by writing in the law: "Nothing in this act shall be considered as conferring any authority to practice medicine and undertake the treatment and cure of disease in violation of the medical practice act of the state of Montana."[195] The bill slowly worked its way through the Montana legislature. By 1912 the Murray Hospital in Butte held graduating ceremony for seven nurses who completed the hospital's three-year nurse training program. In February 1912 the *Montana Standard* read about the training:

> Three years of rigid training and discipline, together with scientific nursing, has brought the training school at the Murray hospital to a very high standard. Splendidly equipped in every way, the nurses are prepared to leave their alma mater, which ranks with the foremost in the state, the comprehensiveness of its curriculum being evident to all who are acquainted with the admirable work performed by the nurses.

By 1913 Montana had ten schools giving training for nurses, but still no state standards of nursing education or qualifications.[196] Graduate nurses in Anaconda and Butte drafted a comprehensive nursing bill to be presented to the legislature in 1913. The bill provided details of standards, qualifications, examinations, and establishing a state board of nursing.[197] The graduate nurses at Columbus and Deaconess Hospitals in Great Falls heartily approved the effort to get state nursing laws passed. By 1917 all nursing applicants had to pass the state nursing board examination.[198] In March 1913 the Montana legislature passed comprehensive legislation providing for examination and registering of nurses. The bill set standards of nursing excellence and education. The *Daily Missoulian* wrote about the bill in March 1913:

> ...It will give a legal status so that the professional nurse will be the registered nurse. It can prevent a probationer, who was not accepted because of her unfitness, or a pupil who was dismissed for cause, from posing as a graduate nurse. It can prevent employees of hospitals and sanatoria who are attracted by a high social position or larger remuneration, from successfully palming themselves upon the public as duly qualified graduate nurses.
>
> ...Graduate nurses do not ask that untrained or unskilled or unregistered nurses should be restrained form following their vocation... Graduate nurses ask that the educational standard of nurses shall be made legal, that coming up to the standard and fulfilling its requirements shall alone constitute a nurse to be recognized as a professional or registered nurse.

Supporting state nursing standards, the *Montana Standard* wrote in June 1916:

> The law in no way interferes with the untrained or practical nurse earning her livelihood, but she must not claim to be that which she is not. The state law fixes the penalty for nurses practicing as trained, graduate or registered who do not hold a state certificate.
>
> The law of 1913 is correcting many abuses which had grown up in Montana...Previously, nurses who had spent a few months in an eastern training school, and who may have been expelled for misconduct or incompetency, migrated to Montana to don the cap and white dress and palm herself off as a graduate from Cook county [*sic*], Johns Hopkins or some other good school, and in many cases they brought discredit upon the profession and disaster to the patient.

Beginning 1913, for nurses to be as a registered nurse in Montana, they had to be at least twenty-two years of age, and a graduate from a training school for nurses connected with a general hospital where at least two years of training was in force. Any person of the required age who had been a nurse for five years prior to the passage of the law, and presented a certificate signed by one physician and two registered nurses, could take the examination to become a registered nurse.[199] Beginning June 1, 1915, all Montana nursing schools had to meet state standards. Among the standards, the school had to be connected with a general hospital having a minimum of twenty-five beds and a daily patient load of twelve patients. The training course for nurses could not be less than two years. Nursing instruction had to include specified subjects. Head nurses and superintendent nurses at the school had to be graduate nurses and registered nurses. Nursing students could not be detailed to private homes. Students were to have at least one year of high school and enter a two-month nursing school probationary period.[200]

In 1913, with the passage of nursing standards in law, the Montana Association of Graduate Nurses changed their name to the "Montana State Association of Registered Nurses." Under state law Montana courts could now prosecute any nurse not registered who was representing themselves as either a "trained nurse," or a "graduate nurse." The law also read any person graduating from January 1, 1890, to July 1, 1917, from a training hospital connected with a general hospital giving a course of at least two-years training, could be registered without an examination from the state board of nursing.[201]

Montana's new nursing laws created a delicate church and state situation. The Sisters of Charity of Leavenworth, Kansas, operated many Montana hospitals, and had sisters of the order who called themselves "nurses." The Sisters of Charity wanted to know if Montana law for nurses applied to them: especially at their hospital and nurses training school in Missoula. The county attorney of Missoula County, D. J. Ileyfron, wrote the Sisters of Charity saying the law applied to them. He also wrote that for Montana to accredit their nurses training school, their superintendent of nurses and all head nurses of had to be registered in accordance with Montana law. If the nurses didn't register, their nursing schools in Montana would not be state approved.[202]

Few questioned Susie Lee Welborn's nursing credentials to become a registered nurse in Montana. Born in Elrod, Somerset County, Kentucky, May 16, 1893, Susie was the oldest of nine children born to Ulysses Grant and Sarah Catherine [Lee] Welborn. In 1904 Ulysses, named for the Civil War general and U.S. president, moved his family to western Montana's scenic Gallatin County and began ranching and farming south of Belgrade. He was a good farmer: his wheat crop in 1904 averaged almost fifty bushels per acre. Susie attended school in the Waterman school district south of Belgrade. Little is known of her upbringing other than she was the oldest child and tended the rest of the growing Welborn household. Susie said in later years, "I diapered the lot of them and washed diapers too."[203] Susie's brother, Harvey Frank, called "Frank," was born a year after Susie. Their siblings came regularly about eighteen months apart.

History doesn't say when Susie decided to become a nurse. She went to Temple, Texas, and attended the Scott-White Memorial Hospital nursing program. Graduating in February 1917, Susie's graduation photograph shows her a pretty young svelte woman, with smooth facial features, and dark hair rolled under her white nurse's cap. She is of medium height and wears a nurse's garb and white cover over her slim and narrow waist. Susie isn't smiling. Her raised eyebrows show a satisfied and welcoming countenance of a professional woman who achieved much. Susie returned to Montana and began her decades-long nursing career at the Holy Cross Hospital in Miles City.

Miles City had been in eastern Montana for a long time. After the Battle of the Little Bighorn ["Custer's Last Stand"] in 1876, the Army built forts in eastern Montana. One fort was at the confluence of the Yellowstone and Tongue Rivers. This fort was known at the Tongue River Cantonment or the Tongue River Barracks. The Army built another permanent fort about two miles west of the mouth of the Tongue River. This fort was named Fort Keogh, after Major M. W. Keogh, killed at the Little Bighorn.

Where Army forts were built in the American West, settlers and camp followers came. Livestock speculation brought thousands of head of cattle to the open ranges of Montana in the 1880s. In time the Northern Pacific railroad followed the Yellowstone River past what was now being called "Milestown," or later "Miles City." Miles City soon was the center of cattle, horses, and commercial business in eastern Montana. [The call letters to the present Miles City radio station are

KATL, pronounced "cattle."]

Miles City is as close to cowboy country as you can get in Montana. Cowboys who wrangled horses, and drovers herding cattle, would in time get hurt. For getting hurt, it was never a question of "if," it was always a question of "when and how bad."[204] Railroad men faced hardships and danger too. In Montana the rich, the poor, the soldiers and cowboys, always had to contend with winter. Winter isn't kind to eastern Montana: fierce screaming blizzards strike the land with a vehemence not seen since the biblical plagues of Egypt. A dogged determination, compelling people to shake their fists in defiance of the Almighty, kept people in Miles City.

Regardless of their grit and steadfast refusal to remove their spurs, these people in time would need medical care. What compelled Susie and other nurses to go to Miles City is lost to history. In the early 1900s, Miles City was a booming cattle town along the railroad: a town with a good hospital. War came. Miles City, the Montana cowboy town, would give much in World War I. When the war toxins sounded, eight Miles City nurses would saddle-up and serve: Bridie Cantwell, Gladys Clayton, Martha Hageman, Johnsie Kell, Ethel Kemmer, Hannah Lee, Louise Lindeberg, and Susie.

The Welborn's of Montana would also give much in the Great War. Susie's brothers, Frank, and Ulysees Marion Welborn, would serve in war. Susie and Frank had their picture taken together, each in Army uniform. Frank, a tall robust Montana man, had a determined countenance. Susie looked guarded and cautious.

Of the eight nurses entering the war from Miles City, Gladys Rozella Clayton was indeed a Miles City hometown girl. She was born in Miles City, August 15, 1894, to Douglas and Mildred [Harrington] Clayton. Gladys grew to womanhood with a father who wrangled cattle on various ranches in eastern Montana.[205] History doesn't say if Gladys was a cowgirl, but living in that part of Montana, saddle soap and rawhide mostly likely rubbed off on her in some measure. She became a war nurse and would serve in four Army hospitals: one in America and three in France.[206] On her veteran's headstone in Fargo, North Dakota, Gladys Clayton Roen ensured a certain flamboyance stayed with her forever. Underneath her name is noted, "Red Cross Nurse, World War I, France. Blue capes with scarlet linings."[207]

Johnsie White Kell, another of the eight Miles City nurses, was a true flower of the South. Johnsie Kell the southern belle, was born April 3, 1874 in Fort Mill, South Carolina. Her father, Dr. Samuel Kell, MD, was a sharpshooter in the Confederate Army. After the war he received his medical degree at the Medical College of Virginia Commonwealth, Richmond, Virginia, and enjoyed a lucrative practice in South Carolina. His son, Johnsie's brother, T. B. Kell, would continue the family tradition of being a medical doctor.[208] Johnsie became a nurse. What compelled this southern belle from the Palmetto State to journey to Montana is lost to history. A journey it must have been. She traveled across green, tree-covered eastern hills, then across the Mississippi and Missouri Rivers, and finally across the vast plains of the upper Midwest to Montana. Johnsie saw an America far from the battlefields of the Confederacy and the genteelness of southern society. Montana lost a remarkable piece of history when no one at the Miles City train station recorded what they saw when Johnsie got off the train and saw the rough and tumble Montana cowboy city for the first time.

Johnsie didn't stay in Miles City. She bought a small ranch near Butte, Montana, and then filed a homestead claim of 320 acres in southern Garfield County: many miles north of Miles City.[209] [210] She would have noticed Montana, especially east of the continental divide, is dry, wind-swept, and in some places quite barren. Southern Garfield County could be very remote. When war came, Johnsie entered the ANC and went to Camp Lewis, Washington.[211] The southern belle would never return to Montana. After the war she returned east and lived in Philadelphia and Atlantic City. Johnsie never married. In 1948 she died in Florida and is buried next to her father in Fort Mill, South Carolina.

Florence Ames arrived at the Northern Pacific Railway station in Billings sometime in 1906. Her mother, older brothers, and sister, Emma, were already in the Yellowstone River Valley. Billings, a growing regional city and soon to be Montana's largest city, needed medical professionals. Florence would be the first known graduate nurse in Billings and began her nearly fifty-year nursing career there.[212] Florence's qualifications and experience stood out. In 1914 she and four other women nurses in Montana, now registered nurses of demonstrated high quality and training, were called to Helena, the state capital, to create Montana's first state board of examiners for nurses. Lucy A. Marshall from Missoula; Mrs. N. Lester Bennett from Butte; Ruby Bohart from Bozeman; Florence Ames from Billings; and Mary Margaret ["Margaret"] Hughes from Helena, comprised and organized the board. They chose a date when all nurses in Montana had to pass state standards. The board also had to compile a list of nurses' training schools, in Montana or other states, whose graduates could be registered in Montana without an examination.[213]

Hundreds of Montana's earliest registered nurses would know of these women. Ames valued her penmanship: the mark of a woman who rose above the hardships of Nebraska's steep farm hills of eastern Nebraska and the many demands of Montana. Ames immaculate written signature, with precise, elegant, flowing letters, perfectly spaced vertically and horizontally, would be for many years among the five original signatures on each registered nurse's certificate in Montana. The governor signed too. Of the five original board members, Marshall, Bohart, and Ames, would set aside their nursing duties in Montana and enter World War I. Marshall, born in Nova Scotia, Canada, and Ames, born in Nebraska, would go to France as Army nurses. Bohart, born in Kansas, would be one of the first Montana nurses to enter the U.S. Navy of World War I.[214]

Hughes organized and coordinated most of Montana's nurses who volunteered for military duty. Hughes had the onerous and formidable assignment to send these Montana nurses into harm's way, and possibly to their deaths. Regardless of where a Red Cross nurse lived and served in Montana, from cities to mining camps and railroad whistle stops, a telegram from Margaret Hughes meant the war was more than a distant thought, the war had arrived at the nurse's door.

Signatures of Marshall, Bennett, Bohart, Ames, and Hughes on the Montana nursing certificate of Elizabeth D. Sandelius. Courtesy James Benbow.

Chapter 5
THE PROFESSION OF CARE

"Calamities and war"

SEVEN REGIONS AND ABOUT FIFTY COUNTRIES MAKE UP EUROPE: the earth's sixth-largest continent covering an area a bit larger than the United States.[215] From ancient times war seemed endemic to this continent with many peoples, cultures, religions, and views living close by. The Red Cross movement began in Europe in the 1860s as a humanitarian effort to reduce human suffering, civilian and military, caused by European wars: especially wars in the mid to late nineteenth century. Henri Dunant, a Swiss, proposed an international conference to create volunteer aid societies for the treatment of the wounded in war, and a universally agreed upon set of rules for noncombatants who would help battlefield wounded.

The treaty also called for the creation of wartime volunteer medical aid organizations having the same status as those treating the military wounded. Dunant's idea led to the first Geneva Convention of 1864. [For his founding of the International Committee of the Red Cross, in 1901 Dunant would be the first recipient of the Nobel Peace Prize.] This treaty read those aiding the wounded [e.g., doctors and nurses] would be noncombatants, be granted neutral status, and would not be the target of intentional hostile gunfire. The volunteers would wear a white arm band with an easily recognizable Greek cross of bright red to show their non-belligerent status.

The United States sent Charles S. Bowles, U.S. Sanitary Commission, to Geneva as an observer to the convention. The United States was fighting the American Civil War and too occupied to consider a treaty created by Europeans whose frequent wars were named after the many years between the first and last shots of anger. Bowles tried getting the U.S. government interested in the first Geneva Convention. For the next twenty years America looked the other way. The U.S. viewed Europe with suspicion and didn't want to get involved in a treaty created by perpetually squabbling people on the other side of the planet. People with unstable governments, monarchies, and a quizzical host of dukedoms, duchies, baronies and associated inbred gold-plated whatnots. After the Civil War, the president of the U.S. Sanitary Commission, Henry Bellows, tried creating an "American Association for the Relief of Misery on the Battlefields," based largely on the models of human relief set forth in Geneva. Bellows' efforts languished as the American government wasn't interested.[216]

Nursing at that time was not a modern order, but held to an old world thought that poor sanitation, disorder, drunkenness, and overall coarseness ruled. Lack of teaching, training, and innovations kept nursing to a rough standard. Women began a slow steady movement to uplift nursing to professional standards of care and compassion. Florence Nightingale wrote of nursing reform efforts: "It may be confidently asserted that never in a modern country has a more useful civic service been performed by women that this regeneration of hospitals by women's boards and nurses during the last three decades of the nineteenth century."[217]

Born in Massachusetts, Christmas Day, 1821, America's Clarissa Harlow "Clara" Barton, a practical nurse not school trained, saw battlefield horrors of the American Civil War and European wars. She testified before Congress on the conditions she saw at the infamous Confederate prison camp at Andersonville, Georgia.[218] Barton took on the mantel of humanitarian work and began efforts to create the American National Red Cross Society: soon called the American Red Cross (ARC). Barton modeled the ARC after European efforts. Under the rules of the International Committee of the Red Cross (ICRC) based in Geneva, a nation's Red Cross society could not gain official status until the host government ratified the articles of the 1864 Geneva Convention. Knowing that America was not interested in international war relief and would not sign the Geneva Convention soon, Barton began advocating the ARC as a disaster relief organization in peacetime "national calamity" emergencies such as floods, devastating fires, disease epidemics, mining and railroad disasters.

This disaster relief concept was an American idea for the world. Americans began thinking of the ARC in terms of local help and benevolence, and not as an international entanglement. To keep the idea alive of war relief and battlefield help to the wounded, Barton said the ARC should be completely neutral in war. Barton looked upon neutrality in war as not refraining from shooting someone, or neutrality as a legal status defined by treaty, but neutrality as providing assistance to anyone, regardless of their station in life: military or not. This neutrality credo became one of the ARC's core principals in peacetime.

In early 1881, Barton, with other prominent Americans, gathered in Washington D.C. to create the ARC, and to draw up articles of incorporation. Part of the articles included volunteer aid as shown:[219]

> IV. In time of peace the committees and sections shall train and instruct volunteer nurses.
> V. In the event of war, they shall organize and place volunteer nurses on an active footing.
> VI. The committees shall send volunteer nurses to the field of battle.

Barton was elected president of the society, a position she would hold for twenty years. America still had to ratify the Geneva Convention of 1864 for the ICRC to recognize the American Red Cross Society. After the assassination of President James A. Garfield in June 1881, Garfield's successor, Chester A. Arthur, agreed to sign the treaty. In March 1882, largely due to Barton's personal lobbying of the federal government and her moral persuasiveness and skillful use of the American press, America signed the Geneva Convention. The ICRC approved the ARC as an entity under ICRC auspices.[220] By the early 1900s, forty-four nations, and America, had ratified the treaty.[221] Although the American government had signed the Geneva Convention treaty, the federal government had yet to officially recognize the ARC. The ARC still needed a charter to operate.

The ARC lived up to its core principle of disaster relief during disastrous floods in America in the 1880s, yellow fever epidemics, and coastal hurricanes in the 1890s.[222] By 1893 Barton had organized a branch of the ARC in New York City. Barton set standards for nursing at the Red Cross Hospital and Training School for Nurses. To become a Sister [nurse] of the Red Cross, the person had to take a regular two years and three months training course at the Red Cross hospital, or present completion certificates from a reputable training school for nurses. The applicant would also have to take six months post graduate work applicable to war or natural disaster. The nurses were required to be on call at all times to respond to emergencies. The nurses would be volunteers and not paid for services.

Barton also ensured nurses knew and understood the ARC was "absolutely neutral and non-sectarian, not ignoring but respecting all nationalities and religions."[223] Deteriorating conditions in Cuba in the late 1890s caused a significant confrontation between Barton's ARC and the U.S. government. Barton wanted to send Red Cross aid to suffering peasants in Cuba, while many prominent men in America wanted to go to war with Spain. Against America's wishes, Barton, under ARC auspices, began sending relief supplies to Cuba. Many in America feared these supplies would fall into Spanish hands and not go where the need was greatest.

While Barton began sending relief supplies to Cuba, America declared war on Spain. America's navy blocked sea-going relief supplies to Cuba. Barton's Red Cross relief supplies could not get through. A loop-hole in the ICRC treaty did not cover combat conditions at sea. The ICRC had no authority to move relief supplies past the American naval blockade. While Barton concentrated on Cuba civilians, America's soldiers, mobilizing for war with Spain, began suffering from effects of disease and the effects of poor sanitary conditions in their training bases in America. Barton seemed to forget the humanitarian needs of America's soldiers heading for war.[224]

By the early 1900s Barton was aging and in ill-health. Others in America wanted a new direction for the ARC, and Barton resigned under pressure. The Spanish-American War showed ARC's ability for war relief, but the effort had challenges. Given its demonstrated organizational and relief abilities, the ARC still did not have a government charter. As governor of New York, future U.S. president Theodore Roosevelt said the ARC "should be as the right hand of the Medical Department of the Army in peace and war, for even the best medical department would always need volunteer aid, and the Red Cross should have a federal organization in every state chapters that should be in close touch with the National Guard, attending to encampments and forming schools of instruction in military methods." Following President McKinley's assassination in 1901, many people concluded the ARC needed a complete reorganization and a new charter. The secretary of war, future U.S. president, William Howard Taft, agreed. Army surgeon general Robert M. O'Reilly, wanted to relook the relationship between the ARC and the Army. As not to impede military operation, the War

Department wanted better coordination of volunteer help from relief agencies.

After Barton's resignation, President Roosevelt was committed to reorganizing the ARC with a new charter. The new charter was drafted and became law in January 1905. In the American Journal of Nursing, July 1905, the ARC printed a circular outlining its plan for organization and operations. The circular read the purpose of the ARC was, "To furnish volunteer aid to the sick and wounded of armies in time of war, in accordance with the spirit and conditions of the Geneva Convention ...." And to "Continue and carry on a system of national and international relief in time of peace and apply the same in mitigating the sufferings caused by pestilence, famine, fire, floods, and other great national calamities."[225]

The charter authorized the president of the United States to appoint the ARC's governing board. The governing body had an eighteen-person central committee whose members served terms-of-office, and a seven-person executive committee that would manage the daily business of the ARC. Many members of these committees came from the federal government. The ARC was now a national corporation under government supervision. The first three presidential appointments to the governing board were all high-ranking retired Army or Navy officers. The new charter allowed other civilian relief organizations to serve America's armed forces, not solely the ARC. The charter also protected the insignia and sign of the ARC. The "red cross" insignia could not be used for commercial advertisement to sell anything or for purposes of trade. The American Journal of Nursing in its February 1906 edition read the Red Cross brassard had restrictions on its use and wear: [226]

> The arm piece or "brassard," consisting of a white band with a Red Cross, may only be worn when on duty under the officers of the Red Cross. No nurse has the right to wear it on any other occasion, nor has any other body the right to give it to her...The laws of all countries rigidly protect the use of the Red Cross as an emblem reserved to the national societies and their workers on the battlefield, or in the camp or hospital in time of disaster."

The ARC began its slow movement toward a semi-governmental body when the new charter read, "the Red Cross was to act in matters of voluntary relief and in accord with the military and naval authorities as a medium of communications between the people of the United States of America and their army and navy."[227] The ARC also became an avenue of American international policy. When William Howard Taft became president of the United States in 1909, Taft and the State Department agreed to allow American diplomatic and consular officials to become ARC members. This wasn't simply symbolic, in case of need overseas the State Department wanted its staff to act as ARC representatives. Because of this arrangement, the ARC became an official conduit of American diplomacy.[228]

From August 1914 to April 1917, the United States maintained an official neutrality position on the war in Europe. However, the war increased in scope, scale, death, and international effect. When America entered the war in April 1917, a fundamental and powerful question loomed: How was the ARC to remain neutral in war, caring for all the world's suffering and military wounded, when its host country, America, was a declared belligerent in the war? Simply said, you change the rules.

In 1911 Taft issued a proclamation reading the ARC would be the official provider of volunteer help to the military in wartime. Federal law passed in 1912 authorized America's army and navy to treat ARC personnel, mobilized with the military, as civilian employees of the armed forces. In 1917 President Wilson appointed an ARC war council. The war council, having many former military officers, suspended ARC's neutrality. The council said, "When war was declared between the United States and Germany, the neutrality of the American Red Cross ended automatically." The ARC agreed it would treat battlefield wounded of any country in accordance with the ICRC treaty, but the ARC withdrew all remaining medical and nursing staff from territory occupied by Germany and the Central Powers. The ARC said it would operate solely in Allied territory.[229] The question of the ARC's neutrality solved with a pen.

At the turn of the twentieth century, nursing remained largely the domain of women. In the ARC nursing was the last remaining bastion of women in an organization led by men. Before the ARC's reorganization in 1905, Mabel Thorp Boardman was the ARC's president after Clara Barton's resignation. Boardman realized that a nursing service should be one of the most important departments in the ARC. She made a strong effort to communicate with established nursing schools and department heads about the importance of nursing in the Red Cross organization. Boardman emphasized ARC's high nursing standards. ARC nursing standards required nurses to be registered in states required registration. Where state law didn't required registration, the nurse had to show a certificate or diploma of graduation from a recognized training school for nurses requiring a course of not less than two years.

In war the ARC supported the Army. By June 1898 Army regulations required "two years residence in hospital training school" for applicants to apply to the ANC. The two-year rule for nursing courses was an Army rule the ARC could not waive. The Army insisted on quality and not quantity.[230] Nurses had to be at least twenty-five years of age, and pass a medical exam by physician every two years. Last, the nurse had to be of good moral character in such manner as the branch society may prescribe.[231] [232]

The ARC had two forms of agreement with nurses: one for volunteer nurses, and one for paid nurses. Volunteer nurses agreed to hold themselves in readiness and to enter ARC service when and where required without compensation, except for transportation and subsistence. Paid nurses agreed to the above, but with compensation of forty dollars per month when on duty in the United States and fifty dollars per month outside the United States, along with transportation and subsistence.[233]

In autumn 1907 the American Journal of Nursing said the ARC Central Committee, state nursing societies, and individual nurses, weren't coordinating their respective efforts. The nursing service seemed not well organized across national, state, and local lines. The Journal wrote editorially: "The question before us is how to bring all of our forces so into cooperation with the Red Cross that prompt and efficient service may always be at the command of that society without delays." These assets included the ARC and the American Federation of Nurses. Challenges existed as to how to organize both into a single body, and how to get mutual cooperation between the two. The Red Cross Central Committee began looking at how to organize a Red Cross nursing reserve force in America.

In April 1908 at the ARC superintendent's convention, the head of the convention asked Mrs. Isabel H. Robb, the first president of the American Nurses Association, to serve as chairman of a committee to look at creating an ARC Nursing Service. That spring the ARC Central Committee had created three ARC departments: War, Emergency, and International Relief. Robb was to look at where the proposed nursing service would fit. She wrote a comprehensive plan to have nurses, regardless of national affiliation, to be members of the Red Cross Nursing Service. The ARC would ask the American Federation of Nurses to supply nurses for the ARC's main nursing reserve force. Robb did not mention or write the idea that the ARC Nursing Service could be the Army's nursing reserve, but the idea began.

In December 1909 the ARC Nursing Service officially came under the ARC's War Relief Board. The surgeon generals of the Army and Navy would serve on the board. The American Federation of Nurses agreed to affiliate with the ARC's Red Cross Nursing Service.[234] A permanent head nurse would be in charge of the Nursing Service. The ARC head nurse organized and ensured proper training of the nursing force. The head nurse would communicate with ARC executive committees on nursing matters and visit and inspect subordinate sectional head nurses.

The Army historically remained a male-dominated bastion of conservative thought and action. A barracks saying is generals are always ready to fight the last war. Forward-looking vision and innovative thought, historically, were not found in the water Army leaders drank, in the air they breathed, or the cigars they smoked. Given the battlefield carnage of the American Civil War, and the demonstrated skill and expertise of many private humanitarian aid societies during the Civil War, especially nursing, the Army did not employ or take into service any nurse from the time of the Civil War to the Spanish-American War: a span of three decades. Federal law at that time allowed the Army to employ women nurses, but at the Civil War compensation rate of forty cents per day and one food ration per day. When the Spanish-American War came the Army, again, needed nurses in abundance.

In April 1898 Brigadier General George M. Sternberg, Army surgeon general, requested authority to employ as many nurses, male or female, as needed. The secretary of war agreed and granted the Army authority to contract for 300 nurses at a rate of thirty dollars per month and one ration per day.[235] Prior to the Spanish-American War, Sternberg had wanted to create a corps of highly trained nurses to serve with the Army in war. Sternberg had previously discussed the idea with Dr. Anita Newcomb McGee, MD. McGee had received her degrees from Columbia University and the Johns Hopkins University. She was also vice-president general of the Daughters of the American Revolution (DAR). At McGee's suggestion, the DAR formed a "Hospital Corps Committee" that McGee chaired. McGee offered the services of this DAR hospital corps committee to the federal government and the government accepted.

A problem existed in federal law: the existing law did not allow contract nurses in volunteer Army units. The Army had several volunteer units going to Cuba. Teddy Roosevelt's Rough Riders, the First United States Volunteer Cavalry, was among the units. The Army surgeon general recommended to Congress that Congress change existing law and approve the DAR as a source of nurses in war. Congress agreed to have the Army employ nurses: male or female. With chapters in every U.S. state and territory, the DAR could get the word out that the Army needed contract nurses. The DAR then became the examining board to ensure nursing applicants had the needed training and experience. The DAR would allow only graduate nurses [nurses having graduated from at least a two-year nursing school] to work for the Army. Nurses did not have to be DAR members; the nurses could come from any organization, and they came from many. The nurses originally had to be between ages thirty and fifty. The lower age limit was soon reduced further to attract more nurses. If the nurse previously had yellow fever, then the nurse was allowed to work in yellow fever infested areas. If she hadn't, the nurse was barred from that area. In time the DAR processed over five thousand applications.

On May 10, 1898, the first six women nurses signed contracts with the Army: two were yellow fever immune. Nurses who signed contracts with the Army were classed as "Nurse Corps (female)," with acting assistant surgeon general Anita McGee as their superintendent. At the height of the Spanish-American War, 1,200 nurses were serving in the ANC. By July 1899, 202 nurses were serving. Less than twenty nurses died in the Spanish-American War: all deaths but two were from typhoid.

In his after-action report about the Army Medical Department during the War, Sternberg, who wanted a permanent Army Nurse

Corps, bluntly wrote:

> ...Prior to the declaration of war [April 21, 1898] no preparation for the approaching conflict had been made by the [Army] Medical Department.... Seven hundred ninety-one men were in the Hospital Corps...and under existing law only 100 could be hospital stewards. The privates had become more or less skilled in litter bearing and first aid work, but had received only a limited amount of training as nurses....
>
> ...As hospitals were established and the sick became numerous, attendants had to be secured by detail from regiments, some of the men assigned to such duty being of good character and anxious to serve, but the large proportion in every respect unfit for nurses....
>
> In the last twenty years the value, the efficiency, and the availability of well-trained nurses has been demonstrated, and it is much to be regretted that this fact was not fully realized by the medical officers of the Army when the war commenced...Our recent experience may justly held to have shown that female nurses, properly trained and properly selected...are of the greatest value. Those who have been serving under contract in our military hospitals, and there have been about 1,500 of them, have with scarcely an exception done excellent work....[236]
>
> Brigade or regimental surgeons were put in charge of the hospitals as they were organized, who as a rule, knew nothing of their duties at first and many could not or would not learn. Those assigned to ward duty often felt that such service was unbecoming the dignity of their rank. Of trained hospital stewards there were very few; rarely did an attendant have any familiarity with the work of a nurse...[237]

In his summary Sternberg wrote harshly [and bravely] of Congress:

> ...The nursing force...was neither ample nor efficient, reasons for which may be found in the lack of a proper volunteer hospital corps, due to the failure of Congress to authorize its establishment and to the nonrecognition in the beginning of the value of women nurses and the extent to which their services could be secured.[238]

After the war McGee testified before Congress and commended the women contract nurses serving in the Spanish-American War. McGee said the contract nurses were better trained and experienced then Army hospital corpsman. McGee mentioned seven organizations that provided nurses: One was the Congregated American Sisters in South Dakota; they provided five American Indian women nurses.[239] Of General Sternberg's efforts to have a trained professional nurse organization during the Spanish-American War, McGee said:

> The surgeon-general [Sternberg] had of his own initiative and without suggestion from anyone asked from Congress and received an appropriation for the payment of contract nurses, either male or female. Had he not done this, the Nurse Corps could have had no existence, and so it should never be forgotten that however much the Surgeon-General may have been assisted by others, the first and fundamental action towards the recognition of women nurses in the army was then by Surgeon General Sternberg.[240]

As her last official act before McGee retired, she wrote the draft legislation forming the ANC. In the Army Reorganization Bill of 1900/01, Section 19 created the ANC, originally called the "Nurse Corps (female)." It read:

> The Nurse Corps (female) shall consist of one superintendent, who shall be a graduate of a hospital training school having a course of instruction of not less than two years, and of as many chief nurses, nurses and reserve nurses as may be needed, provide that they

shall be graduates of hospital training schools and shall have passed a satisfactory professional, moral, mental, and physical examination.

On February 2, 1901, President McKinley signed the bill with Mrs. Dita H. Kinney as the new head of the ANC. Kinney, from New York State, had experience in peace and war, and was trained at Massachusetts General Hospital.[241] McGee also helped in drafting legislation creating the Navy Nurse Corps. The Navy Nurse Corps soon followed. The first effort to pass a bill in Congress creating the Navy Nurse Corps was in 1903. Congress passed the bill in 1908. In 1908 the Navy Nurse Corps became part of the Navy Bureau of Medicine. Navy rear admiral William C. Braisted was then the Navy surgeon general. Esther Voorhees Hassan was the first superintendent of the Navy Nurse Corps. The Act of May 13, 1908, read largely the same as the Army:

> The Nurse Corps (female) of the United States Navy is hereby established and shall consist of one superintendent, to be appointed by the secretary of the navy, who shall be a graduate of a hospital training school have a course of instruction of not less than two years, whose term of office may be terminated at his discretion and of any many chief, nurses, nurse and reserve nurses, as may be needed.

Hasson resigned from the Navy Nurse Corps in January 1911, Lenah Sutcliff Higbee took her place. A naturalized citizen from England, Higbee was trained a nurse in New York City. She served at New York's Bellevue and Allied hospitals. Higbee enrolled in the ARC in May 1912. Higbee was a woman of strong but quiet personality; she was highly regarded in the Navy Nurse Corps. Enrollment in the Navy Nurse Corps was stricter than the ANC. The lower age requirement for the Navy Nurse Corps was twenty-two years; the Navy, even in war, did not waiver this.

The other strict requirements for the Navy Nurse Corps were the applicant had to be a U.S. citizen, and physically fit. The Navy used an existing Naval Reserve force regulation to enroll the women nurses in the Navy Nurse Corps.[242] The regulation was enrollment of persons in the Naval Coast Defense Force, class 4; or volunteer naval reserve for duty in the Naval Coast Defense Reserve, class 4, in the Naval Reserve Force. The regulation read "persons," and did not have a gender restriction or gender requirement. This would greatly aid the Navy in the next few years when the Navy needed women yeomen for administrative work when male sailors took to sea during war.[243]

At the turn of the twentieth century, Jane Arminda Delano, born March 13, 1862, Montour Falls, New York, had not seen war and wasn't an active ARC member. From 1902 to 1904 Delano was superintendent of nurses at Bellevue Hospital, New York City. A disciplinarian and professional woman, she kept, and insisted upon, high standards of nursing competence and personal behavior. Delano became secretary of Red Cross nursing enrollment for New York State, where she sent an appeal to every nurse in New York State to join the ARC Nursing Service. Her competence, leadership, and high standards, were soon noticed at governing levels of the ARC. Delano was almost single-minded in her pursuit of excellence in those women wanting to enter the Red Cross Nursing Service.

In December 1909 Delano was named head of the newly created Red Cross Nursing Service, in the Red Cross War Relief Board. Congress had created the ANC largely due to Army surgeon general Sternberg's strong recommendation. Sternberg needed a chief nurse of the ANC. He asked the head of the ARC, Mable Boardman, for a recommendation. Boardman said Delano would be Boardman's pick. Delano would be both chief nurse of the ARC Nursing Service and superintendent of the ANC. Boardman said Delano would unify ARC and ANC efforts.

At the time of Delano's appointment as superintendent, ANC, the Army had about eighty nurses in the Army Nursing Reserve. Delano recommended eliminating the Army Nursing Reserve and have the ARC Nursing Service be the Army's nursing reserve. Sternberg agreed. Delano also insisted and got, greater pay, cumulative leave, laundry of uniforms, first-class transportation for all nurses and improved living quarters for nurses in the Army Nursing Reserve. Delano's successor as superintendent of the ANC was Isabel McIsaac: a graduate of the Illinois Training School for Nurses.[244] [Florence Ames, graduate nurse, Billings, Montana, was a graduate of the Illinois School.]

Delano was superintendent of the ANC for two years. Her efforts increased the number of nurses enrolled in the ANC to about three thousand. In her resignation letter of March 11, 1912, to the Army surgeon general, Delano wrote she wanted to develop a working connection between the ARC as the Army's nursing reserve, and to put the ANC on a solid basis. She wrote she had believed she had done this. Delano concluded she would now devote her volunteer time to the Red Cross Nursing Service to keep it as a reserve for the Army.

Beginning 1910, Delano, in her position as chief nurse, ARC, began a comprehensive plan of organization, training, recruitment, and improvement for ARC nursing in America. One of the first priorities was to create State Committees on ARC Nursing Service. Each committee would have between five and ten members, the members had to be affiliated with a nurses' association. Montana was in the northwestern section of the ARC Nursing Service. The head of this section was Linna G. Richardson, in Portland, Oregon. Richardson would oversee the state committees of Oregon, Washington, Idaho, Wyoming, and Montana.[245] The Montana state ARC Nursing Service committee was in Helena. Later the ARC would reorganize its geographical divisions and put Montana in the northern division: along with Minnesota, North Dakota and South Dakota. The director of the ARC Nursing Bureau for the northern division would be Edith A. Barber. Barber was serving on the faculty of the University of Minnesota, nurses training staff. Margaret Hughes, Helena, would be the head of the ARC Nursing Service in Montana.

America's local, state, and national leaders continued to face challenges never before seen to the magnitude needed to wage global war. The military looked to men and women having mastery of precision crafts and professional skills. Regardless of the craft or life-saving skill, someone had to prepare, write, type, send and file, something as innocuous as a piece of paper. In the Great War, America's navy found an unusual challenge surrounding the dull, uninviting grind of paperwork. The Navy had to solve this challenge—and fast.

Chapter 5
THE YEOMANETTES

"The keys of victory"

ENSIGN EUGENE J. FRIEDLANDER, U.S. NAVY, got his official orders from Thirteenth Naval District, Puget Sound Naval Yard; Bremerton, Washington. An electrician and radio qualified naval officer at Puget Sound Naval Yard, he wasn't going to sea, he was going to Montana.[246] A native of Minneapolis, Minnesota, the twenty-eight-year-old officer had crossed Montana on the Great Northern Railway going west to Seattle and his assignment to America's fabled sea service. The Navy needed men and wanted to recruit east of Washington. In mid-April 1918 Friedlander was going back east: not to Minnesota, but to the Montana cities of Billings, Butte, Helena, and Great Falls. The Navy assigned him to lead a five-man "traveling enrolling party," or mobile naval recruiting team into Montana, and enlist highly skilled men for ships at sea and naval bases on shore. The five-man team accompanying Friedlander had an assistant surgeon, a chief quartermaster, two yeomen, and a hospital corpsman. The Navy wanted to recruit three thousand men from Montana. Friedlander had to deliver. The Navy needed seamen, corpsmen, mess attendants, stewards, mechanics of all kinds, boilermakers, blacksmiths, coppersmiths, carpenters, masons, and radio operators.

By end of April, Friedlander had spent two weeks in Billings, Great Falls, and Bozeman. His successful recruiting had enlisted 300 men for the Navy.[247] Friedlander was also sending forty men a week from Montana to aviation school to learn the many skills of keeping fragile airplanes flying.[248] Barnstorming aviation began a mystic aura lasting as long as young boys, after seeing their first airplane overhead, would spread their arms and run across hills and fields flying in their minds. Montana men wanted to fly too, but for every pilot in the air many men were needed on the ground keeping those delicate paper and wood creations of Wilbur and Orville Wright ready for war.

Friedlander was good at his job, he later served in World War II and retired as a Navy captain.[249] Due to his successful recruiting in Montana, the Navy told Friedlander to stay two weeks longer. He and his mobile recruiting team headed to Butte. Butte men began eagerly enlisting for a life on the water versus breaking their bodies digging for copper ore a thousand feet underground in dangerous mining tunnels. The men would get a guaranteed monthly pay check in the Navy rather than punching a time card coming out of the mines. In the mines of Butte if a man got hurt and couldn't work, he was out of a job. If a man got hurt in the Navy, a regular paycheck still came while the Navy provided the finest of medical care for injured sailors. Butte men also faced the draft, signing up had its advantages rather than waiting for a draft notice to come. All-in-all, not a bad deal for military eligible men from Butte. On Thursday, May 30, by 9:00 a.m. men lined up at the federal building in downtown Butte for their chance to sink the Kaiser's navy.

The Navy had a surprise for Friedlander. A few days before, while he continued enlisting men, the Navy told him he had to enlist two qualified women stenographers. In the Navy a yeoman is a clerk-typist who does clerical and administrative work. The Navy needed women yeomen for shore duty at Puget Sound Naval Yard. The women had to be between eighteen and thirty-five, of good character, and neat appearance. A high school diploma with business or office experience were preferred but not required.[250] The women had to be proficient in typing, shorthand, letter writing, and spelling. The Navy didn't have a marriage restriction for women enlisting. The women could be married, and even have children. The Navy's view was the family situation was the woman's business and not the Navy's. The woman couldn't bring her husband or family at the Navy's expense, but she could commute back and forth if she wanted. If the woman got pregnant during her Navy service, she could ask for a discharge that the Navy generally granted.[251]

Friedlander had to make interview questions, and a typing and shorthand test. Twenty-five typed words per minute error free was considered entry-level typing proficiency. He also had to determine how to give these women required physical examinations. Word got around fast in Butte that the Navy was enlisting women. Women answered enthusiastically. That same Monday when Friedlander arrived at the Butte federal building to enlist more men, he found twenty women besieging the building for a chance to enlist in the Navy as women yeoman. The women may have heard that Navy pay for a yeoman third class was $32.60 per month with other monthly allowances of $30.00 per month. Promotions increased the pay. A chief yeoman would make about double the pay.[252] Navy yeomen Fred Henry, and H.E. Anderson, traveling with Friedlander and the recruiting party, began processing the twenty women and determining how to give these women typing and shorthand tests.[253]

Vera May Elder and Helen Sherry heard the recruiting call for Navy yeomen. They were among the twenty women waiting for Friedlander at the federal building in Butte. Nineteen-year-old Vera Elder grew up southeast of Butte at Grace, Montana. She lived in the Meaderville area northeast of Butte: an immigrant community near barren cut hills and headframes above dangerous mine shafts. She worked at Butte Water Company as a stenographer. Elder was an accomplished musician at Butte College of Music where she studied fine arts and music. Elder sang contralto solos in many events and concerts. She was looking to be a music teacher in Grace.[254]

Twenty-seven-year-old Helen Sherry was from Fort Benton: northeast of Great Falls along the Missouri River. Established 1846, Fort Benton wasn't named after anyone from Montana. The Army bought the fur trading post at the site from Auguste and Pierre Chouteau, Jr. and named it after Missouri senator Thomas Hart Benton. Fort Benton is the oldest continuously inhabited white settlement in Montana. You can argue that Fort Benton is the farthest inland seaport in America, as the Missouri River became the main water route for westward expansion during the nineteenth century. Given a shallow-draft steamboat, a capable ship's captain who knew every turn, sandbar, snag, and rock on the Mississippi and Missouri Rivers, could go from the Gulf of Mexico, up the Mississippi and Missouri Rivers and into Montana. Upper Missouri River boat traffic stopped at Fort Benton. Boat captains could go no farther. Lewis and Clark followed the Missouri twice: going and coming. They discovered the Great Falls of the Missouri River upstream from Fort Benton. The falls were a natural block for river traffic, the traffic stopped permanently at Fort Benton. As late as 1908 riverboat traffic still faced challenges at Fort Benton. On Sunday, May 31, 1908, the fully loaded steamboat *O.K.* a freight and passenger boat owned by Captain George H. Stevens, misjudged distances and height of the draw bridge at Fort Benton. The stern of the boat struck the bridge and caused considerable damage, but no injuries to passengers.[255]

You wouldn't think Montana a seafaring place or a place for watermen, but Montana men and Native Americans had been on the water for a long time: especially on the Missouri and Yellowstone Rivers. The Navy and Coast Guard have named thirty-one ships and submarines for people, cities, rivers, and tribes with ties to Montana.[256] Given that, the Montana Naval Forces Monument was dedicated June 28, 2008, at Fort Benton. A few hundred feet from the Missouri River, the monument has separate ornate oval plaques in a large circle for each ship or submarine named for someone or something from Montana. Fort Benton gave much in Montana's shoreline history: including two women in the Great War, Helen Sherry and Elizabeth Patterson.

Born Christmas Day, 1890, in Neenah, Wisconsin, Helen Sherry moved to Fort Benton with her family around 1901. She lived in Fort Benton with her parents, James and Ellen Sherry and three older brothers. An outstanding school student, Helen received awards for perfect attendance and a state scholarship for the highest grades in her high school class of 1908 at Fort Benton. At her commencement, Helen gave a speech entitled, "The American Woman."[257] In February 1909 Helen was earning her living as a stenographer. Less than a year removed from high school, she returned to join the Fort Benton High School Literary Society's winter program and entertainment. Part of the program, be it serious or fun, was she and a fellow high school graduate, Kate Lee, debated the question of marriage. Helen and Kate's positions were women should be allowed to make marriage proposals, and the present custom of waiting for the man to make up his mind was bad. The opposing male team of Woodford Dimock and Eugene Sullivan had the other position that men should always propose first. Newspaper accounts don't read of laughs, harrumphs, or guffaws from the audience. Given Sherry's high academic marks in school, she probably argued her position well. Feminist thoughts were not to be that night; Dimock and Sullivan won the debate. Men at Fort Benton would continue being the ones asking for a lady's hand.[258]

Helen Sherry continued her employment as a stenographer. She worked in Helena when the state legislature was in session, then in the northern Montana towns of Havre and Choteau to transcribe county records. She went to Butte to begin her nearly life-long career as a legal secretary. In Butte she worked for Fred J. Furman, attorney-at-law, and lived in the Bank Hotel.[259]

Common names given to geographic folds in the land can tell you where a person is from in the American West. In the southwest, a higher flat plain on the horizon is called a "mesa;" in Wyoming a "butte;" in Nebraska, "the table land;" or in Montana, "the bench." John Fulford Patterson, born 1861 in Harford County, Maryland, came west at age eighteen and homesteaded on the bench sixteen miles southeast of Fort Benton. His land was along the Big Sag and Shonkin Creeks near the Highwood Mountains. History doesn't record why Patterson decided to become a sheep rancher, but he did, and he was good at it.

The catastrophic winter of 1886/87 in the high plains, however, almost did him in. In a fierce Montana blizzard on the windswept bench, one of Patterson's sheep herders struggled to Patterson's ranch house to tell him the sheep had stampeded and the other herder couldn't be found. Patterson and another herder mounted their horses and began the search in near-lethal winter conditions. Before he left his ranch house, Patterson said they would make every effort to find the lost herder even if that meant all the sheep had to die. Riding fifteen miles Patterson found the wayward sheep and the herder, turned them, and began the desperate effort home. Snow, high winds, heavy drifts, and lethal cold, can kill a Montana man sure as a bullet. The three men and herd stopped at a distant ranch for safety in the storm. For three days and nights in the coldest weather known on the bench, Patterson and the two men survived and brought their sheep herd home. On the long drive home, Patterson lost ten head of sheep.

Of Patterson's effort, the *Fort Benton River Press* wrote: "We are not often called upon to record such wonderful pluck and endurance as was shown by Mr. Patterson and his men."[260] That same year Patterson would winter a band of 7,500 sheep on the Sun River range west of Great Falls. As years passed he would sell up to three thousand lambs and load twenty-four rail cars at Fort Benton heading for Minneapolis-St. Paul.[261]

Patterson became a prominent citizen in Montana's Choteau County. He ran for public office as county treasurer, and then county commissioner 1888. In 1901 Patterson was elected to the Montana House of Representatives as a Republican.[262] Patterson was also deputy sheep inspector for Choteau County and detected a serious livestock disease. To stop the disease, he eventually treated over forty thousand head of sheep.²⁶³

Patterson started a family with a son and two daughters. His daughter, Elizabeth, born February 1893 on her father's remote ranch, grew up on the bench and received her schooling in Fort Benton. Montana soon exacted its price from Elizabeth's capable and resolute father. He began having breathing problems; doctors diagnosed pleurisy or possibly tuberculosis. They recommend John Patterson move to California: maybe the better and warmer weather would cure him. In 1905 he sold his livestock and moved to San Diego for treatment. His family, with Elizabeth, stayed on their Montana ranch. Warmer weather didn't help John Patterson, he died in San Diego on March 7, 1905. Family and friends brought his body to Fort Benton.²⁶⁴ He is buried in Fort Benton's Riverside Cemetery with an ornate dark granite headstone.

Fatherless at age eleven, Elizabeth and her surviving family stayed at Fort Benton. She graduated from Chouteau County High School, class of 1911, three years after Helen Sherry. Elizabeth then began finding her way in life. She first went to Shattuck-St. Mary's Academy, an Episcopal mission school in Faribault, Minnesota. Elizabeth then studied nursing for a short time at Columbus Hospital, Great Falls, Montana, but never graduated. She went to secretarial school in Spokane, Washington, and moved to Seattle to become a secretary. When war came, Patterson went directly to the Navy Training Camp at Seattle and enlisted as a yeoman. She served for less than a year and achieved the rank of yeoman second class. In time she would return to her native Montana and continue her life.²⁶⁵

In Butte, Vera Elder and Helen Sherry took the Navy's proficiency test given to the twenty women who applied. Elder and Sherry had the highest scores of the twenty women at the Butte federal building. Elder and Sherry enlisted for four years or the duration of the war: whichever came first. The Navy called up Elder in July 1918, and Sherry in August 1918. Both went as stenographers for the duration of the war to the Thirteenth Naval District headquarters, Puget Sound Naval Yard, Bremerton, Washington. A week before Elder departed for the Navy, she received two farewell dinners and parties. Mrs. Cora Lenniger and Mrs. Gilbert of Butte, gave Elder a farewell party, and Mrs. Charles Ornsby gave a farewell dinner in Elder's honor at the well-decorated Ornsby house.²⁶⁶ ²⁶⁷ It is not known if Sherry got a sendoff of any kind.

Sherry never married or had children. Her service echoed her skills and intelligence. In time she would become one of two Montana women who achieved rank of chief yeoman: the highest Navy rank available for female yeomen of World War I.[268]

Other Montana women began hearing of the Navy's requirement for women, and enlisted apparently without fanfare, parties, or sendoff dinners. Five other Montana women are known to have went directly to Puget Sound Naval Yard to enlist as female yeomen: Esther Hervin, from Great Falls; Vida Nerlin, from Joliet; Violet Smith, from Shelby; Irma Wright, from Denton, and Gertrude Zerr, from Lakeview. The youngest was nineteen; the oldest, thirty-two. Their average age was twenty-three. Of Montana's women who enlisted in the armed forces of the United States, by validated date of entry, Irma Myrtle Wright, Navy service number 187-43-99, is Montana's first female military veteran who was not a nurse. Yeoman Third Class Wright entered the Navy on March 3, 1918.[269]

At the beginning of World War I, America's navy needed many men and right away. The men would sail America's fleet into harm's way. More ships needed more men. Secretary of the Navy Josephus Daniels, faced a tremendous challenge: when the fleet sailed, who would remain on shore to manage the many administrative support functions needed to keep the Navy working? The Navy had many male yeomen on duty in the department of the Navy, naval yards, and naval training stations. Regulations at that time allowed enlisted men serve on shore duty for no more than six months. Then the male sailor had to serve on ship. This meant enlisted men in the Navy could not be permanently stationed on shore.[270] Secretary Daniels was running out of sailors; he needed a solution and fast.

Born in Washington, North Carolina, 1862, Daniels became a powerful newspaper owner of the *Raleigh* [NC] *News and Observer* by fundamentally changing the role of newspapers in American life. He started a publishing dynasty that would last one hundred years. He was a progressive Democrat and an ambitious man who became active in politics through his newspapers and financial fortune.[271] A prohibitionist and family man who could show independence on occasion, by age thirty Daniels was a significant power-broker in Raleigh, North Carolina.[272]

He was looking to expand his influence nationally, and the

election of 1892 gave him that chance. Grover Cleveland, a Democrat and former U.S. president, returned to the presidency in 1892 by defeating the sitting president, Benjamin Harrison. In the election the Democrats also won control of the U.S. House and Senate. Daniels saw his chance. Daniels went to Washington D.C. and through his political connections looked for a job in the Cleveland administration. At the time of Cleveland's election, the federal government had eight cabinet positions. The head of the Department of the Interior was important as it managed government and military pensions. It was also the human resources hiring office for other federal departments. Cleveland appointed Daniels to head the Department of Interior's Administrative Division. Daniels, a patient and calculating man who never ran for or held public office, would personally manage the hiring of the government's civil service positions. Cleveland and others noted Daniel's ability to organize, manage, and have creative thought on how to solve problems.[273]

Grover Cleveland was America's only president to date to have two non-consecutive terms in office. After Cleveland's second term, Daniels returned to North Carolina and tended his newspaper business. When the 1912 presidential campaign had Woodrow Wilson running as a resolute Democrat, Daniels saw a chance to return to Washington D.C. Supporting Wilson, Daniels worked campaign strategy for him. Wilson handily won the 1912 election with an overwhelming electoral vote over former president Theodore Roosevelt, who ran under the Progressive Party or "Bull Moose," banner.[274] As a reward for Daniels' support, Wilson offered Daniels the position of secretary of the navy. Daniels readily accepted. Daniels took over a conservative and narrow-minded navy. The Navy lacked a modern organization and was a technologically backward force with arcane and inhibiting traditions. America's involvement in the Spanish-American War showed the value of naval power with heavy guns. At the beginning of the twentieth century, Europe began designing and building early versions of the modern battleship. Collectively an upheaval of naval thought and organization had begun.[275]

America's navy was preparing to sail for war. Daniels needed naval personnel for permanent shore duty. From his experience managing the administrative division of the U.S. Department of the Interior, Daniels knew he didn't have the budget or time needed to hire civilian civil servants to replace Navy yeomen going to sea. Daniels also needed the authority to quickly move personnel by force of military orders wherever the need. Daniels couldn't do that with civil servants. That meant enlisting more yeomen into the Navy. From his long-held societal progressive views, Daniels looked to enlisting women for administrative support on shore. Previous laws and regulations prohibited women from joining the Navy or other regular military forces. Through his chief counsel, Daniels found the answer in a vaguely worded Navy regulation. The regulation was for enrollment of *persons* [italics added] in the Naval Coast Defense Force, class 4 reserve duty.

The first three classes required previous sea-going maritime experience or being a crewman on a ship destined for naval war service. This meant only men in the first three reserve classes. The regulation read "the enrollment of all persons who may be capable of performing special service for coastal defense." The regulation did not have a gender restriction or gender requirement.[276] This seemingly minor administrative loop-hole gave Daniels authority to enlist women yeomen into the Navy. He also got officer and enlisted pay increases for the Navy to equal the Army. Enlisting women into the Navy, Daniels insisted on, and got, equal pay for the women as the men.

On March 19, 1917, less than a month before the U.S. entered World War I, the Navy's Bureau of Navigation [forerunner to the Navy's Bureau of Personnel] alerted each naval district that the district could begin enlisting women into the Naval Coast Defense Reserve. Prior to World War I the Navy assumed women would not be in the naval service, and the Navy didn't have procedures or process to receive women in uniform. Holding to a male-only tradition of the sea, the conservative Navy brass of the day didn't want women in the naval service. The order to enlist women came from the secretary of the navy himself, and that settled it. The first recognized woman to have enlisted in the Navy was Loretta Perfectus Walsh, born 1896 in Philadelphia, Pennsylvania.[277] By date of entry into the Navy, Walsh is also recognized as the first woman to serve in the armed forces of the United States in a non-nursing capacity.[278] In time, 11,880 women enlisted in America's World War I navy.[279] Seventeen women are known to have enlisted from Montana in the World War I Navy.[280]

To enlist as a Navy yeoman, the women couldn't be black or "colored" as the word was then. America's black women had no shortcoming of zeal and ability when wanting to serve in the war effort. Daniels was a progressive, but he saw the progressive agenda as a Democratic Party platform and not Republican Party. Being born during the Civil War and living through the Republican Radical Reconstruction period of the South, Daniels looked upon black voting rights and black growth in political power as a result of Republican Party policies. This Daniels, a staunch Democrat and a native son of North Carolina, could not abide.[281] This may have influenced greatly his negative views on black enlistments in the Navy.

Women enlisted in the World War I Navy as yeomen, but they could be used largely in any rating or job not requiring them to serve aboard ship. Therein the challenge: how to ensure women, especially those with gender non-specific names, weren't assigned to sea duty on ship. The Navy, never expecting women to ever enlist, had no procedure to identify women in the Navy and ensure they weren't assigned to sea duty. The Navy solved this by officially adding the suffix (F) behind the Navy rank "yeoman," to denote female: or yeoman (F). How would the Navy and others refer to these women? Were these women "sailors" if the Navy wouldn't allow them sea duty? If these women were called "yeomen," would that confuse gender identity needed to keep women from sea duty?

In time the nickname "yeomanette" surfaced. Legend and lore exists as how this nickname came. One idea is if you quickly pronounce yeoman (F) as "yeoman-eff," it sounds like "yeomanette." The nickname probably came from feminizing or reducing the stature of the noun, colloquially or mockingly, with "ette." Navy brass objected strongly to the words "yeomanette," "yeowomen," "yeo-girls," or even "Liberty Belles." Rear Admiral Victor Blue, chief of the Navy's Bureau of Navigation, had responsibility for Navy personnel matters. He rejected informal nicknames. In his letter to all Naval districts, Blue clearly and without discussion, ordered the end of the informal and unapproved practice of calling women yeoman "yeomanettes," "yeowomen," or "Liberty Belles." Blue ended his letter stating, "The official designation of these young ladies is 'Yeoman (F)'; and it is hereby directed that the use of these unofficial titles be discontinued."[282]

Officers may command the military, but enlisted men and women run the military: even in the Navy. In spite of Blue's orders to stop the name "yeomanette," the word became a badge of honor to the World

War I women wearing the navy-blue uniform with the crossed quill pens and red chevrons on their sleeves. This wouldn't be the first time in America's military history that enlisted ranks would informally tell officers what manner of bilge the brass could drink. For America's women who served with distinction in the Navy of World War I, the title "yeomanette," proudly remains.

In his syndicated column of the day, Frederic J. Haskins, a newspaper correspondent for several newspapers and whose information column appeared in over one hundred newspapers, wrote of the yeomanettes:

> The young woman who is eager to enlist and wear the uniform can have her wish fulfilled by enrolling in the United States naval reserves. These women are not enlisted to climb ropes, drill, or do any of the sailor's jobs. In all probability they will never mount a ship's deck in an official capacity. They are enrolled as yeomen, and are employed, most of them, at the peaceful work of taking down shorthand notes and making them intelligible by way of a typewriter.
>
> Such duties do not appear thrilling or even of great importance, but many of these girls, who have demonstrated ability to carry out orders quickly and effectively, to handle confidential correspondence and transact business requiring a high degree of executive ability. Some are holding positions heretofore have been considered men's jobs exclusively.
>
> Admiral McGowan, chief of the naval bureau of supplies and accounts, declares that the women serving in his department are more satisfactory than the men. "They are more ambitious and capable and less dissatisfied with conditions and pay," says the admiral. "They are my right-hand men, and my only trouble is in getting enough of them...."[283]
>
> Among the specialized women workers in the navy department are five finger print experts. To these young women is entrusted the important and difficult work of taking finger prints of enlisted men. Other women classify and file the records, and so complete

is the filing system that prints of any man in the naval force of 450,000 can be located in from three to five minutes. The navy relies on its finger print system to identify men in case of casualty…

Some of the women are expert translators. Others are cable decoders and still others are draftsman. No radio operators are recruited as few naval radio operators are employed on shore duty, and the navy is firm in its decision on shore duty only for its women….

The great need of the navy as regards to woman power is stenographers, typists and bookkeepers, especially stenographers. The head of one navy bureau states that he could use nearly 300 stenographers now, while other bureaus set no limits.[284]

In May 1918, a year after America entered the war, the *Great Falls Tribune* reported on Alice Johnson, a young woman from Great Falls working as a stenographer who was now a yeomanette:[285]

Miss Alice Johnson has joined the navy [*sic*]. This does not mean that she will scale the ropes like a real honest-to-goodness sailor, but she is a yeoman or rather a yeomanette just the same. Her duties will be clerical and stenographical in the Bremerton navy yard, taking the places of men who are needed to man the guns of the fleet. When told of the possibility to go to France and serve in the American navy yards overseas, Miss Johnson gasped a second and exclaimed: "Oh, wouldn't that be the most perfectly wonderful thing in the world?"

The Navy didn't send Johnson overseas, they sent her and many Montana yeomanettes, to Puget Sound Navy Yard, Bremerton, Washington.[286] About forty yeomen (F) nationwide were sent overseas: mostly to the Hawaii territory. Five were sent to France to work with the Navy's Bureau of Medicine, and others were sent here and there.[287] No yeomanette known from Montana served overseas.

The U.S. Marine Corps would go to war too. Until 1947 with the passage of the National Security Act, the Marines were part of the Navy and directly subordinate to the orders of the secretary of the navy. [After 1947, the Marines had equal standing with the Army, Navy and Air Force.] By 1918 when two brigades of Marines were sent to France and with other force commitments worldwide, the Marines saw the need to get more administrative help in uniform. Knowing that Secretary of the Navy Daniels had authorized enlisting women, the Commandant of the Marine Corps, Major General George Barnett, asked Daniel's permission to enlist women into the Marines. Daniels agreed.

The requirements for women in the Marines were largely the same as the Navy's: between ages eighteen and forty, excellent character, neat appearance and have experience as a stenographer, typing, correspondence, and general office work. Major General Barnett also gave the death blow to anyone calling women Marines, "marinettes." Barnett said emphatically the women would be called "women marines."[288] Navy enlisted personnel ignored the edict about banishing the name "yeomanette." Marine enlisted personnel knew they ignored their commandant's order at the Marine's own peril. The Marines didn't press the recruiting very hard, and by war's end a little over 300 women enlisted.[289] The Marines sent a recruiting party to Montana to enlist women, but no Montana women known served in the World War I Marine Corps.[290] Opha Mae Johnson, Kokomo, Indiana, is the first known female Marine in American history. In World War I she enlisted as a clerk in the Marine Corps reserve on August 13, 1918.[291]

Montana's newspapers of the day were very accepting of women entering America's World War I Navy. Although no Montana headline banners trumpeted local women going to the Navy, many articles complimented the women. When Yeoman (F) First Class Artie Cullop, Missoula, Montana, returned to Missoula on furlough in November 1918, the *Daily Missoulian* reported:

> Shake hands with Missoula's only yeomanette. At first you may not notice her uniform. You may think the hat band around her natty hat is something borrowed. But that's just because you aren't used to seeing yeomanettes. Take a look at the sleeve beneath the blue cape with the regulation buttons and the black braid of the sea forces.

On that sleeve is a red chevron of three stripes. "Do we drill?" Yeomanette Cullop smiled. "Yes we do," she answered. "And no play drill at that. We differ from the sailors only in the actual method of service. We do our fighting on a typewriter."

Another challenge, among many facing the Navy with women recruits, is the Navy didn't first have a military uniform for women. In May 1918 the *Great Falls Tribune* printed a photograph of Alice Johnson in Navy uniform, but Johnson was wearing a modified naval officer's uniform. Johnson wore an officer's hat, with black band beneath an unstiffened white crown. The emblem of an officer had been removed and replaced by an anchor denoting an enlisted man. Johnson's uniform coat was an officer's coat without rank insignia. This was common in the first months of women in the Navy. The Navy used what it had with available uniforms. Beginning April 1917, the Navy began designing a women's uniform, with a single-breasted jacket, with rank and rating badge on the left sleeve midway between shoulder and elbow. Skirt hems would be eight inches from the ground. Standard Navy neckerchiefs would be tied under shirt collars. Plain black high top or low-cut shoes were worn. Women's hats would be straight brimmed felt or white straw with brims three inches wide with a crown four inches high. The words "U.S. Naval Reserve" were printed on the front of the hat above the brim. White gloves complimented the uniform. The women also had a summer white uniform. For winter and cold weather, the Navy latter issued the yeomanettes a stylish navy-blue cape with grey gloves.

The Navy needed time to fully integrate the women's uniform into the Navy's standard uniform issue. Contracts for women's uniforms would take time. The Navy sent uniform specifications to Naval Districts and women were free to make their uniforms or have local tailors make the uniforms, as long as the uniforms met precise Navy requirements.[292] Tailor shops made the women's uniform for about $25.00 and the cape for about $30.00: more than a month's pay.[293] The women also received a monthly allowance to replace or repair uniform items. The Navy women's uniform became widely accepted and the Navy Nurse Corps copied the uniform design, and added a scarlet lined cape. The Navy designed a different styled hat and a double-breasted jacket.[294]

Elizabeth Kelly, yeoman (F), entered the Navy in Portland, Oregon. Her sister, Mrs. Joseph R. Jackson, lived in Butte, Montana. In November 1918, the *Montana Standard* wrote Kelly's thoughts:

> Of course, the nicest thing about a uniform is its time saving. You don't lose a minute getting it on. You don't have to decide in the morning what you will wear. It's your uniform with a clean white blouse. You know it has to be kept in order. Laundry bills of shuddering size come from a white blouse every day. I think that women will be in the navy [*sic*] after the war. Women were rather jeered at when the ruling was first made admitting them, but they proved very satisfactory, I understand. Why not? Give a woman anything to do and she can do it.

Gertrude Alice Zerr, indeed, accomplished much. A remarkable woman whose love for Montana would forever be written in national lore and publications, was born in Keokuk, Iowa, February 18, 1886, to a large Catholic family headed by John and Mary [Spring] Zerr. Gertrude became an educated and independent woman. She had wanderlust and wanted to live in and write about Montana. Zerr became a school teacher. By 1912 Zerr had taught school in Livingston and Cooke City, Montana. In a letter to her friends in Livingston, Zerr wrote that her trip from Gardiner, Montana, to Cooke City was made by stage, horseback, and a dog team: with the latter part of the trip made entirely by dog team. Zerr would remember the deep snow at Cooke City and write of it in her literary series, "Trails to Tiny Towns:"

> It's funny about snow: there's so much of it-and it's such an impalpable, sinister, relentless, merciless thing, insistent, senseless, intangible, elusive, and so *white*!.... [Italics original.]
>
> Another month, and still it falls, but the tenderness has become a mockery. Another space of time, and it stings and bites venomously. Week after week, month after month, it falls, and falls, and falls.

The Yeomanettes 85

The August 1923 edition of *Harper's Magazine* published her four-part non-fiction literary series of Montana, "Trails to Tiny Towns." Of Zerr's writings, the editors of Harpers wrote:

> This is...a series of remarkable experiences of a woman school-teacher in the sparsely settled districts of the West. In these "far places" – remote from town and railroad- a rugged and picturesque life is being lived to-day [*sic*]...For ten years Miss Zerr has here found the role of school-teacher an extraordinary adventure, and her graphic chronicles is a moving and intensely human story.

By 1914 Zerr had received a University of Montana scholarship in mathematics with a $100.00 stipend.[295] In 1915 she was a school teacher in South Moiese, Montana: northwest of Missoula. By 1918 she was living in the remote area at Lakewood, Montana: west of Yellowstone National Park. When and how she learned of the Navy's recruiting efforts for yeomanettes, history doesn't say. In May 1918 at age thirty-two, Zerr departed Lakewood and went directly to the Puget Sound Naval Yard. She enlisted as a yeoman (F). Zerr contributed much to American and Montana. She would be one of two Montana women in World War I who would achieve the rank of chief yeoman (F). After the war Zerr would return to her adopted home of Montana, and continue writing of its people, challenges, dangers, romance, and culture.

Though far less in literary merit compared to Zerr's writings, a 1917 published poem "Yeomanette" by Tom Terry reads:

The Yeomanette

The manly clerk is free at last
To hurry to the front.
The yeomanette assumes his tasks,
Is glad to bear the brunt.

Her work is not spectacular,
She wields no sword or gun,

But tasks like hers must be fulfilled
Or else no war be won.

She pounds the keys to victory,
She types the orders quick
That spell disaster to the foe,
That make the Kaiser sick.

Though one time frightened by a mouse
Which fled across the floor,
She bravely does her duty now
While thund'rous cannon roar....[296]

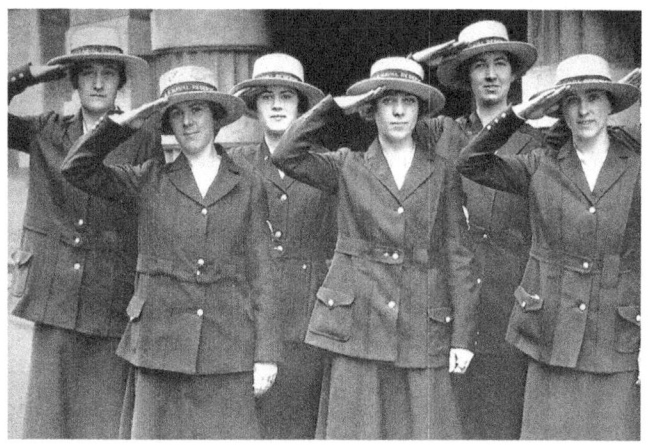

Navy yeomen (F), San Francisco, CA.
Courtesy National Archives and Records Administration

Chapter 7
THE CALL

"Clouds of war reach Montana"

IN OCTOBER 1919 THE *Conrad* [MT] *Independent* had a banner headline reading: "[She] has Often Fought Death in the Wilds. Pioneer Montana Nurse has a Wonderful Record of Saving Lives." Irene M. Cumming wrote of Margaret Hughes, Montana Supervisor of Nursing for the American Red Cross:

> ...[Hughes] is one of the best known and most beloved women in the state. For the past 20 years she has been relieving the suffering of Montana citizens and, although her home...has been in Helena, Miss Hughes has been called to all parts of the state to care for sick patients.
> At one time...[during] a typhoid epidemic, Miss Hughes nursed seven patients at an isolated ranch miles from a railroad. The doctor was able to make but one visit during the ten weeks of Miss Hughes' stay. The patients were all seriously ill, and four of them owe their lives to the plucky little nurse who cared for them...snatching but a few hours sleep weekly....
> She is a resident nurse for the sick in their homes. She gives instructions to prospective and young mothers...[and] inspects school children. She organizes clubs and classes...in home care for the sick and is a valued assistant to the health officer... in prevention of tuberculosis, typhoid, and other diseases.

In 1917 at age forty-five, Hughes, was a diminutive woman at five feet two inches tall, 120 pounds, with brown hair and brown eyes. She had a compassionate, but resolute countenance.[297] She wore her hair short with a simple style. Her face wasn't full but it offered a welcome expression to those in serious medical need, and there were many in need in Montana in the late nineteenth and early twentieth centuries. As years passed, her shallowing cheeks and thinning face weren't loyal to her and showed the years of hardship and toil she endured in Montana.[298]

Hughes was born June 30, 1871, in the small community of Smithville, Grimsby Township, Lincoln County, Ontario, Canada: about halfway between Niagara Falls, New York, and Hamilton, Ontario. Smithville was a few miles south of Lake Ontario's shore.[299] Society didn't consider nursing a respectable profession then, and family discouraged Hughes from being a nurse. She kept trying. A local Smithville doctor noticed Hughes' ability in giving nursing care in a home health setting. The doctor encouraged Hughes to follow her desire to be a nurse and gave her ideas on what to read and how to prepare her for further study.

At twenty-three, Hughes entered the Mack Training School for Nurses at the General and Maine Hospital, St. Catherines, Ontario, Canada. Hughes completed a two-year course of study in nursing, and graduated November 1896. Early in 1897 Hughes was a private nurse in Niagara Falls, Ontario. A former superintendent of the Mack Training School, "Miss Hutchinson," had moved to Helena, Montana, and worked at St. Peter's hospital. Hutchinson wrote Hughes about nursing opportunities and challenges in Montana. To meet that challenge in Montana, Hughes took postgraduate nursing study at the Women's Hospital in New York City. In 1898 Hughes moved to Helena and began working at St. Peter's hospital. In 1906 Hughes renounced her Canadian citizenship and allegiance and fidelity to English King Edward VIII. As required on the Declaration of Intention form from the U.S. Bureau of Immigration, Hughes also certified in writing she was not a polygamist, an anarchist, or believer in polygamy.[300]

When Hughes arrived in Helena, she saw St. Peter's hospital lacked a competent and trained nursing staff. The hospital superintendent of nurses had no modern nursing experience, and only three graduate nurses and an untrained assistant were available for each patient floor. Untrained nurses were assigned to the night shift. Hughes tried improving the nursing staff at St. Peter's, but got nowhere.

Hughes resigned from St. Peters and entered private nursing care in Helena and surrounding areas. Private care nurses were also expected to do house work for the patient they served. Hughes, a graduate nurse with credentials, told Montana doctors she refused to do house work for patients and would take only acute cases. Through her work, skilled nursing care in Montana gained respect. Hughes returned to Ontario, Canada, in the early 1900s, but Montana beckoned again. Returning to Helena, she established the Lewis and Clark County Association for Nurses. With other graduate nurses coming to Montana, more county nursing associations began. In 1911 Hughes helped create the Montana State Graduate Nurses Association. This association successfully lobbied the Montana state legislature to create state nursing standards. In 1913 Montana governor Samuel V. Stewart appointed Hughes as an original member of the Montana State Board of Nursing Examiners.[301]

Clouds of war began early for Hughes. Her native country, Canada, a member of the British Commonwealth, entered World War I in 1914, but Hughes stayed in Montana. As war loomed closer to America, the ARC began organizing and mobilizing. The ARC had thirteen regions in America and needed state coordinators. Given Hughes' qualifications, abilities, and "pluck," she became the chairman of the Montana State Committee on Nursing Service for the ARC. Hughes' responsibilities began extending beyond Montana's vast skies, prairies, and mountains. Beginning spring 1917, she had to learn and learn fast, the formidable and grave task of counting, organizing, and preparing for war, many of Montana's nurses.

America has never been a martial society with a deep-seated military tradition. America has traditionally thought a large standing army in peacetime is counter to the goals of a representative democracy. Vast oceans east and west, with friendly nations bordering north and south, protected America from any threat of continental invasion, [Pancho Villa and his banditos notwithstanding]. Large standing armies and navies are also very expensive to keep, man, and operate. If you aren't threatened with invasion and you have no territorial ambitions, then why keep a large military force? The thought of protection through isolation began to fail. In the late nineteenth century America had fought Spain and other forces overseas. America began sending expeditionary forces outside the continental borders of America. Modern-for-their-day warships could cross vast oceans with speed previously thought unworkable. Submarines, airplanes, and wireless communications made quick work of distances and barriers.[302]

The challenge to America in history is preparedness to fight when all means of diplomatic solutions to a potentially lethal international conflict have failed. America historically concluded its militia, and later National Guard troops, were a sufficient force, easily mobilized for national emergencies. Powerful forces in America at the turn of the twentieth century didn't agree. It can be troubling when a nation thought capable and ready, draws its collective pistols and sabers to find the armaments rusted with no ammunition at the ready, or call for men to find few exist. Good intentions will take you so far, then you have to ignite your abilities. For America, its matches of war were found initially wet.

On April 6, 1917, at 1:18 pm, President Woodrow Wilson signed the declaration of war against Germany. Newspapers and radios relayed the message throughout America and the world. America began its slow inexorable movement from a pacifist nation to a nation at war.[303] U.S. Army general Peyton C. March, chief of staff of the American Expeditionary Force [AEF] in Europe would write in his post-war report: "The entry of the United States into war on April 6, 1917, found the nation about as thoroughly unprepared for the great task which was confronting it as any great nation which had ever engaged in war.[304]

At the beginning of World War I, America's army had almost 5,800 officers and 122,000 enlisted men: a negligible and tepid force. America's National Guard, still under state control, had just over 100,000 men: many on the Mexican border chasing, but never catching, Pancho Villa.[305] In 1916 Congress authorized the construction of 157 warships with an appropriation of over $300 million dollars: mostly spent on large ships. At the beginning of the war, America's military had seven troop ships and six cargo ships. The Army didn't have enough infantry rifles. The Army used modified British Enfield rifles. Of fledgling aviation, America had 300 airplanes of various types and manufacturers.[306] American naval leaders failed to comprehend the escalating role of submarines in modern warfare, and the need to build many lighter, faster, destroyers in anti-submarine combat. And always, America needed time to build its new modern ships. Sailors had to be found and trained. The Marine Corps began the war with just over five hundred commissioned officers and thirteen thousand enlisted men.[307]

Gone were simple armaments and short-range, inaccurate weapons.

Munitions and cannon significantly improved. Artillery became an efficient and accurate killing machine. Black powder gave way to high power smokeless powder. Lethal and hideous war gas appeared. Flamethrowers came. On the fields of France, machine guns were killing and maiming hundreds of thousands of Allied soldiers ordered to advance straightaway at the enemy with centuries-old massed infantry battlefield tactics. Modern, technically advanced armies and navies, needed large support infrastructures. This included organized and effective medical support to treat the wounded soldiers having all manner of ghastly wounds and battlefield suffering.

Major General John J. "Black Jack" Pershing, age fifty-seven, a career soldier from Laclede, Missouri, assumed command of the AEF on May 12, 1917. A capable leader, soldier and statesman, Pershing faced a formidable challenge in forming, training, and moving to Europe, a large American fighting force. He formed a staff for the organization of forces to be sent to France. The early assumption was the AEF would need roughly a half-million men. In time the AEF would need a million more. Beginning 1918 Pershing was fortunate to have as his surgeon general, Army major general [Dr.] Merritte Weber Ireland, MD, from Indiana. Ireland had fought in the Spanish-American War, the Philippine War, and the Pancho Villa expedition. In 1903 Ireland was commissioned a surgeon in the Army Medical Corps.[308] Pershing would write of Ireland:

> He is abounding in vitality, mental and physical, quick and accurate in decision, and prompt in action once the decision is made. He understands men and knows how to work with them for the common end. He has a thorough knowledge of the organization of the army and the medical department's place in it. He is…unusually able in administration. He is courageous in…avoiding error. He has an attractive personality and diplomatic…mind. …The goal of his ambition…is to make his [medical] department more useful not only to the army but to the profession in general.

Ireland would receive many distinguished awards from governments and the medical profession. He would be the president of the America College of Surgeons, a fellow of the American College of Physicians, and the president of the National Board of Medical Examiners.[309] He would die at age eight-seven in Washington D.C. in 1952 and be buried in Arlington National Cemetery.

Shortly after America declared war, Ireland presented a comprehensive report to Pershing on the needs of the AEF medical service. Based on an estimated force of over one million soldiers for France, Ireland reported the Medical Department [also called "Sanitary Service"] with doctors, dental surgeons, veterinarians, chemists, and female nurses, would need over 118,000 personnel, or about 10 percent of the AEF force. Ireland estimated hospital bed strength at one bed for every four enlisted soldiers in the AEF: equaling over 240,000 beds. For medical officers, over 9,200 were needed. Last, and compelling, Ireland calculated he needed 22,340 nurses in Europe: roughly one nurse per ten hospital beds. The Army estimated the ratio of one nurse per ten beds was a conservative estimate and didn't leave room for epidemics or a mass casualty event, such as a natural disaster.[310] At the beginning of World War I, the Army wasn't prepared for the medical reality of the coming war. Among its many shortages in materiel and personnel, the Army had 235 regular nurses and 165 reserve nurses in the ANC. Ireland needed volunteer nurses, the call began.[311] [312]

By 1916 President Wilson began seeing the inevitable and endorsed efforts to mobilize America for war.[313] The possibility the United States would enter the European war, and with border incursions by Mexico's Pancho Villa, led America to relook its organization for war. This included how the separate states would support a war effort through state militias: collectively called the National Guard. Questions existed about who had authority over the National Guard, and could the National Guard, a state force, be used outside the boundaries of the United States? The regular Army and National Guard could not agree on the National Guard's role in war. The National Guard wanted to be the national military reserve, while the regular Army, not assured the National Guard was ready, willing, and able to answer the call, wanted a federal militia to be the Army reserve.

Congress solved this with the National Defense Act of 1916. This act specified rolls, responsibilities, and procedures for mobilizing

America's military for war and federalizing the National Guard. The act also increased the size of America's military, and created an officer training program now called the Reserve Officers Training Corps or ROTC.[314] The appropriations bill supporting the National Defense Act had a rider to it creating the Council of National Defense (CND) and an advisory commission. The CND was composed of the secretaries of War, Navy, Interior, Agriculture, Commerce, and Labor. The law creating the CND gave the government authority to form other agencies. The seven-person CND had detailed knowledge of industry, public utilities, natural resources, or other subjects of national interest and importance. The goal was to organize America's ability to advise and assist, in a coordinated effort, to conduct a large-scale war overseas and how to support the effort in America. But the CND was not an executive body and lacked authority to accomplish things. Who had authority and who didn't, quickly blurred. The CND served as a clearing house of information to advise established executive agencies on matters supporting the war.[315] Its sole force was public advocacy and little else.

At the turn of the twentieth century the role of America's women in the national arena and the national conscience grew in importance. Women began actively supporting the mobilization for war. Women had over time created many societies and organizations to advocate the rights of women. How these women were to be organized, mobilized, and used for the war effort, no one really knew. America's women of that day did not have a fixed, universally agreed-upon status in society.[316] The energy, initiative, and willingness of women to support the war effort was readily apparent, but no one yet had a plan to create a systematic national women's effort.

When war preparedness came, the CND created a Woman's Council/Committee to coordinate the many varied and focused national women's organizations and societies. The Women's Council was the first American governmental body staff solely by women. The council, led by eleven women of national prominence, would in time have as its members the presidents of seventy-three women's organizations in America. Coordinating this many organizations, with their diverse focus and agendas, was largely impossible. President Wilson authorized the Woman's Council, with Dr. Anna Howard Shaw, MD, as chairman. Secretary of War Newton D. Baker, said of the Woman's Committee: "The Woman's Committee was the leader of the women of America. It informed and broadened the minds of women everywhere, and with no thought of propaganda it made an argument by producing results."

The Woman's Committee drew up a plan of organization that provided a temporary chairman in each state. Mrs. Tylar B. Thompson, Missoula, Montana, was the chairman of the Montana Woman's Committee: later succeeded by Mrs. Henry L. Sherlock, Helena, Montana.[317] Montana's vast expanses of prairies and mountains challenged the best of organizer to communicate with citizens about any war support plan. In time the Woman's Committee graded each state as to the state's effectiveness and abilities to mobilize and use women for the war effort. The grades were A, B, and C. Montana received a C rating.[318] A vital question lingered: "What are we [women] supposed to do in the Woman's Committee?" To clarify the role of the Woman's Committee, Shaw wrote the secretary of war and reported:

> When I asked the Secretary of War just what was to be our particular function, he said the Woman's Committee was to be the clearing house through which women's work shall be coordinated and in which women shall cooperate so that any line of work taken up in the state shall be carried on along similar lines; and when more than one agency is doing the work, if there is one that has the machinery to do it better than the other, then the organization with the best machinery shall be instructed to push the work along and all other societies similarly employed shall cooperate with them."

The Woman's Council agreed to look at subjects where women could influence national policy supporting the war: areas of food, industry, labor, education, morale, and special training for service.[319] The CND had a General Medical Board to advise and assist on medical matters. On June 24, 1917, this board created a committee on nursing. State committees on nursing had been formed under the Woman's Committees of the State Councils of National Defense in twenty-seven states. In other states the Committee on Nursing functioned through the state associations of graduate nurses. These nursing committees saw their primary function as to promote nursing education and increase the supply of student nurses and help the ARC to increase the enrollment of graduate nurses to meet war demands. The Committee on Nursing sent letters and circulars to universities and institutes of higher learning to appeal to young educated women to enter the nursing profession, and to encourage nursing schools to increase their ability to train nurses.

The Committee on Nursing began a voluntary national census on trained nurses in America. This was an outgrowth of the Woman's Committee wanting to take a national census of women and what abilities the women had. By September 1917 this voluntary census had been done in twenty-four states. This census was done through the American Nurses' Association. The Committee regularly conferred with the ARC on matters concerning both organizations.[320] However, at the end of the day, organizations in war needed executive authority to be effective. The CND and Woman's Council never had that. The War Department and the ARC did. People looked to the War Department and ARC to support the war effort home and abroad.

As part of the preparedness movement two years before America entered the war, the ARC began organizing, manning, and equipping preconfigured hospitals that could be transported when and where needed. The idea for a preconfigured, ready-to-deploy hospital, began in 1914 by Dr. George W. Crile, MD, of Lakeside Hospital, Cleveland, Ohio. Former Ohio governor Myron T. Herrick, asked Crile to provide support for the volunteers of the American Ambulance service in France during the early stages of the war.[321] Crile then looked at providing hospital support, and offered the idea to the Army. The ARC also supported the idea. Under the direction of Army colonel Jefferson R. Kean, Army Medical Corps, the ARC's Military Relief Department began asking Red Cross chapters nationwide to provide trained civilian personnel, doctors, and nurses available for rapid response hospitals in time of war or national disaster. The hospital would have a capacity of 500 beds and have all needed equipment for immediate operation. Three hundred medical personnel would operate the hospital. Only the larger civilian hospitals in the major cities of America had staffs of sufficient size to organize these hospitals called "base hospitals" (BH).

In spring 1916 the ARC began buying, storing and having ready for immediate transportation, nonperishable medical equipment and supplies supporting these hospitals. For the minimum amount of equipment, the ARC needed about $25,000 privately raised per hospital. The federal government wouldn't fund the hospitals. The ARC estimated seven railway freight cars would be needed to transport the hospital's equipment. The ARC agreed to ready the hospital for Army use when needed. If the Army called the hospital for duty, the Army would pay the salaries and transportation of the hospital staff going with the Army.[322] The volunteers for the base hospital would also keep their jobs with their parent hospital.

In April 1917 British and French representatives arrived in Washington D.C. and requested immediate medical support for the British Expeditionary Force (BEF) in France. The British needed six American base hospitals and 116 extra medical officers. The War Department agreed and tasked the ARC to furnish the base hospitals for immediate transportation to France. The hospitals selected were to sail from May 8 to May 25, 1917. In order of sailing the hospitals were, BH No. 4, Lakeside Hospital, Cleveland; BH No. 5, Harvard University, Boston; BH No. 2, Presbyterian Hospital, New York City; BH No. 10, Pennsylvania Hospital, Philadelphia; BH No. 21, Washington University, St. Louis; and BH No. 12, Northwestern University, Chicago.[323] The base hospitals had sixty-five nurses each. [In time the number of nurses per hospital would increase to one hundred.][324]

BH 10 mobilized May 6, 1917, in Philadelphia, and sailed for France, May 19, from New York City.[325] BH 10's contingent of nurses looked over their shoulders at America maybe one last time as the ship sailed from the docks at Hoboken, New Jersey, through the narrows and lower bay, then out to sea. Helen Fairchild, a nurse from Pennsylvania in BH10, wrote many letters home describing vividly, the realities of nursing in combat conditions in France.

Another of BH10's nurses was far from Butte, Montana, where she was born, and the scenic Big Hole basin where she grew to womanhood. Alice Hough Ralston, born in Butte, Montana, December 30, 1884, was the daughter of William Alexander Ralston and Francis L. "Fannie" [Cox] Ralston. William and Fannie had three sons and one daughter. Born in Pennsylvania, William Ralston had moved to Montana and married Fannie in 1878. He became a wealthy cattleman in Montana's

Big Hole basin.[326]

Alice attended local schools near Butte. A graduate of Montana State University in Bozeman, she went east to become a nurse and graduated from the Pennsylvania Hospital's nursing school in Philadelphia.[327] In 1911 she relocated to Coeur d'Alene, Idaho, to take charge of a nurses' training school.[328] By 1914 Alice had returned to Philadelphia. In April 1914 she entered the Navy Nurse Corps, and worked at either Navy Base Hospital 5, [Methodist Episcopal Hospital], or the Naval Station Hospital [St. Agnes Hospital]: both in Philadelphia. In June 1914 Ralston's parents were killed in an automobile accident south of Butte. In October 1914 Ralston resigned from the Navy and returned to Montana.[329]

By 1917 Ralston moved east and lived in New York City. When war came in 1917, she was affiliated with the Pennsylvania Hospital as a nurse. She joined BH 10. When the Army activated BH 10, Ralston enrolled in the ANC. She would serve in the Navy and Army as a nurse. By date of entry into the Navy Nurse Corps in April 1914, Ralston is the first Montana female known to have officially entered the military as a graduate nurse, and the first known Montana nurse to go overseas in war as a member of a military unit: BH 10. She would serve two years in France in war: the longest overseas tour-of-duty of any Montana military nurse in World War I.[330]

ARC nurses began serving as instructors and educators in many medical subjects. In early 1917 the ARC decided nurses were needed elsewhere in direct support of the military. To release nurses and organize women to take over medical support training, such as making bandages and packaging non-perishable hospital supplies, the ARC created two organizations: the Women's Advisory Committee, and the Women's Bureau. In 1917 Jane Delano wrote:

> This reorganization served two purposes: it released… nurses…from being instructors…[in non-medical subjects]…it marshalled the forces…of women volunteers…[and] the great army of volunteer workers throughout the country…It left the Nursing Service free to deal with its purely professional duties.

Immediately after America entered the war, more nurses applied for ARC membership. From January 1 to October 31, 1917, over seven thousand American nurses enrolled. By October 31 the ARC had over fourteen thousand nurses.

Delano determined the ARC needed a comprehensive national census and survey of specialized skills of ARC nurses. Beginning June 1917, the Nursing Department of the ARC did an exhaustive survey of all hospital training schools in America. The survey was done by writing to the Board of Nursing Examiners in each state for a list of all accredited and non-accredited nursing schools in the state. The letter sent to the Board of Examiners read: "The Red Cross is making every effort to anticipate the demands that will be made for nurses not only in Europe, but in our own country should the war be of several years duration...It may be necessary to supplement the nursing service both in military and civil hospitals..."

From this list the ARC sent surveys to the respective schools asking for detailed statements of standards and nursing resources. From this survey the ARC classified the nursing schools that responded, into one of five categories: Class A, schools meeting all ARC requirements; to Class F, schools deemed "undesirable." From the survey of the nurses' skill levels, Delano would write letters to nurses advising them what further training the nurses needed to meet ARC nursing standards.

Delano then began a national census of nurses not at nursing schools. Through nursing volunteers who conducted the census, by summer 1917 Delano reported America had almost eighty-four thousand registered nurses.[331] Montana conducted a nurses' census. By year's end 1917, Margaret Hughes reported Montana had 697 nurses registered in the state: fifty-four of the 697 were ARC nurses. Hughes reported Montana had thirteen accredited hospital training schools with 261 students enrolled in nursing school.[332]

Immediately after the war began, the ARC and the Army weren't very successful in recruiting nurses. Whether the word wasn't getting out, or the realities of war hadn't arrived, may have contributed to the lack of enrollment. Major recruiting drives for ARC nurses wouldn't being until late 1917 and early 1918. When a nurse joined the ARC nursing service the nurse had to indicate where she wanted to serve. The choices were, wherever needed; anywhere in the United States; or in her own locality.[333] "Wherever needed," included overseas in war.

The Call   99

The ARC also wanted nurses to know that mobilization for war was serious business not to be taken lightly.

Montana, even with its vast expanses of prairie and mountain, can act as one big small town with many miles between general stores. In Montana self-reliance meant survival; prairie hubris came from facing hard challenges and enduring. Shared hardship in Montana's forests, rivers, mountains, railroads, and deep underground mines, with women supporting their menfolk, formed bonds lasting forever. In this region, where toughness wasn't vainly boasted but showed quietly through grit, and where women carried newborn children while tending calves and lambs, word began trickling out among the few hundred registered nurses about the need for nurses to go to war. Virginia Flanagan, Great Falls, Montana, heard the call.

Virginia Elizabeth Flanagan was born September 1, 1876, in Fort Benton, Choteau County, Montana, to Michael A. and Elizabeth [McKinley] Flanagan. Michael and Elizabeth would have four children: three daughters, [Virginia, Grace, and May] and son, Frank. Michael came to Virginia City, Montana, from Dubuque, Iowa, in July 1866. He moved to Fort Benton and worked as a bookkeeper for T. C. and J. W. Power & Brothers: general merchandise men and riverboat agents. In 1875 Michael returned to Iowa and married Elizabeth. They returned to Fort Benton where he founded the first drug store in Fort Benton. In 1880 he became the postmaster in Fort Benton: serving for seventeen years.

Virginia was educated at the DeSalles Convent in Dubuque, then returned to Fort Benton and entered nursing school at the Columbus School of Nursing at Great Falls. She graduated with the class of 1911.[334] Flanagan moved to Minot, North Dakota, and worked at St. Joseph's hospital. She later returned to Great Falls and worked as a private nurse. She occasionally worked with the Columbus hospital. Flanagan because a registered nurse in accordance with Montana law. She enrolled with the ARC in 1916.[335] Hearing the ARC call for war nurses, Flanagan answered. She wrote in her memoirs:

> When war was declared in April 1917, the American Red Cross immediately began the recruitment of nurses for the armed forces. I was among the first to enlist, and the first nurse to answer the call to service

from Great Falls, Montana.

My Oath of Allegiance was sworn before Charles N. Pray, Notary Public, on June 28, 1917. Mr. Pray was a long-time friend of the family, and now is better known as Judge Charles N. Pray, retired Federal Court Judge [sic].

I left the dear old City of Great Falls, Montana, on June 30, 1917, amidst the tears and cheers of loyal friends and relatives. Even though I was the first nurse to answer the call from Great Falls, I felt it was much ado over nothing as I was only doing my duty as a loyal citizen, and as I was one of the older nurses in the state, it was only fitting that I should be the first to go.

My destination was the Letterman General Hospital in San Francisco, and I was to travel with two other nurses from the state, but we missed connections, so I traveled alone, and found it very lonely.[336]

A loyalty oath was required of nurses when they enrolled in the military. Montana nurses had to find a person empowered to give the oath. The nurses raised their right hand and recited the oath, or signed a paper having the oath. The oath as Flanagan recited was:

I, Virginia Flanagan, of Great Falls, Montana, in the County of Cascade, and state of Montana, do solemnly swear (or affirm) that I will support and defend the Constitution of the United States against all enemies, foreign and domestic; that I will bear truth faith and allegiance to the same; that I take this obligation freely, without any mental reservation or purpose of evasion; and that I will well and faithfully discharge the duties of the office which I am about to enter. So help me God.[337]

Virginia wrote she was one of the older nurses in the state—she may have been too old and perhaps knew it. At the beginning of World

War I, the Army required nurses to be between ages twenty-five and thirty-five. On Flanagan's official military service record card, she gave her birthdate as September 1, 1881, making her thirty-five years old when she departed for Army service. This met the Army's upper age limit.[338] But her passport application and Montana death certificate read she was born September 1, 1876: making her forty years old in June 1917, and too old for Army nursing service.[339] Virginia never mentioned or explained the discrepancy.

Other Montana nurses were among the first to enter service with Virginia. The other nurses scheduled to travel to their military duty assignments with Virginia, but missed connections, were, Elizabeth Sterling, from Missoula, Montana; and Violet Hodgson, from Baker, Montana. Sterling, born December 16, 1884, in Brooklyn, Iowa, had graduated from nursing school in Des Moines. She had received postgraduate training at the Women's Hospital in New York City, and the Iowa State University. Sterling had worked in Missoula as a nurse for eight years. Missoula doctors said she was remarkably competent and capable.[340] Violet Virgie (Hoffman) Hodgson was born March 19, 1888, Sunbury, Pennsylvania. She was a graduate nurse from the Presbyterian Hospital, Philadelphia, Pennsylvania, class of 1912. She married Joseph Hodgson in 1916 and they moved to Baker.[341] An attorney-at-law with law degree from the University of Michigan, he practiced law in Miles City and in Baker.

Other nurses would soon answer the call to serve. The early trickle of Montana women going to war soon became a steady stream.

Chapter 8
A TELEGRAM FROM MARGARET

"Help that wouldn't come"

IN MAY 1844 SAMUEL FINLEY BREESE MORSE, an early American painter and inventor, finally showed the feasibility of the telegraph for people to communicate over distances. From the Supreme Court chambers in the basement of the U.S. Capitol building in Washington D.C. he tapped on a telegraph key the famous words, "What hath God wrought." The telegraph line went to the Baltimore and Ohio railroad station in Baltimore. He would struggle for years for patent recognition from the U.S. government. Telegraph lines followed the transcontinental railroad across America. Western Union Telegraph Company completed the transcontinental telegraph in October 1861 at a cost of a half million dollars [in 1861 money]. Where the railroads went, so did the telegraph. Telegraph users initially paid a dollar per word to send a telegram.

The telegraph began arriving in Montana in the late 1860s and early 1870s. The main telegraph line to Montana came north from Salt Lake City, Utah: a stop on the transcontinental railroad. The telegraph followed the north spur line of the Union Pacific railroad. By 1874 the telegraph had reached Montana with stations in the western part of the state at Virginia City, Helena, Bozeman, Deer Lodge, Fort Shaw, and as far north as Fort Benton.[342] In time every town, city, and railroad stop along the rails in Montana, had a Western Union telegraph station.[343] The lines followed the rails to give instructions, train orders, report derailments, delays, or schedule changes. Aboveground telegraph lines could break in bad weather; following the rails made locating the break easier. For a telegram at government rates, Western Union charged twenty cents for twenty words or less. This was for a telegram sent within a set distance from the sending station. After receiving a message, the station operator would print or type the message, fold it, and put it in a yellow envelope for delivery to the recipient. Government telegrams had priority over business messages.[344]

Not everyone in Montana lived down the street from a telegraph station. Homesteads and ranches could be many miles distant, or the recipient didn't come to town often. When World War I began, government messages crisscrossed America. In Helena, Margaret Hughes, began using the telegraph often. Montana's nurses knew a small yellow envelope with a telegram from Hughes meant the war had arrived.

Most ARC nurses used the same process to enroll in America's military. By some manner the nurse learned the ARC was the nursing reserve for the ANC. The nurse would contact the nearest ARC office for information. The ARC would begin correspondence with the nurse or schedule an interview. If the nurse was still interested, the nurse would complete paperwork, and be scheduled for a physical examination. The nurse would receive a typhoid inoculation during the physical examination. The chairman of the local ARC office, or the state director of the ARC Nursing Service, would get and verify the nurse's credentials, certificates of inoculation, her address, and date of availability. The state director then sent the information to the ARC divisional office. The director of national ARC nursing, or the War Department would, in time, notify the nurse that she had to report for duty. Montana nurses would receive the telegram, either direct from national ARC nursing, or through Hughes in Helena. For Lucy Walters, the telegram might have read:

> Lucy Walters, Reserve Nurse, Army Nurse Corps, now at Glasgow, Montana, will proceed without delay not later than November 2, after having taken the oath of office, to Camp Lewis, American Lake, Washington, and will report to the Commanding Officer, United States Army Base Hospital for assignment to duty. Travel is necessary in the Military Establishment.[345]

The nurse's home address had to be accurate. If the nurse was not at the given address, the War Department would revoke the orders and the nurse would not go. Someone then had to take her place. The ARC said a nurse had to send a confirmation telegram to the ARC before the nurse's papers could be sent to the War Department. Clara Noyes, director of ARC nursing, sent a letter to all nurse organizing units emphasizing the need for accuracy, timeliness, and resoluteness for nurses reporting for duty. Noyes wrote to organizing offices [in

Montana, Margaret Hughes] that the office had to confirm the nurse's address and that the nurse was ready to go. The state ARC office ensured the nurse knew it was impossible to release the nurse from her obligation to the War Department unless of grave illness. If the nurses who were called to serve lived near each another, the ARC wanted those nurses to travel together. If Montana's nurses lived in distant towns they would have to travel at their expense to a designated city in Montana where the nurses could proceed together. If this wasn't possible, the nurse [e.g., Lucy Walters and other nurses in Glasgow, Montana] would receive separate travel orders and a government transportation order for a train ticket from the nurse's home.[346]

Patriotic fervor, community accolades, sense of adventure, philanthropy, and hubris, faded instantly when many Montana nurses began receiving small yellow Western Union envelopes. The message read the nurses were to go to distant places unknown to them and serve in war. The telegram didn't guarantee the nurses would return. When they were called, the nurses weren't given much time to get ready. The *Billings Gazette,* October 1917, read two Billings nurses, Clara Peterson and Emily Covert, had received orders to report to eastern hospitals for intensive training before being sent to France. Two other nurses in Billings, Minnie Barrow, born in New York City and working for Dr. W. A. Waters in Billings, and Dora Mecklenberg, born in Minneapolis, Minnesota, also received orders to make themselves ready to report for duty on short notice. The *Billings Gazette* ended the article with a sober, "All [four women] expressed anxiety to enter the service." Clara Noyes said of the task confronting America's nurses:

> As I stand facing you tonight, sister nurses, under the shadow of war, we know not what we as nurses shall be called upon to do…You may be called upon to give fully, to make great personal sacrifices, but we know you are prepared, we know that you are ready, we know that we can depend upon you… wherever our Army and Navy may be sent…It must be written upon the pages of history for all time that our Red Cross nurses were prepared, that in this war our soldiers…were not neglected and that they were properly nursed.[347]

A Telegram from Margaret

With the draft underway, thousands of America's men began moving to basic training bases and camps across the nation. The Army began building sixteen training camps for the National Guard and sixteen camps for the Army. By September 1917 these bases began receiving over 400,000 recruits. Each camp would have a 1000-bed hospital. The nearest soldier basic training camps to Montana were, Camp Lewis, near Tacoma, Washington; Fort Riley near Junction City, Kansas; and Camp Dodge, near Des Moines, Iowa. The Army rapidly built barracks for arriving soldiers. As soon as the Army built barracks, recruits filled them. As thousands of soldiers arrived, they brought disease or quickly fell to the rigors of Army basic training.

The Army established Camp Lewis training base in July 1917. Construction of the base hospital began in mid-August. A tent hospital was used in the interim. Minor surgical cases were tended in the tent hospital, major cases went to Tacoma General Hospital. On September 10, 1917, the first wards of the base hospital were ready for use. All wards were one story buildings. Quarters for doctors and nurses were also built. Camp Lewis had two buildings for nurses with sixty-seven rooms. The Army Medical Department reported 200 nurses overcrowded the nurses' quarters. The overflow of nurses would stay in the officer's hospital ward, and later in a two-story hospital ward building. The camp had adequate utilities, water, and electricity, but laundry never kept up to demand.[348] Camp Lewis could get dismal, it had two seasons: three months of summer and nine months of rain.[349]

In July 1917 the base hospital at Camp Lewis had forty-nine patients. By December the hospital will have treated over four thousand patients. Treating these four thousand sick and injured soldiers, the Camp Lewis base hospital medical support staff had forty-four medical officers, and 383 enlisted men. By the Army's planning figure of one nurse per ten patient beds, Camp Lewis should have had 400 nurses by year's end, 1917. In December 1917 the hospital had eighty-two nurses.[350] Of the eighty-two, two were from Montana: Lucy Walters and Grace Gibson. Gibson, born December 30, 1891, in Worden, Montana, was a 1916 graduate of the Montana Deaconess Hospital's training school for nurses in Great Falls.

In early November 1917 Margaret Hughes notified Walters and Gibson to report for duty.[351] Since Walters and Gibson were from different Montana towns, they most likely didn't travel together to

Camp Lewis. Whether they got acquainted at Camp Lewis isn't known. Given the desperately short number of nurses at Camp Lewis, Walters and Gibson most likely met. Walters had time to write a letter to the Valley County, Montana, Red Cross chapter, in Glasgow, Montana: her adopted home. It read of conditions and work at Camp Lewis:

> It is so sweet and so thoughtful to send me the jelly and the candy...I gave a Montana boy from Butte one of the jellies. His name is Private Keegan.[352] He is here with a broken leg. I never knew him before, he's just a thorough Montanan...And the remainder of jelly we eat at our table. Within 15 minutes after receiving the candy it was all gone. Oh! It was good.
>
> I live in a dormitory with twelve other nurses. New quarters are under construction and we hope to be better cared for. A patient made a desk for me and another gave me a trench mirror...I have a good single or three-fourths bed with a good mattress, blankets and linen, and we have a few chairs and our trunks in the dormitory. I am part of the old quarters they have for each room a set of drawers and mirror and chair....
>
> We hope that when the new quarters are finished that will do away with dormitories as living rooms. There are now ninety-four nurses here and I understand that our capacity is 120 nurses. We now have a capacity of 1,500 patients, and the base is nearly full most of the time. I have been head nurse in my ward since ten days after arriving, but [I] have served one month night duty during that time.
>
> ...We haven't the eight-hour [shift] system yet, which the government allows...for there are not enough nurses [to cover all shifts].[353]

By January 1918 Camp Lewis had received over 46,000 recruits: the most of any national training camp at the time. Of these recruits, medical staff at Fort Lewis would reject over five thousand as being medically unfit. The largest reason for rejection, by far, was poor eyesight, followed by bad teeth. Why these weren't detected at the local draft board physicals became a national concern.[354]

In her letter, Walters, the self-sufficient independent woman, the graduate nurse born in the deserts of southern New Mexico Territory who was cited for bravery in Kansas City, the tough and adventurous nurse on the high plains of northeast Montana who volunteered for war, was quietly pleading and trying to soften the blow for help needed for the soldiers and for her:

> ...I wonder if there aren't some more graduate nurses in Valley county [sic] whom some of you could induce to be patriotic enough to volunteer for...the war? ... We always have good times and have four hours off duty when the work permits, which would give us 8 hours on duty...I'm sure the ladies of the Red Cross chapter at Glasgow are patriotic enough to nurse each other if need be and send the graduate nurses to the [military base hospitals]....[355]

Throughout the war the Army would assign twenty-seven Montana nurses to Camp Lewis. Seven of those would soon go to France.[356]

Lucy's plea for nurses became America's plea. As war planning grew, and the number of men entering the Army increased, the need for nurses approached the unbelievable. Using Army major general Ireland's planning numbers of one hospital bed per four soldiers, and one nurse per ten beds, a proposed 1.5-million-man army in France would need over 37,000 nurses.[357] By August 18, 1917, Jane Delano reported the ARC had slightly over 66,000 registered nurses and almost 18,000 non-registered nurses in America: a total of about 84,000 nurses. She also reported America had over 14,000 students enrolled in accredited nursing schools.[358]

In France alone, the Army estimated the need for over 40 percent of all America's nurses. At the peak of America's involvement in wartime France, the Army would get less than a third of the numbers needed for American nurses in France. America's war nurses would have to reach within themselves to depths they never knew possible, to work until near exhaustion, in some of the harshest conditions known, many times under enemy fire, to care for wounded, injured, and sick

Americans in uniform. Many of these nurses would never come home.

The ARC had to make a plan for nurse recruitment, nurse training, and a proposed idea of volunteer help. Doctor S. S. Goldwater, MD, superintendent of Mt. Sinai Hospital, New York, and chairman of the Committee on Hospitals of the Council of National Defense, wrote in report on nursing help:

> I come finally…to the safest and best way out, in fact, the only way out, namely, the training of a large number of non-professional, voluntary, war nursing aides, enlisted for the period of the war, and composed of a class which will not take up nursing professionally…but [are] willing to give…hospital service during the emergency…They [are available], they are strong, healthy, patriotic, and willing. *They are the only labor reserves that the country possesses, and they can be brought into the nursing field without lessening the available supply of workers for any essential industry*…[italics original][359]

America's registered nurses initially opposed the idea of volunteer nursing aides in war. Registered nurses thought nursing aides would lessen nursing standards and return America, again, to earlier less professional standards of nursing care.[360] America and the ARC had to balance the need for trained professional nurses, and untrained American women who wanted the chance to serve through the ARC. The needs of war came first; America was out of options. The ARC began a three-prong effort for World War I wartime nursing support: recruit existing nurses, establish nurse training, and look to volunteer nursing aides. America had no choice.

The ARC had no nursing schools and didn't have time to create any. The ARC recruited from civilians. Its first recruiting drive was in late 1917. To show the national need for nurses and ARC workers, the ARC organized a massive parade in New York City on October 4. Between twenty to twenty-five thousand ARC workers and nurses marched down Fifth Avenue at noon. Estimates were over 300,000 New Yorkers watched the parade. Guests and dignitaries, civilian and military, reviewed the parade: the first women's parade in city history.

Led by the famed marching band leader, John Philips Sousa and his band, thousands of women in white uniforms, with white hats having the distinctive red cross emblazoned on the hat, marched in formation. Reports read Fifth Avenue was a sea of Red Cross red. Five divisions formed the impressive parade. Leading the second division was Mrs. Addie Bagley Daniels, the wife of the secretary of the navy, Josephus Daniels. Daniels decided earlier that year to enlist women in the Navy. Of the parade, Daniels said, "They are magnificent women."[361]

The national enfranchisement of women grew louder. Women demonstrated their abilities, readiness, and power to become part of the national effort in war and in society. The right to serve and go into harm's way was immediately apparent. The right to vote in federal elections was still far off but women were rapidly closing the gap.[362]

Even with a great display of patriotic intentions, nurse recruitment lagged at year's end, 1917. The ANC had 3,800 nurses. Each Army and National Guard training camp in America needed at least sixty-five nurses in each camp's base hospital. The Army needed 371 nurses to fill immediately the base hospital need in America. Troops in the American training camps had priority.[363] The first American soldiers began arriving in France in November, 1917. One of the first American battle casualties was Lieutenant [Dr] William T. Fitzsimons, MD, U.S. Army Medical Corps. Fitzsimons, age twenty-eight years, a graduate of the University of Kansas and faculty member there, was killed-in-action on September 4, 1917 when German bombs fell at BH 5 in France.[364] Fitzsimons Army Hospital, Denver, Colorado, would be named in his honor. American soldiers in France began dying. Nurse recruiting in America was running out of time.

The Women's Committee, Council of National Defense, conceived a plan for the ARC to enroll 25,000 student nurses to replace the depleted national supply of trained graduate nurses. The idea came from the Surgeon General's office early in 1918 in estimating future nursing needs. The government began a national campaign for thousands of student nurses to join the United States Student Nurse Reserve. These student nurses would have to agree to be ready to train as nurses when the government called. The requirements for these student nurses were, they had to be between ages of nineteen and thirty-five, intelligent, and responsible. College education was a plus. The women could enroll in three ways: agree to accept assignments to nurses' training schools in civilian hospitals until April 1, 1919; agree to be candidates for the Army Nursing School [established in 1918]; or agree to accept Army assignment to a civilian nursing school.

Montana governor Sam Stewart publicly declared:

> I am confident that in the state of Montana there are very many young women who will be willing and anxious to have some share, even though it is indirect, in carrying on the tasks of war and the work the war entails; and I am convinced that there will be generous and gratifying response from [Montana's] loyal young women...[365]

The *Great Falls Tribune*, August 11, 1918, sounded a patriotic call for "young ladies" to enroll in the Student Nurse Reserve. The *Tribune* wrote:

> There has been no patriotic call...made upon...Great Falls or Cascade County...where there has been a failure to meet or go beyond the quota [needed]. There should be very little delay in securing 100 young ladies who are called for to complete our enrollment in the nurses' reserve...There surely could be no stronger appeal....There are surely many girls who are here, no one dependent upon them, who are not engaged in essential employment and who possess the qualifications required to enter upon this work for their government.
> ...It is about as necessary to have sufficient number of nurses to properly care for wounded and dying soldiers as it is to have adequate ammunition and guns.

Governor Stewart's call worked. Montana would be *the first state in America* [italics added] to fill its quota of candidates for the Student Nurse Reserve by sending from 260 to 270 completed applications. Mrs. H. L. Sherlock, Montana's state chairman of the Women's Committee of the National Council of Defense, received a national congratulation for Sherlock's efforts.[366]

Many national management and administrative challenges existed in operating the Student Nurse Reserve. The high educational standards [two years minimum of high school] to enter the program, rejected a high percentage of applicants. Roughly two-thirds of applicants were rejected. In all, eleven thousand women nationally were accepted in the Student Nurse Reserve.[367] The nurses' training would vary from two to three years depending on the nursing school the woman attended. The nursing school had to meet state nursing board requirements. Five qualified Montana nursing schools agreed to the program.[368] The government would pay for the student's room, board, and tuition. The students would also get a text book and uniform allowance.

The government said if war ended while the student was in school, the student could complete her training at government expense. The student nurse had to complete the training and be a graduate nurse before she could accept an assignment in the military.[369] The student had to declare an assignment preference: either preferred or deferred. The preferred option meant the student nurse would accept an assignment wherever the need; the deferred option meant the student nurse wanted to go to specific hospitals: mostly a nearby hospital.[370] History doesn't record what preference Agnes Talcott desired, but she wanted to serve.

Agnes M. Talcott was born June 19, 1892, in South Dakota to Albert M. and Hattie Talcott. By 1915 they had lived in The Dalles, Oregon, and then moved to Billings, Montana. Agnes began her nurse training in Billings. A handsome young single woman with smooth elegant features, Talcott enrolled in the Student Nurse Reserve. She left Billings and enrolled in the Methodist Deaconess Hospital, Bozeman, Montana, to complete her nursing training. She never did. She died of influenza in Bozeman on November 1, 1918. Her family at her side.

On Memorial Day, 1924, Billings would honor Agnes when a white stone mausoleum was dedicated at Mountview Cemetery in Billings. The *Billings Gazette*, May 31, 1924, wrote the mausoleum was a "magnificent structure and one of the most modern and enduring structures in the state." A beautiful east-facing stained-glass window rests high above the main entrance to the mausoleum. The morning sun brilliantly illuminates the window as viewed from within. The window measures five feet by five feet with a square base and oval top. Hebe, the goddess of youth, holds a raised lamp shedding rays of light over rugged fields in the foreground marking the graves of forty Yellowstone men who died in France. In Hebe's left arm, she bears a tablet with a single star on it in honor of Agnes who died wanting to serve in war.[371] Talcott is buried between her parents in Mountview Cemetery.

Montana was in the ARC's northern division, and the ARC assigned the northern division a recruiting quota of 1,165 nurses.[372] In December 1917 the ARC notified Margaret Hughes to alert Montana's nurses who volunteered, that the nurses might be needed on short-notice. Hughes told the nurses to have passport photographs taken, get copies of birth certificates, but not quit their regular jobs. The Military Intelligence Department would investigate the nurse volunteers for personal loyalty to the government.[373] Hughes didn't know exactly how many Montana nurses would be called or when.[374]

By year's end 1917, thirty Montana nurses had gone to war: the majority went to training bases and camps in America. The Army did send a few American nurses directly to France, such as the six base hospitals in May 1917, but sending nurses first to basic training bases had priority. The nurses would serve six months at stateside military hospitals. This ensured nurses were well-trained and physically and psychologically fit for the rigors of war. If the nurses wanted, and were deemed capable, the Army sent them overseas. Military patients in stateside base hospitals during 1917 and early 1918 were mostly the sick, accident cases, and other non-battle related medical needs. America's combat wounded in France would not begin arriving in America for months to come.

Jessie M. Turnbull, in her October 1917 article "Will You Be A War Worker?" in the American Journal of Nursing wrote of war as she knew it would come:

> ...Women want to equal men in achievement, all for the war. Our sisters have gone into many fields as chauffeurs, truck drivers, munition workers, conductors...to take the place of men called to the firing line. Each [woman] has a place of duty, the personal character being often the deciding factor.
>
> "I'd love to be a trained nurse" is an expression common enough. Let us consider it...The United

A Telegram from Margaret   113

States hasn't felt any real war suffering [yet]. Sickness... from ordinary causes, with every convenience at hand is no great hardship. Wait till [*sic*] our men are sent back to us, then realization of war horrors will come as our Allies know it. To nurse the ordinary sick with the best of equipment is trying, to nurse the wounded tests nerves of steel. Have you that strength?...Men do not want a doll ambling around; they want a nurse with a backbone in her....

Know thyself and knowing, enter the highest and most specialized branch of woman's endeavor—nursing, with loyalty and sincerity of purpose to succeed.

On October 20, 1917, five Montana nurses received orders to report to Fort Riley, Kansas. These five nurses, the first to report as a larger group, [and the first from Montana to go to Fort Riley] represented a cross section of the state: Anna Christensen, from Livingston; Cora V. Craig from Glasgow; Annabelle Frey from Butte; Emeline Gonczy from Great Falls, and Louisa Lindeberg, from Miles City. Henrietta Vineyard, a Butte hometown girl born March 6, 1892, was a nurse at Butte's St. James Hospital. She would receive telegraphic orders to report to Fort Riley on October 25. In World War I, Butte, the gritty Montana mining town, would send more women [thirty-seven] to war than from any place in Montana.[375]

In 1853 the Army established Fort Riley, named after Major General Bennett C. Riley, who led military escorts along the Santa Fe Trail. In 1887 the Army established its cavalry school at Fort Riley. Fort Riley, had almost twenty thousand acres of land. This gave the fort plenty room for a basic training base for soldiers. Beginning with World War I, the Army built Camp Funston on Fort Riley. Camp Funston had few semi-permanent buildings and did not have a permanent hospital. The Army built its hospital at Camp Funston using simple lumber construction. The hospital was ready for patients on September 27, 1917. Fort Riley had extreme climate with hot summers and cold winters. The hospital officers stayed in Randolph Hall. The hall had two-room apartments and ten sets of quarters. For nurses, the Army built two-story, standard wooden barracks buildings, completed in January 1918. With the expanding number of soldiers at Camp Funston, the Army built a separate mess hall [dining room] for nurses. In October 1917 this mess hall fed ten nurses at a time. Later, a small mess hall was specially built for the nurses in the contagious disease ward allowing the nurses to remain and work in the isolation ward. Camp Funston did not have laundry capabilities until November 1917. Camp Funston sewage drained directly, untreated, into the Kansas River. Livestock manure was piled on the flat land near the camp and burned.

Beginning September 1917, Camp Funston had treated 124 patients, by December, 1,574. In September the camp hospital recorded no patient deaths, by December it recorded seventy-nine. When the five Montana nurses reported to Camp Funston, October 1917, the camp hospital had twenty-eight nurses. By year's end 1917, the hospital would have slightly over one hundred nurses. From 1917 to 1919, the hospital never have over three hundred nurses at any time.[376]

The Army looks to unit cohesion. Keeping people together who came from the same town, the same state, or the same geographical region has benefits. The people [now soldiers] kept together were most likely to be acquainted, have the same culture, background, and outlook: a certain clannish nature in life. Many of the Army's infantry divisions in World War I were formed from National Guard units in a state. The Army also tried to keep nurses together who came from the same location: even as widespread as Montana. The five nurses from Montana who went to Camp Funston, Kansas, were called the "Montana Nurses' Unit." Anna Christensen was the head of the unit.[377] No letters or diaries of the five nurses have been found recording their experiences at Fort Riley/Camp Funston. Ethel Haigitt, an Army reserve nurse from Toronto, Canada, wrote of her nursing experiences at Fort Riley. She and others arrived at the fort in late November 1917.

> …[We] arrived at the fort at 5:20 a.m…daylight was beginning to show…with thick fog…The train… stopped out in freight yard…we had a considerable distance to walk to the little depot. Each had a heavy suitcase, to say nothing of numerous boxes of candy, which we piled into a sweater, tying it up like a bundle

of clothes. We had not notified the Chief Nurse…of our expected arrival…consequently the usual [nurses' transportation] was not there…

We [did not know] how to get to the nurses' home…[But a lieutenant] offered [to take us there]… [Arriving at the nurses' home about 6:15 a.m.] we heard the maids getting breakfast and very soon nurses commenced coming in…We were recognized as new arrivals and all kinds of questions were showered upon us, as to where we came from, what unit we were from, etc…The girls seemed a jolly lot and pleased to see us.[378]

Haigitt's letter continued with, yet again, another sobering reality:

I soon found out how badly more nurses were needed, so maybe this was why their [the nurses already there] pleasure at seeing us was so great; it was not long before I was receiving newcomers with open arms….

They were very busy on the wards, so we were asked to be ready for duty by nine o'clock…[At the isolation ward] I found two nurses and a head nurse…this section, though full of patients, probably 140, [had nurses who had been there] for about two weeks….

…As you may judge, we were very short of nurses through all the Fort…During the first two weeks…I was very tired.[379]

Henrietta Vineyard reported for duty at Fort Riley, November 1917. She wrote home about Fort Riley:

Today I had a bunch [of patients] handed me. I was put in charge of section I. Each ward has been separate, but things have not been going right in some of the wards, and the sergeant in charge of the section asked Miss Harding, chief nurse, to put me in charge of the section to straighten this out…

I have had it mighty easy for the last week and I took advantage of it, but I am in the harness now.

There are six wards in the section, averages 30 to 45 patients in each ward; and such a variety. All of our patients [that can walk] have a ribbon band on their left arm with their diseases on it. This is to keep them from associating with other patients having different diseases. The diphtheria patient has a blue ribbon...scarlet fever, red ribbon...general medical meningitis carries yellow; German measles, white, and [tuberculosis], pink....

I have 17 nurses besides myself, twelve [nurses] on days and five [nurses] on night duty. I hope to get things straightened out...by the last of the week.[380]

The Army did give Vineyard time off. She wrote she shopped in Topeka and went broke buying a black suit, shoes, and hat.[381]

Another Montana nurse, Alice Emelia Becklin, born in Arapahoe, Nebraska, November 15, 1891, entered the ANC at Red Lodge, Montana, on October 22, 1917. The Army sent her to Fort Riley where Becklin served for about a year until October 1918. The Army then sent her to France. Becklin would stay in the ANC as a career officer and nurse. She would retire in 1945 after twenty-eight years of service with rank of lieutenant colonel: the highest military rank for a nurse of that day.[382] Becklin never married but adopted a daughter later in life.[383] By war's end, the Army would assign twenty-two Montana Army nurses to Fort Riley/Camp Funston. The Army would later send sixteen of the twenty-two to France.

In World War I the Army sent many Montana nurses to permanent military hospitals in America. In 1898 the Army built Letterman General Hospital at the Presidio of San Francisco. The hospital received patients and war wounded from the Philippines. It also received patients from the Hawaiian Islands and Alaska. Originally called "General Hospital, San Francisco," in 1911 it was renamed "Letterman General Hospital," for Jonathan Letterman, who served as medical director for the Union Army of the Potomac in the American Civil War.

At the beginning of World War I, the hospital was well-established with a 400-bed capacity. In the war the Army would build twenty-

A Telegram from Margaret 117

six new buildings: mostly for patient wards. By January 1918 the hospital had 1,100 beds. America's war wounded from France would not begin arriving at Letterman until August 1918. By year's end 1917, the hospital had twenty-eight medical officers, 362 medical enlisted men, and seventy-four nurses.[384] Nurses stayed in two dormitories and twenty-four separate rooms. The nurses shared two baths, six washstands, and six toilets. When more nurses came, the Army had to erect extra tents to house the nurses.[385]

Virginia Flanagan was one of the first Montana nurses to enter the ANC of World War I. She received orders to report to Letterman General Hospital. She was supposed to travel to Letterman with two other nurses from Montana, but she missed connections and had to travel alone. Riding the train from Great Falls to Spokane, Washington, then to Portland, Oregon, she arrived in San Francisco the morning of July 3, 1917. No one met her at the San Francisco train station. She soon found transportation from the city to the scenic Presidio on the south promontory overlooking the entrance to San Francisco Bay.

Flanagan wrote of the Presidio:

> ...Our home at the Presidio was beautiful, we had every convenience...and the place was very well managed. We had a Chinese cook, and a Japanese head waiter...there was nothing that could be improved upon in the culinary department.
>
> Letterman General was very orderly and well managed, it certainly didn't seem much like going to war...The hospital was badly over crowded, so several two-story emergency buildings had been erected to accommodate the additional patients.
>
> I was...assigned to...a surgical ward...I had 40 patients, and most of them were very sick; the head nurse was very over-bearing and exacting, but I love the work, and the soldier boys who are so very grateful for everything. Baker was my corpsman on night duty, and I have never had a more cheerful and competent person to work with....
>
> I had my days of joy and days of sorrow; sorrow one day when a young lad was [dying] and mistook

me for his mother because I was there to comfort him. After times such as this, we would go to the city to forget...[386]

Elizabeth Ellen Sterling, a Missoula, Montana, nurse was supposed to travel with Flanagan to Letterman General Hospital, but travel arrangements got confused. Sterling eventually arrived at Letterman. She and Flanagan met and worked together. The Army would eventually assign twenty-three Montana nurses to Letterman. Twelve of the twenty-three would later go to France.

The Army organized Camp Dodge, Iowa, north of Des Moines, on August 28, 1917. It was a basic training base. America is a nation of immigrants. Many recruits didn't speak English well or not at all. The Army began English lessons at Camp Dodge for the soldiers unable to speak English. One of the pamphlets issued to recruits read:

> Make up your mind to learn English, if only a few words a day, as it will help you in the service. Remember, you stay in the service even though you never learn to speak one word of English. Therefore, learn to speak English for your own sake.[387]

History doesn't say if the pamphlet to recruits was written in English: a language they presumably couldn't speak or read. Illiteracy was not a reason to keep a soldier from shooting the Kaiser.

Elmer Olson, a 30-year-old Army recruit from Anaconda, Montana, wrote about basic training at Camp Dodge:

> This sure is the life; if it don't [sic] kill me, it will make a man of me. I am in a company close [sic] to 400 men, and our lieutenant is some driver, but one of the finest fellows you ever saw....
>
> This is sure some camp. There are [a lot of men] here just now....
>
> ...I don't know how many tents there are [here], but it looks like a million. All the new men in the last draft are staying in this camp. We will move to the barracks in about two weeks....

All the new men are from Montana, North and South Dakota, and Nebraska—all western men, and they sure are a husky-looking bunch....We are in quarantine two weeks until they find out...if we are diseased in anyway. Tonight we are going to have a broncho-busting [sic] contest between South Dakota and Montana, and believe me we will be...pulling for Montana...[388]

During the war Olson would never be promoted beyond private, and he would stay in America.[389] History doesn't say if Olson made a living in Montana busting broncos.

If arriving recruits didn't pass medical inspection, the Army would quarantine them in a base hospital. The Camp Dodge base hospital had two, two-story buildings: one used as administration and officers' barracks; the other as a patient ward. As soldiers arrived for basic training, sick or diseased patients were rapidly admitted to the camp hospital. This created a severe shortage of hospital beds and ward space. Existing barracks buildings became hospital wards.

By October 1917 workers had built nineteen ward buildings. When the Camp Dodge base hospital opened, the hospital officers stayed in three barracks that had outside latrines. The nurses stayed by themselves in a building attached to the hospital by an enclosed walkway. The nurses' building had bedrooms, a mess hall, and kitchen. In April 1918 more patients arrived. However, a fire destroyed the nurses' quarters. The Army built other nurses' quarters, but this did not provide sufficient space for 225 nurses eventually on duty. The overflow of nurses went to an old officers' barracks previously closed.[390] By the end of December 1917, Camp Dodge base hospital had over two thousand admissions. To manage this patient load, the hospital had fifty-eight officers, 320 enlisted men, and sixty-three nurses. By November 1918 the base would have 376 nurses.[391]

In June 1918 Dr. Donald Campbell, MD, president of the Murray Hospital in Butte, Montana, stopped at Camp Dodge after attending the American Medical Society convention in Chicago. The Army had assigned three nurses from Butte to Camp Dodge. These three nurses, Nellie Oldhouse, Kate Boles, and Ella Hornkey, had graduated from the nursing school at Butte's Murray Hospital. Campbell reported that mothers of the soldiers in training at the camp shouldn't worry about the medical treatment of their sons. Campbell said Camp Dodge had about fifty thousand soldiers and one hospital having 2,200 beds with fifty beds in each ward.[392] Twenty-nine Montana nurses would eventually serve at Camp Dodge: more than any one place in America during World War I. Of the twenty-nine, five would later go to France. Among them Florence Ames, Billings, Montana: an original member of the Montana State Board of Examiners for Nurses.

In July 1918 six graduates of the Columbus Hospital Training School for Nurses, Great Falls, Montana, decided to stick together: thick or thin, war or not. They were Wilhelmina "Minnie" Hume, Mary Gregory, Margaret Thompson, Alma Hutton, Lydia Fousek, and Mina Aasen. These six yearling nurses would travel to Camp Dodge in a roundabout way. Private Elmer Olson may have enjoyed becoming a man at Camp Dodge, but Fousek would discover how merciless the camp could be. For Aasen a different rendezvous waited for her decades later on a jungle-covered strip of mountainous land in the Philippines: a rendezvous with hell at a place called Bataan.

Chapter 9
THE GREAT FALLS SIX

"Thick or thin, hell or high water"

THE PRISONERS LINED UP FOR ROLL CALL THREE TIMES A DAY, every day: 8:00 a.m., 5:00 p.m. and 8:00 p.m. They gathered around the old university building built centuries before. They were a vanquished people, starving, sick, and diseased people who had to bow deeply from the waist in homage and obeisance to their captors. She would say in later years: "Oh, how I hated to bow to them!" In the crowded nurses' dormitory-style barracks, eighteen nurses stayed in one room with barely enough space to get around. Sanitation failed in rainy seasons, sewage overflowed and ran throughout the compound. Food dwindled to a ration of watery rice soup, starvation began slowly, inexorably. Hope teetered, boredom stupefying, help not coming, and people dying.[393]

Standing in line those days and every day for almost three years at Santo Tomas Internment Camp (STIC), Manila, Philippine Islands, Mina ["Meena"] Andy Aasen, second lieutenant, ANC, was a "lifer." A career Army nurse, she was a long way from Millmar, Minnesota, where she was born; Minot, North Dakota, where she grew to womanhood; and Great Falls, Montana, where she became a nurse. Born April 19, 1894, at forty-eight years of age in the Philippines, Aasen was one of the "old gals." This was Aasen's second tour-of-duty at Sternberg Hospital in Manila. The Army had assigned Aasen to Sternberg from 1931 to 1933. The Army renamed the General Hospital, Philippine Islands, to "Sternberg Army Hospital" to honor Army brigadier general George Sternberg, who helped create the Army Medical School and the ANC.

Manila cast an exotic oriental spell under a tropical sky. The workload wasn't hard, the evenings social, recreation abundant. Easy travel to China and other oriental ports-of-call. Tropical Philippine weather was more bearable that blinding blizzards and lethal cold of North Dakota and Montana. Aasen had been in Manila before, why not go back? She did. She sailed from San Francisco, June 5, 1941 and arrived in Manila, June 24.[394]

When Aasen arrived in Manila at Sternberg hospital, she probably reported for duty to another Montana nurse: Captain Elizabeth Valine "Valine" Messner, ANC. Born in Utica, Montana, December 7, 1890, Messner was one of three children, all daughters, of Martin and Mary Messner. Utica, about forty miles west of present Lewistown, Montana, was cowboy country, and in the early 1880s, headquarters for the Judith Basin Cattle Pool. Utica was also Charley Russell country, many of Russell's paintings show life around Utica. Russell even had a homestead in Pagel Gulch above Utica.[395] For eighteen years Martin Messner had been a successful cattle rancher along the Judith River in north-central Montana. People thought highly of him. Montana cowboys don't scare easy, but when someone says, "typhoid," the room gets quiet. That's what killed Martin Messner the first part of November 1907. Valine was almost seventeen years of age when she helped bury her father in the Utica cemetery. Martin left Mary and daughters, Valine, Zella, and "Jo," an estate valued around $25,000.[396] The daughters would get an inheritance when they became of age. Mary sold the ranch and livestock, then moved the family to Lewistown where Mary bought real estate and made a living off the rent.

Her own woman now, Valine took her inheritance and went to Spokane, Washington, where she received her nurse's training at St. Luke's Hospital and School of Nursing. She entered the ANC on June 6, 1916, in Moore, Montana. The Army gave her a rating of chief nurse in November 1917. During World War I Messner would serve in many stateside hospitals. She did not serve overseas in World War I. Messner would nurse wounded and sick soldiers in two world wars and beyond. Regardless of her assignment, Messner would be the chief nurse of her duty station.[397] She, like Aasen, would be a "lifer." The Army would be Messner's home for the next thirty-one years. Messner, Aasen, and Alice Becklin, never married. These three women with ties to Montana, made the ANC a career in two world wars.

Messner may have met another Lewistown nurse: Joan Nicholson Ray. Born in Northumberlandshire, England, August 16, 1885, Nicholson had married Charles O. "C.O." Ray, in November 1913 in Moore, Montana: west of Lewistown.[398] [399] Charles and Joan lived in the Judith Basin near where Messner grew to womanhood. In 1913 Joan was a nurse. Life didn't work out for Joan, and in January 1915 she divorced C.O. for abandonment.[400] A future treasurer of Judith Basin

County, C.O. also had his hand in the Judith Basin till. Convicted of embezzlement in 1929, he would go up another Montana river to Deer Lodge and spend a year as a guest of Montana taxpayers at the Montana state penitentiary.[401]

Joan Ray entered the ANC early in 1918. Ray would serve stateside in the war. After the war Ray stayed in the Army. The Army assigned her to Sternberg Hospital late in 1921. Ray and Messner served together for about a year at Sternberg.[402] After a tour-of-duty in the Philippines, Ray returned to America and served in Army general hospitals for a few more years. She resigned from the Army in May 1927. Ray then moved to southern California and, like many Montana women veterans of World War I, faded into history.[403]

After World War I Messner's military nursing service continued with assignments in the Philippines, in Tientsin, China, then back to America to several Army general hospitals.[404] Messner returned to the Philippines and Sternberg Hospital where she was chief nurse of the Philippine Command. In 1941 Messner was at Sternberg when Aasen arrived. Messner's regular three-year tour-of-duty at Sternberg ended October 1941. Messner handed the reins of chief nurse to Captain Maude C. Davison, ANC. Messner's 51st birthday, ironically, was December 7, 1941. Davison, Aasen, and many other Army and Navy nurses remaining in the Philippines, would not be celebrating anything for a long, long time.

Mina hated bowing physically to her captors and wanted history to remember. Aasen was one of the sixty-six ANC nurses held prisoner-of-war by the Japanese in the Philippines in World War II. In the annals of American history, where the exploits of courageous men and women are trumpeted loud and with honor, these women will forever be known as the "Angels of Bataan." These were courageous indomitable women in uniform who endured unimaginable hardships in the steaming, disease-infested jungles and open-air makeshift hospitals of the Bataan Peninsula. Struggling against increasing terrible odds, fading hope, and discouragement, Aasen and the other nurses had to find strength, energy, and force of will to keep wounded and sick American and Filipino troops alive in the desperate opening days of World War II far from America.

At the end of December 1941, the Japanese had invaded in great strength, the Philippine island of Luzon at Lingayen Gulf. Japanese forces moved south to Manila.[405] To avoid massive civilian casualties and needless destruction of Manila, Allied command declared Manila an open neutral city: meaning the Allies would not defend the city by force of arms. All American military personnel, including American nurses, had to evacuate Manila and move to the narrow, mountainous, and inhospitable Bataan Peninsula across Manila Bay. By some mistake eleven Navy nurses were left behind in Manila. The Navy nurses began to think they were expendable. By January 1942 the Army estimated Bataan held over 100,000 people with fourteen thousand Americans among the many. On Bataan Peninsula the nurses operated two open-air field hospitals for wounded and sick allied soldiers: the first American military open-air hospitals since the Civil War.

Starving and without support, Allied and American forces on Bataan could fight no more. They surrendered April 9, 1942. The infamous "Bataan Death March" began for the American and Allied prisoners. After the war the Allies estimated of the 72,000 men who began the Death March, less than half survived. Before the surrender of allied forces on Bataan, the American command ordered nurses to evacuate Bataan and go to Corregidor Island: the fortress guarding the entrance to Manila Bay. The wounded and sick Allied soldiers in the two open-air field hospitals had to be agonizingly left behind.

On Corregidor Island the nurses operated a hospital in deep, dark, and dank tunnels. Corregidor surrendered May 6, 1942, and the Americans and nurses became prisoners-of-war. The Japanese moved the male soldiers to brutal prisoner-of-war camps in northern Luzon. The nurses were taken back to Manila and into STIC. In time the Japanese would crowd almost four thousand military, civilians, men, women, and children, into the old high-walled Spanish university founded by Dominican fathers, over 300 years before. Over three years would pass before the American promise of help and liberation would finally come, and Mina and the other Angels of Bataan would breathe again the sweet air of freedom.[406]

Mina was born April 19, 1890, in southern Minnesota to parents of Norwegian ancestry. In 1896 Mina's father, Sigurd Olsen Aasen, moved the family to a homestead ten miles north of Minot in north-central North Dakota. Sigurd had put all the family belongings, even livestock, into a single railroad car for the journey west. Mina, her two brothers and three sisters, rode in the passenger coach; Mina's parents rode with the livestock.[407] In time Sigurd, an excellent carpenter, made a home for his family on his homestead land. Mina later said she found how demanding farm life can be on the open plains north of Minot. Mina said she would never marry a farm boy. She knew her mother did twice the work her father did in cooking, sewing, washing clothes, helping with the milking and tending livestock, caring for children, spinning wool for clothes, and keeping the fire going in winter. Mina was sixteen years old in 1906 and had finished eighth grade. She would never complete high school.

After she finished schooling, Mina moved to Minot and lived with her sisters. Laundry was the only work available for girls. Mina would say, "We washed everything by hand, using a rub-board and strong soap…Our hands were rough and dry." In North Dakota's severe winters Mina carried the wet laundry to the attic and hung the laundry on lines in the unheated space. She was determined to show everyone she could work and make her way. Mina loved to dance and traveled miles to attend barn dances. No man's ring ever adorned her hand. She decided life had better things to offer than being an old farm woman by the time she was thirty. She said, "I didn't want to marry a farm boy, so I stayed aloof after a few dates when any young lad wanted to go steady."

In 1914 Mina's sister, Ida, had married. Ida and her husband homesteaded at Brady, Montana: located between Havre and Great Falls. Mina and sister, Anne, visited Ida. From Brady, Mina and Anne decided to go to Great Falls for work. They went to Columbus Hospital at Great Falls, and asked the Mother Superior if the hospital needed workers? The Mother Superior told Mina and Anne the hospital needed nurses. Mina and Anne enrolled in the Columbus Hospital School of Nursing. Soon Anne left the nursing school but Mina stayed. Anne ran a cook-car to feed wheat threshing crews in the vast grain fields of north-central Montana near the Canadian border. One threshing season Mina took time off from her nursing studies and helped Anne. Mina soon discovered cooking for many men wasn't what she had in mind for her life's work. Mina said, "Anne was an excellent cook, but I could care less about preparing food." Mina summarized her experience that year during threshing season:

It was nice to have a 'vacation' from nursing school, but I was happy to return to the hospital in Great Falls when the threshing season was over. That was my one and only experience in the cook-car and I knew for sure I wanted a career in nursing instead of a life of cooking and washing dishes.[408]

Mina entered Columbus Hospital School of Nursing at Great Falls in 1916. This would be the hospital's last nursing class where students didn't need a high school diploma to enroll. The Sisters of Charity of Providence opened Columbus School of Nursing in 1892. Named after the Italian explorer, Christopher Columbus, the hospital soon had many patients from Great Falls: a city of about ten thousand. By 1894 the Sisters had built a hospital building and began seeing patients.[409]

The Sisters of Charity began a nursing school. The graduating class of 1917 had thirteen women: Mina Aasen, Anna Curran, Bernice Friend, Lydia Fousek, Katherine Welter, Mary Gregory, Susannah and Evelyn Rackham, M. Alma Hutton, Wilhelmina Hume, K. Elsie Peterson, M. Margaret Thompson, and Sylvia Kyte. The hospital held graduation ceremonies for the new nurses, May 27, 1917: a few weeks after America declared war in World War I.[410] The new nurses had formal photographs taken in immaculate white nurses' uniforms with creased hats and rightfully earned Columbus Hospital nurses' pins below their left shoulder. As World War I progressed and the need for nurses increased, six of the thirteen, Aasen, Hume, Gregory, Thompson, Hutton, and Fousek, decided to sign up with the Red Cross and go to war together. [One of the thirteen, Anna Curran, had already entered the ANC and was assigned to Vancouver Barracks, Washington.] This notion of going to war together is what Jane Delano, director of the ARC had in mind.

Clara Noyes, ARC director of nursing, wrote to superintendents of America's nursing schools and urged the superintendents to form ARC training units within the nursing schools. Challenges of war, relocation, traveling to new and perhaps formidable places, seem less daunting when you go with someone you know and have worked with. None of the "Great Falls Six" were Montana natives. Of the six, "Minnie" Hume, was from Dundee, Scotland. Three were from North Dakota: Aasen, Hutton, and Thompson. Lydia Fousek was born in Minnesota.

Her father, Albert J. Fousek, a cigar maker, was mayor of Great Falls.[411]

The ARC organized these training units within the senior classes of the nurse training schools. The ARC soon found "young, adventure-loving, brave and eager group company of [women] almost all were of recognized dependability and skill."[412] The ARC numbered each training school unit with a numerical designation intentionally set to a high number. This numbering system avoided confusion with base hospitals and other hospital units. The ARC formed the first nurse training unit in North Carolina with designation T. S. Unit No. 500. By summer 1918, 1,362 nurses volunteered for war service from 307 nurse training units in America.[413] Nurses at Columbus Hospital, Great Falls, Montana, formed Columbus Unit 511, organized by Sister Remi. More nurse training units formed in Montana: St. John's Hospital Unit 606, Helena, formed by Sister Mary Charitina, R.N.; St. James Hospital Unit 607, Butte; formed by Maude E. Lally, R.N.; Montana Deaconess Unit 620, Great Falls, formed by E. Augusta Ariss, R.N., and St. Peter's Hospital Unit 671, Helena, formed by L. Van Luvance, R.N.[414]

On June 1, 1918, seven nurses from St. John's Training Unit 606, Helena, went to Letterman Army General Hospital, San Francisco, California: Fannie Larson, Julia Martin, Margaret Martin, Katherine O'Donnell, Mae Opp, Erma Stabler, and Frances Vollmer. On July 9, 1918, seven nurses from the St. James Hospital Unit 607, Butte, went to Camp Pike [Camp Robinson], Arkansas, a basic training base near Little Rock: Margaret Cariher, Josephine Dolan, Mary Duval, Catherine Melia, Katherine Small, Mary Strutzel, and Bertha Thompson. On August 8, 1918, six nurses from Montana Deaconess Hospital Unit 620, Helena, went to Camp Custer, Michigan, a basic training base near Battle Creek: Aimee Doerr, Bell Menzies, Dorothy Miller, Cloe Peters, Elta Reed, and Elizabeth Shortreed.[415] The ARC training unit concept was successful in Montana.

By summer 1918 the Great Falls Six waited for orders to report for duty. The call for nurses never diminished, and the six nurses from Montana wanted to go to France. Near the end of June they probably received orders to report for duty. On Monday, July 1, 1918, Mayor and Mrs. Fousek entertained the six eager new ARC nurses at the Fousek home in Great Falls. The Fousek's invited many guests. Mrs. Fousek elaborately decorated the dinner table with baskets of peonies and roses. Entertainment and music filled the evening. Door prizes were a hand-painted china basket for the women, and a box of cigars [probably rolled by Mayor Fousek] for the gentlemen.[416] The six nurses raised their right hands and took the loyalty oath on July 11, 1918, in Great Falls. They were on their way—or so they thought.

History doesn't say why the six went first to Washington D.C., but they did.[417] Aasen, along with several other nurses, began working in Walter Reed Army Hospital. Minnie Hume reached New York City waiting to go to France, but the Army changed Hume's and the other's assignments.[418] The Great Falls Six had to report for duty at Camp Dodge, Iowa. It would almost cost Lydia Fousek her life.

America's World War I military training bases held tens of thousands of men. This rapid expanding and transporting people across America built a highway for spreading diseases. The Army put recruits in overcrowded barracks and tents. Avoiding overcrowding is not always practical in military life: especially in World War I training camps. Men with communicable diseases ended up in temporary hospitals. Water supplies came from wells or streams near rudimentary sanitation. Open sewers, untreated sewage dumped in rivers, burning manure, mounds of garbage, and large herds of nearby livestock, and pigs, destined to feed soldiers, added fuel to the fire of disease.

Sanitary engineering existed in the Army, but engineers on duty acted much as advisors and lacked authority to mandate standards.[419] The Army's belief of "keeping things clean" had merit, but with the urgent need of training soldiers for war, the Army voluntarily accepted less than sterling standards of sanitary conditions for soldier wellbeing. The Army surgeon general's office, sanitary inspection team, reported in August 1918, that Camp Dodge, Iowa, where Montana's "Great Falls Six," reported for duty was "…the most unsanitary place…in any of our Army camps. The garbage station is very badly managed…This filth is almost a solid mass of…maggots."[420]

Epidemiology, the study and methods used to find causes of diseases and outcomes on the human population, was in its infancy in the nineteenth century. By early twentieth century doctors had a basic understanding of what caused many communicable diseases, but lacked a systematic societal plan [or modern antibiotics and vaccines] to contain and treat the disease before it reached epidemic proportions. "Cleanliness and good air" seemed universal treatments.

The Great Falls Six 129

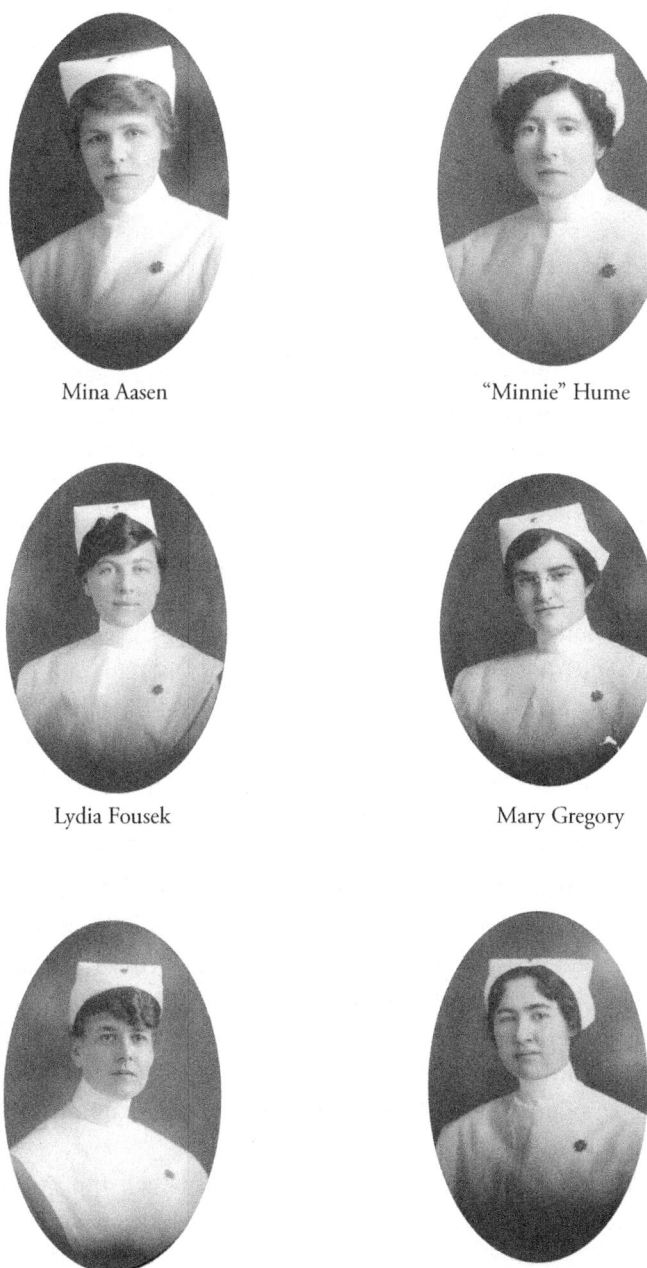

Mina Aasen

"Minnie" Hume

Lydia Fousek

Mary Gregory

Alma Hutton

Margaret Thompson

The Great Falls Six
Courtesy The History Museum, Great Falls, MT

In America's thirty-two World War I training camps, doctors kept detailed records of medical challenges and conditions. In spring 1918 many camps began reporting influenza outbreaks. As soldiers came and went through east coast ports, the first cases of influenza were reported in Boston at the Commonwealth Pier.[421] The first Army authenticated case of influenza in the autumn epidemic was at Camp Devens, Massachusetts, September 8, 1918. The Army surgeon general first did not require telegraphic reports of influenza and did not know of outbreaks. When the outbreak was eventually confirmed at the end of September, the Army quarantined Camp Devens. The camp could not receive new recruits or allow soldiers in camp to leave. The Army reported Camp Devens had ten thousand men more than it could house. The Army tried blocking or slowing troop movements between camps, but this wasn't always possible. Influenza spreads fast. By end of September 1918, eighteen Army training camps were heavily infected and the disease spread. The Army surgeon general recommended all draft calls to those infected bases be canceled, and transfers from one camp to another be limited.

By September 26 the Army surgeon general reported Camp Devens had 45,000 men and over twelve thousand cases of influenza.[422] By September 28 the War Department began giving specific instructions to all Army training camps on how to fight the disease. Calling the disease a "crowd disease" the Army mandated at least fifty square feet of space per non-infected soldiers in barracks, hospitals, and tents. For infected soldiers, the Army mandated one hundred square feet per soldier. At the end of the message, the Army surgeon general's office gave a sobering warning: "Sufficient trained Medical Department [personnel] are not available for transfer [to help]." On October 5 the surgeon general's office categorically reported: "...Influenza is so widespread throughout the country, it is impossible for medical officers to state with any degree of safety that any particular command is free from infection."[423]

The epidemic wasn't contained on shore. When the troop ship *Leviathan* carrying U.S. soldiers to war, arrived in Brest, France, October 7, 1918, eighty-five men aboard had already died, with 366 cases of pneumonia and almost 600 cases of influenza still active on board. One percent of the entire ship's convoy arriving at Liverpool, England, on October 8, had died at sea. The situation was serious, and the Army classified secret its influenza reports to the Army chief of staff. This hid facts from the public—and the enemy—about influenza's effect on U.S. troop ships and at basic training camps.[424]

At Camp Lewis, Fort Riley/Camp Funston, and Camp Dodge, hospital admissions in January 1918 were about three thousand patients at each camp. In January few patients died. By October 1918 at the peak of the influenza epidemic, patient admissions at each camp soared to over three times the number in January; patient deaths were in the hundreds and higher. In October the Camp Dodge hospital had admitted over eleven thousand patients with over 700 deaths.[425] One of the patients was Lydia Fousek, nurse, ANC, Great Falls, Montana. She wrote to her parents, Mayor and Mrs. A. J. Fousek in early October 1918: "…Had quite a high temperature but worked every day. My throat is very sore and I cough."[426] She continued saying of the hundreds of nurses at Camp Dodge, more than 100 were hospitalized due to influenza. She wrote extensively, and the *Great Falls Tribune* published her entire letter on October 20.

> This is my second day up and I am learning to walk all over again…many maimed and disabled nurses [are] walking around again. We have 475 nurses now on duty and 100 sick ones. The nurses must be living under lucky stars, very few of them have had pneumonia. One poor little girl died last night. She was to have graduated in the spring and came from Council Bluffs [Iowa] to help during the epidemic. Words cannot picture some of the things that have happened here…These poor boys being brot [*sic*] in by that never-ending stream of ambulances so sick that they could not sit up, just falling on the ground… Two weeks ago…I had received my orders to prepare my ward for influenza, they were hauling them in, not one or two at a time but seven and 10 and 12….
>
> Now we have 53 patients in our 38-bed ward. There are a good many deaths and some of the scenes are heartbreaking. Poor mothers, they get so tired looking for their boys among all these thousands of patients…One poor white-haired lady looked for

> her boy for six hours and when she finally found the ward where he was he had been dead 10 minutes and calling for her all afternoon. They knew she was in camp and could not find her....
>
> While I was sick my patients...sent me some beautiful roses...from Des Moines...The first patient I admitted sent me a box of candy when I was ill and the afternoon I received it he died. I did not know [that] for a few days....
>
> Good old Great Falls [Montana]. There is no place like you on the map!

Lydia Fousek needed a long time to recover from influenza at Camp Dodge. None of the Great Falls Six would go overseas in World War I. Except for Mina Aasen the rest of the six would leave the Army after World War I ended.

Influenza struck Montana hard beginning October 1918. Montana newspapers wrote of daily battles against the epidemic. By end of October, the Montana state board of health reported 861 deaths, by November an estimated one thousand deaths.[427] The United States Public Health Service sent five doctors from Oregon to help Montana. By mid-October the Montana board of health reported two thousand cases of influenza in Montana. No one knew the exact number of cases. Montana and America could do little to fight the disease. Influenza vaccine was still in experimental stage and not recommended for general use.[428] The Army developed a pneumonia vaccine in August 1918, but it had not been widely tested.[429]

The Montana state board of health received telegraphic reports of influenza conditions across the state. Cities closed schools and theaters, canceled church services, and prohibited public gatherings. Anaconda barred public gatherings even at funerals, only family could attend.[430] The bars in Butte were an exception. The Silver Bow County board of health said if America won the war, in spite of the epidemic, saloons in Butte could remain open and sell drinks over the bar. This assumed Butte wanted to celebrate: always a foregone conclusion. Butte miners were going to test a theory that whiskey and ale could cure influenza.[431]

Butte turned the high school and Finlen Hotel into hospitals for influenza patients. The city estimated the two places could hold twenty-five hundred cases if needed.⁴³² Thirty-three people had died in Butte from influenza by the third week of October. One family, the O'Meara's, lost the husband, wife, and daughter, within twenty-four hours of each other.⁴³³ At the beginning of the epidemic in Butte, physicians thought inhaling the dust from Butte's many unpaved streets and mine dust had something to do with the influenza epidemic. Given that theory, Butte fire brigades got busy and soaked all Butte streets.⁴³⁴ It didn't help with the epidemic, but at least Butte cleaned its streets.

Many Montana newspapers printed county-by-county reports of influenza conditions.⁴³⁵ Official death totals were not known because not all cases were reported. Montana's many smaller towns suffered due to lack of help and lack of nurses. Permelia Clark, superintendent of the Frances Mahon Hospital, Glasgow, where nurse Lucy Walters had worked, reported to Margaret Hughes that influenza conditions in Valley County were "dreadful to say the least." Clark improvised a hospital at Wolf Point: east of Glasgow. The hospital had one trained nurse to care for patients. Clark recruited twenty volunteers, aides, and helpers to care for influenza patients. In Malta, west of Glasgow, twenty people died in ten days from the disease. Clark canvassed Malta to find anyone with nursing training. She found one person, not a graduate nurse, but the person had some training. A few other well-intended, untrained people helped. Montana fought influenza but lacked nurses to travel the great distances in the state to care for patients. More people died.⁴³⁶

The Montana state board of health and Public Health Service needed energetic and innovative means to fight influenza in the vast spaces of Montana, and with few remaining nurses. The *Great Falls Tribune* on October 19, 1918, called the plan the "Flying Corps." A small group of volunteer doctors and nurses would remain on call to respond to any location in Montana needing immediate medical help. This medical team would be paid $200 a month, plus travel expenses, and $4.00 per day subsistence allowance. The team could quickly respond to communities in need. What few graduate and trained nurses remaining in Montana that autumn in 1918 faced a terrible dilemma: enter the military nurse corps to help America's sick and wounded soldiers, or stay and help friends, neighbors, and citizens in Montana who were dying of influenza.

Army brigadier general James "Jimmy" Guthrie Harbord, was

chief of staff of the growing AEF in the early days of the war in France. He would later successfully command troops in the field. This included commanding the Marine Corps, Fourth Brigade at Belleau Wood. The previous Marine Fourth Brigade commander, Brigadier General Charles A. Doyen, came down with influenza in France, and General Pershing, AEF commander, needed an officer to immediately take command of the 4th Brigade. Pershing chose Harbord. [Doyen would soon die of influenza in October 1918.][437] On October 3, 1918, Harbord, chief of staff, AEF, sent a message to the Army chief of staff and Army surgeon general about influenza conditions in France. Harbord wrote:

> ...Influenza exists in epidemic form amongst our troops in many locations in France accompanied by many serious cases of pneumonia. Requests coming [from] all quarters for additional members of the Army Nurse Corps. In all probability conditions will not improve but will grow worse during the winter. Request 1,500 members of the Army Nurse Corps... be sent to France as an emergency requirement at the earliest practicable date for duty at camp hospitals and to make up shortage.[438]

Nurses were in short supply. In March 1918, before the influenza epidemic struck, Jane Delano reported on the shortage:

> ...If we [ARC] are to meet the needs of the Army and the Navy with registered nurses alone, it will necessary to withdraw [from civilian service] not far from fifty percent of the total number of graduate nurses [in America]. Even though we include all graduate nurses who are not registered, placing the total at about one hundred thousand, at least thirty-three percent of the entire number [in America] must be secured if we are to provide nursing care for our Army and Navy.[439]

Sadness and irony affect a soldier's heart in ways not spoken, but seen in their eyes. Virginia Flanagan would write of her nursing experiences at Camp Kearney, San Diego, California: "The poor sick

The Great Falls Six   135

boys at Kearney were very patient, but felt they were sacrificing their lives for no good purpose as so many of them died in camp of the flu."[440]

In July 1917 the ARC thoroughly reviewed the entire challenge of nursing needs in the civilian sector and in war support. President Wilson's War Council brought together all nursing advisory committees to create a plan to address nurse shortages. The committee agreed the ARC was barely meeting nursing needs early on in the war. The committee expressed concern on how to meet the need for nurses in the coming months as the war progressed. The committee recommended five major initiatives: Hospital training schools change curricula to meet war conditions; change nurse age requirement to twenty-one to forty years; early graduation of nurses; train nurses' aides and use public health nurses more. The officers of the ARC Nursing Service approved the recommendations.[441]

Montana implemented the recommendations. By August 1917 Montana's university system began a two-semester preparatory course for nurses. This was designed to shorten the three-year nursing school course to two years. This shortened curriculum wasn't working.[442] By 1918 the University of Montana offered an intensive ten-week summer school replacing a full year of nursing preparatory training. Applicants had to have at least two years of high school before entering the nursing program. The state board of nursing examiners agreed to this accelerated training. After the accelerated training, the nursing students had to complete a year of supervised training at a hospital before the students could take the registered nurses examinations. Arrangements were made at the major hospitals in Montana to support this.[443] Professor W. G. Bateman, University of Montana, agreed with the accelerated nursing training saying, "We do not want to repeat the experience of England where a great number of trained nurses were drained from civilian hospitals and private service, and there was distress among the civilians as a result."[444]

"Slacker," a biting and derogatory term, appeared in America's World War I vocabulary. The word meant someone deemed less than supportive of the war effort, less willing to serve, or downright cowardly. Tom Davis, of the Camp Lewis Young Men's Christian Association, was speaking in Butte, Montana, when he defined "slacker":

> A slacker is like a custard pie—yellow through and through with not enough crust to go over the top… and a slacker is a man who will not 'come through' for the war chest and stand squarely behind the boys who are fighting his fight, my fight and your fight. He is a dog—no, I must apologize to some dogs—he is a dirty yellow dog.[445]

America was getting desperate for nurses. The term "slacker nurse," appeared. The growing thought was a nurse should support the war effort or support the public health effort: especially in the influenza epidemic. Private nursing, a nurse hiring exclusively to a family and not serving the public or the military, began looking as a spineless easy way out. The head of a New York nurses' training school said:

> In the time of war it is a disgrace for a trained nurse to be employed in a private family in the capacity of companion or to look after healthy children…Strong able-bodied women…should be working in hospitals or serving their country, I wish it could be made impossible for private nurses to get work.[446]

Jean Kynoch, a registered nurse wrote from Fort Harrison, Indiana:

> Don't be a slacker [nurse]. Do not the nurses realize that if they do not come in now they will spend the rest of their lives offering apologies and excuses for not serving the most ideal county in the world—the U.S.A.? I shall not envy the private duty nurse, and I do not envy her now…I feel as the public does about the slacker nurse, and sincerely hope it will not be influenced to condemn the whole nursing body because a few lack common sense, and the greatest of all, do not realize where their duty lies.[447]

The American Journal of Nursing in its January 1918 edition editorialized about "Are We Slackers." The editorial argued women nurses were not entering ARC service and war service because the nurses' families didn't want them to. The Journal said if women are old enough to be on their own and earning a wage, then they are old enough to decide for themselves about where to serve. The Journal summarized its position in saying: "Do not let it go down in history that when the young men of our country were called into service in defense of the democracy of the world, the nurses held back, because of financial reasons or because they shrink from the hardships of war service."

America needed more nurses, and the subject of enrolling black or "colored" nurses came to the ARC. As early as December 5, 1911, at the meeting of the National Committee on ARC Nursing Service, held at the Continental Hall of the Daughters of the American Revolution, a motion was made and carried not to enroll "colored nurses" in the ANC. "…owing to the impossibility of securing proper quarters for them [black nurses], it has never been the policy of the Surgeon General's office to consider the appointment of colored nurses."[448]

Jane Delano originally considered the idea of enrolling black nurses. A black nurses' unit, the Lincoln Base Hospital unit, New York City, was formed. Within a year of the hospital's activation, it was dissolved apparently without explanation. Delano recommended black nurses be sent to Camp Dodge, Iowa, and care for black soldiers arriving there. The surgeon general's official reason for not enrolling black nurses was the Army didn't have resources for building separate quarters, mess halls, wards, etc., for black nurses. In spite of the immediate need for trained and graduate nurses, and the demonstrated skill, expertise, and patriotic service of America's black nurses, especially during the influenza epidemic, the Army and the ARC were reluctant to fully cross the racial barrier line.[449]

The racial barrier line did not stop American Indian women from serving as war nurses. Fourteen were previously known to have served as nurses in the World War I ANC. Two of the fourteen were known to have served overseas.[450] [451] One of the fourteen was from Montana. Regina McIntyre-Early was born near Missoula, Montana, April 14, 1895. Her mother was Alphonsine Nordgren: an enrolled member of the Confederated Salish-Kootenai Tribes. McIntyre-Early's father, Hugh McIntyre, was Canadian. McIntyre-Early attended the Sisters of Charity School at St. Ignatius Mission, Montana, and also the Holy Names Academy at Spokane, Washington. She graduated from the

Sisters of Mercy Hospital, nursing school, Kalispell, Montana, in 1917. On February 5, 1918, McIntyre-Early entered the ANC, and the Army assigned her to Fort Riley, Kansas. In September 1918 the Army sent her overseas where she served in three separate base hospitals in France until July 20, 1919. After her war service she stayed in New York City and married Joseph C. Early in November 1919. She was a handsome young woman with a pleasant smile.[452] McIntyre-Early survived war, but died of pneumonia in New York City, January 29, 1923. McIntyre-Early's family returned her to her ancestral homeland in Montana. She is buried next to her father in Polson, Montana.

Graduate nurses, or registered nurses, were professional women with credentials, but their military pay didn't reflect that. The military would pay nurses fifty dollars per month, or if the nurse served overseas, sixty dollars per month. In 1917 this put the military nurses on the same pay scale as a senior sergeant.[453] If the nurse worked for the state of Montana at detention hospitals, the nurse would earn one hundred dollars per month. If the nurse worked at an emergency hospital in Montana, she would earn five dollars a day.[454]

Informal wage and price controls for nursing in Montana began. Margaret Hughes wanted Montanans to know an appropriate pay scale for ARC nurses. Hughes recommended for graduate nurses, one dollar for the first hour and fifty cents for each additional hour. For undergraduate nurses and nurse's aides, fifty cents for the first hour and twenty-five cents for each additional hour. Hughes said volunteer nursing service would be provided for families unable to pay. The fixed fees would be turned into a general nurses' fund and the nurses paid at a monthly rate established by the ARC.[455]

The Army and Navy nurses received the same pay regardless of hours worked. They didn't punch a time clock. They didn't get paid by the patient, or paid by untold miles they traveled by car, horse, train, or walked, to care for sick in Montana. They certainly didn't go overseas in war for a paltry ten dollars extra per month. Regardless of where the military stationed these women in America, where they cared for tens of thousands of American soldiers in the many basic training camps, and earning less money than at home, the nurses began to think, talk, and write about "going across."

The Great Falls Six

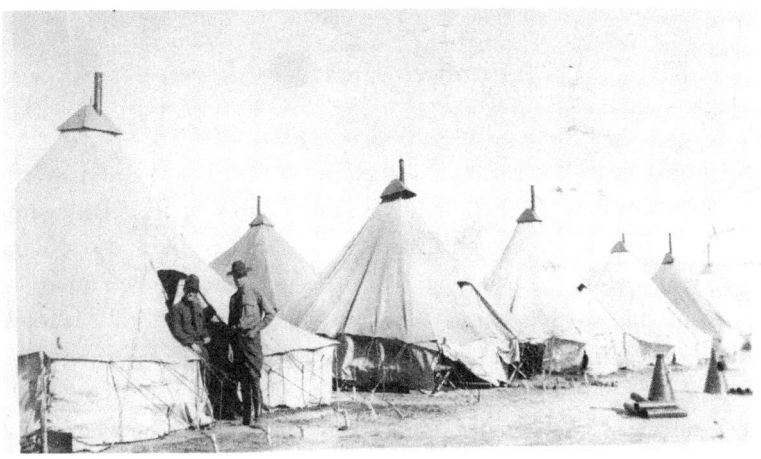

Recruit tents, Fort Riley, Kansas.
Courtesy James Benbow.

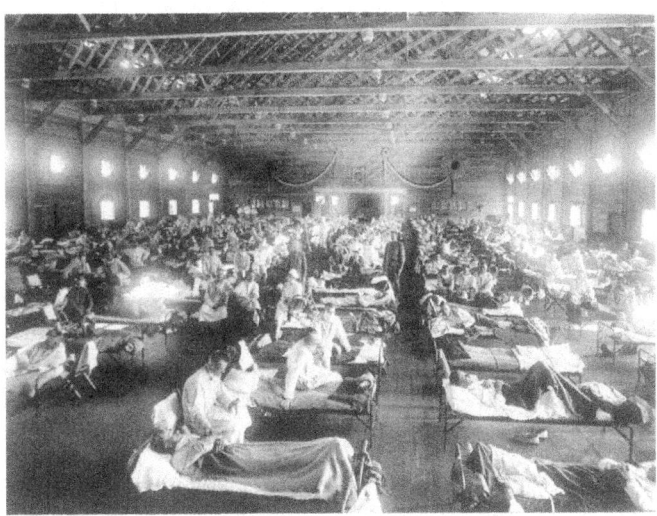

WWI Camp Funston, KS, influenza ward
Courtesy National Archives and Records Administration

Chapter 10
GOING ACROSS

"The only cowards were...."

NURSE LUCY WALTERS SCREAMED. THE SHIP'S DECK WAS LISTING and she was desperately grasping at anything to keep from falling into the icy waters of the North Atlantic. She could swim, and in Kansas City years before she had gone into the water to rescue two drowning women. The North Atlantic Ocean was different and deadly. It wasn't a small river in Kansas City, and the enemy was a German submarine: a submarine with one purpose, blow ships from the water with deadly torpedoes and accurate deck guns. This June day, 1918, the German submarine's captain and crew on the high seas were handsomely earning their pay.

As late as November 1915, seventy-eight-year-old Navy admiral Thomas Dewey, the "Hero of Manila Bay," wrote: "The submarine is not an instrument fitted to dominate naval warfare...the battleship is still the principal reliance of navies, as it has been in the past."[456] The myopic Dewey was blind to coming reality. After World War I ended, a new reality existed for the Navy and America. Secretary of the Navy Josephus Daniels, in his annual report to the president for fiscal year 1919, began looking beyond conservative and perhaps biased naval thought of centuries. Naval battle tactics historically were massing of ships and meeting the enemy head-on in attack formation. Daniels finally and reluctantly opened the door to new ideas and vision. He gave the submarine credit. Daniels wrote: "...the submarine (an American invention) was the stiletto [knife] of the sea...which became the most destructive agency of maritime warfare the world had ever dreamed."

Navies of the world for centuries concluded the larger the ship and heavier the gun meant control of the seas. Large warships became more a symbol of national pride and power. These coal-burning warships, sometimes more a showpiece than a versatile and economically sustainable weapon of war, were expensive to build, man, and operate. These massive and powerful warships pulled national resources needed to support land forces. The ships required extensive support bases throughout the world with larger port infrastructures providing coal, provisions, and crew support. Refueling a ship with tons of coal could take between three to eight days depending on laborers involved.[457] In early twentieth century, large warships with heavy caliber armaments and steam turbine propulsion were called "dreadnoughts": the forerunner of modern battleships. Countries built these ships for one purpose—sink other ships. Many dreadnoughts and battlecruisers reached speeds of twenty-five knots [twenty-nine miles per hour]. Sustaining these speeds required herculaneum effort from the ship's "black gang": the coal stokers and firemen covered in coal dust deep within the bowels of the ship.

Germany didn't need large dreadnaughts for national survival. Unlike England, Germany wasn't an island nation depending on unencumbered sailing on the high seas for food, commerce, and protection. Without its navy, England was instantly vulnerable: especially with trade and commerce.[458] In early twentieth century England imported two-thirds of its food.[459] From 1905 to 1917 Great Britain built sixty-two warships in sixteen classes of dreadnoughts and battlecruisers. In that same time Germany built eight battlecruisers.[460] In World War I German and English dreadnoughts fought a single sea battle: The Battle of Jutland off Denmark's west coast from May 31 to June 1, 1916. With loss of ships and men, both sides claimed a pyrrhic victory. England had far more warships than Germany. With fewer warships, Germany knew it would lose a prolonged naval surface ocean war against England. Germany looked to other means for deadly hit-and-run naval tactics. If Germany couldn't defeat England on the seas, then Germany would go under the seas. The German unterseeboot [underwater boat] or U-boat began.

When World War I began, Germany had about fifty U-boats of various types. Maintenance and repairs meant many weren't seaworthy. In September 1914 a U-boat attacked and sank three much older British warships.[461] U-boats weren't heavily armored; well-aimed gunfire could sink or disable U-boats. U-boats faced great odds attacking British war ships. Attacking unarmed and slower Allied merchant ships proved a more effective [and survivable] means of warfare on the high seas. On February 8, 1915, Germany declared the seas around Great Britain a war zone. The German navy said it would attack any Allied or neutral country merchant ships in these waters. The *New York Times*, May 1, 1915, published the German embassy warning: "Travelers intending to embark on the Atlantic voyage are reminded that a state of war exists between Germany and her allies and Great Britain and her allies... [and] vessels flying the flag of Great Britain, or any of her allies are liable to destruction...and that travelers sailing in the war zone on ships of Great Britain or her allies do so at their own risk."

Days after publishing the warning, on May 7, 1915, a German U-boat torpedoed the British passenger ship *Lusitania*.[462] The American press said the sinking was murder on the high seas; Germany didn't think so. Germany said the *Lusitania* was a British flagged ship [it was] and carrying war materiel [it was]. The *Lusitania's* full cargo manifest of war materiel and small arms munitions would not be publicly released until 1965.[463] In early months of World War I, fewer than five U-boats were available to patrol the entrances to the Irish Sea where the U-boats did most damage.[464] In April 1917 U.S. Navy rear admiral William S. Sims met with the British admiralty in England for talks on the naval situation facing both countries. The British situation stunned Sims. Britain's First Sea Lord, Admiral Sir John Jellicoe, revealed a closely guarded secret: German U-boats had sunk over 800 Allied ships while losing ten submarines. Jellicoe emphatically said Britain could not sustain its sea losses and could not hold much longer.[465]

By September 1915, bowing to international pressure and condemnation for "murder on the high seas," Germany limited its U-boat warfare to blockading of shipments to belligerent nations. If a nation declared a naval blockade, that nation through right-of-search, could stop ships bound for an enemy harbor and inspect the ship's cargo for contraband. If military specific contraband supporting only military use was found, the blockading nation could seize the contraband or destroy it. Food could not be seized.[466] All this had too many rules. German naval command disagreed with this new limitation policy and argued to the Germany government that if a ship was an enemy flagged vessel, then disregard the limited policy and sink the ship. The German navy's argument swayed the Kaiser. The German Reichstag announcing unrestricted submarine warfare would begin February 1, 1917.[467] Unrestricted submarine warfare meant Germany would not stop and search ships; it would sink them—and it did. German U-boats sunk ten Allied ships on February 1.[468]

When America entered the war, civil and military leaders understood they needed troop transports to carry over one million men to France. Naval fighting ships are not built or outfitted as transport ships, civilian ocean liners are. Early in the war the Army chartered passenger ships directly from the ships' owners. The United States Shipping Board, originally created in peacetime for regulating shipping and promoting the American merchant marine, now faced war. On June 15, 1917, Congress gave the Shipping Board extended war powers with authority for acquisition and operations of sea vessels and regulation of shipping and shipbuilding. The Shipping Board, through its Emergency Fleet Corporation, could build ships, charter ships, and commandeer foreign vessels.[469]

By September 1, 1917, the Shipping Board seized ninety-nine German ships: eighty-seven were seaworthy. Of the ninety-nine German ships, the U.S. government seized the passenger liner, *Vaterland*, and renamed it SS *Leviathan*. The *Leviathan* was the largest ocean liner of its day and could carry thousands of troops.[470] Other interred German ships became American vessels: the *Kaiser Wilhelm II* was renamed *Agamemnon*; the *Hamburg* renamed *Powhatan*; the *Rhine* became *Susquehanna*.[471] Many times American troops and nurses sailed on British and French flagged ships. Soon the blood of thousands of Americans would stain red French land and rivers and would keep Britain from the hands of the Germans. America held the hand of fate for France and Britain. In spite of this, America had to pay these countries almost $100 per soldier, per person, per nurse, for these Americans to sail on French or British flagged ships, as if the soldiers and nurses were tourists on a pleasure cruise.[472]

An American ship, built with American steel, American sweat, and in an American shipyard in Philadelphia, would hold many records for transporting troops. The SS *Great Northern* was built in 1914 as a joint venture with, among other companies, James J. Hill's Great Northern Railway.[473] In 1917 the Navy acquired the ship through the United States Shipping Board. The SS *Great Northern* served as a troop transport ship beginning 1917. The ship bears the following records: more men per day transported than any other ship; fastest round trip from New York to Brest, France, [fourteen days, three and one-half hours] and most economical run, taking on no water or oil on the other side.[474]

Facing tremendous shipping losses, Sims recommended the British and Allies begin a convoy system for ships crossing the Atlantic. A fleet of merchant ships and troop ships, sailing in formation guarded by destroyers and other war ships for protection, had better chances of survival against submarines. The British dismissed the idea outright. Their view was a convoy system needed many escort ships for guards, ships Great Britain could ill-afford to divert.[475] Beginning June 1917, with hastily assembled cruisers, transports, and armed merchant vessels, the first transatlantic convoy sailed from America to France.[476] With destroyers sent to Europe for escort duty, convoys could sail at five to seven day intervals depending on convoy speed.[477] The convoy theory began working, losses due to submarine attacks dropped.[478] U-boats never sunk an eastbound transport ship carrying soldiers, doctors, or Montana nurses.[479]

Montana state senator James M. Burlingame, from Great Falls, had a bit of a little boy fun streak in him. On January 17, 1917, Burlingame was in Helena on state business. C. D. Greenfield, Montana's commissioner of agriculture and publicity, was having a party at Greenfield's house on Spruce Street [present Holter Street] in Helena. Burlingame attended. Burlingame had long supported improving Montana's nursing standards, and successfully introduced legislation in Montana in 1911 to set nursing standards in law. Six years later he was going to need a nurse and soon.

During a break in Greenfield's party, several of the women attending suggested free-wheeling down Spruce Street on a child's street coaster. Burlingame offered to act as the coaster's pilot. Five adults crowded on the coaster, they pushed off and headed east down the street northwest of the Montana state capitol building. Gathering speed down the east-sloping Spruce Street, Burlingame and the women were going too fast make a turn at the bottom of the hill. Burlingame tried steering the coaster from impending doom, but failed. Burlingame and the others crashed into a stone wall in front of the Anton M. Holter residence: petticoats and coattails a 'flying. Burlingame flew over Holter's stone retaining wall and landed hard: breaking Burlingame's leg. The women on board Burlingame's out-of-control frolicking flying carpet were mostly uninjured. While Burlingame's luck in driving gave out, he was fortunate to have on board that day, Miss Gertrude Sloane, nurse. She sprained her ankle in the crash but tended the injured. Burlingame was rushed to a local downtown medical office. His leg was set and he would spend the next two weeks in Helena's Placer Hotel recuperating.[480]

Gertrude Sloane was born September 2, 1878, in Camp Missoula, Montana, to John L. and Lizzie [Mansfield] Sloane. The Army, bowing to local citizen's insistence the Army protect them apparently from Indians, built the camp in 1877. The fort never built a perimeter log enclosure around the camp. People easily came and went. Born March 27, 1847, in New York City, John Sloan had served in the Union Army of the American Civil War with the colorful Fifth New York veteran volunteers, Duryea Zouaves. In August 1864, during the fierce battle of Weldon Railroad south of Richmond, Virginia, enemy fire wounded Sloane four times in one day. Promoted to rank of lieutenant, Sloane decided to go west and seek his fortune. He served with the Second California Volunteer Cavalry until 1866 when he was mustered out of the Army. In 1871 he and Lizzie married in Wichita, Kansas. She bore him seven children. In 1877 the Sloanes moved to Missoula, Montana. Sloane became a judge. A highly respected jurist, citizen, community leader, husband and father, Sloane held many civic and governmental positions. He died in Seattle in 1914 and was buried in Missoula.[481]

Sloane's daughter, Gertrude, grew to womanhood in Missoula. In 1909 she graduated from St. Luke's hospital nursing school, St. Louis. Gertrude worked as a surgical nurse in St. Paul, Minnesota, until 1913 when she returned to Missoula to care for her ailing father. In Missoula she gained a reputation as an efficient and well-respected nurse. In 1913 she was elected president of the Montana State Association of Graduate and Registered Nurses.[482] After World War I began, Gertrude became chairman of the Missoula Women's Navy League.

Sloane left no record of her decision to join the ARC nursing service and becoming a nurse in the ANC. By September 1917 Sloane had enrolled in both, and decided to go to France and help the war effort. She departed Missoula, Wednesday, September 26, 1917, and traveled east to New York City, her father's home town, to begin the transatlantic journey to war.[483] Sloane sailed on the RMS *Baltic* with a hospital contingent of twenty-one doctors and sixty-five nurses. Launched in 1903 by Harland and Wolff in Belfast, the *Baltic* was the world's largest ship until 1905.[484]

Sloane would write letters of her 14-day voyage going across, but her family in Missoula wouldn't get her letter for weeks. To her sister, Mrs. Tyler B. Thompson, Missoula, Sloane wrote not as someone going to war, but as a tourist on a new adventure:

> October 17 [1917], We are way out at sea and really enjoying the trip. Strange to say I have only been sick one day, but we have had a wonderfully smooth trip. When I tell you we have 500 men on board and 19 women, you know we are having much attention...
>
> We have lifeboat drill every day and run around all the time with our "preserves" as we call them. In our convoy are nine ships, three tanks [sic], three armored cruisers, two transports, and our line, which is the flagship. Our captain is a retired admiral of the British navy and would make a wonderful Santa Claus.
>
> Yesterday morning we had dense fog and two ships [were lost to visual contact]. It all cleared this morning we all got together again and are a happy family once more. On one of the ships, the *Megantic*, there are over 5,000 Chinese coolies being taken over to the trenches. The scope of the war is tremendous...
>
> We have French [language] lessons each day...and various boat drills.[485]

As the RMS *Baltic* neared the Irish coast the U-boat menace increased. Sloane wrote:

> Thursday. Today at noon we were ordered to put on life belts and wear them the rest of the trip...We carry our life belts everywhere we would go and sleep with them at night. At night we slept in heavy woolens and had our things ready to put on in a moment's notice. We said we were preparing to go subbing, but it was a terrible strain.
>
> ....Our convoy [disperses] Saturday and we then pick up...destroyers [for submarine escort].[486]

Not fully realizing the depravities of war she would soon face, Sloan was critical of the *Baltic*'s amenities while sailing the North Atlantic. She wrote: "Some boat [this is]. Chocolate candy is $1.75 per pound."

Sloane arrived safely in Liverpool in October 1917. By year's end 1917, three Montana nurses, Gertrude Sloan, Clara Brunelle, and Alice

Ralston, would be in France. America would soon need more nurses "over there," and desperately. More nurses wouldn't come for months.

On June 11/12, 1918, seventeen ocean vessels began marshalling in lower New York Bay off Staten Island. The ships were to sail in convoy across submarine infested waters, then through the Irish Sea to Liverpool, England. Two ocean liners, the SS *Missanabie*, and the SS *Megantic*, would be taking on passengers: either at Hoboken, New Jersey, across from New York City or from the piers on the east side of the Hudson River at New York City. The *Megantic* wouldn't be carrying thousands of Chinese coolies this time. Waiting for the tide, the two ships prepared to sail with the convoy.

The *Missanabie*, built 1914 and operated by Canadian Pacific Ocean Lines, and *Megantic* built 1908 and operated by White Star Line, were British flagged passenger vessels. Each ship carried one hundred nurses of the ANC and about one hundred doctors, corpsmen, and medical troops destined for the AEF. On the *Missanabie* four Montana nurses waited with their thoughts: Effie Louise Fowler, from Great Falls; Harriet Marie O'Day, from Billings; Elizabeth "Sandy" Sandelius, from Cokedale; and Harriet Vineyard, from Butte. On the *Megantic* were Virginia Flanagan, from Great Falls; Grace Gibson, from Worden; and Lucy Walters, from Glasgow.[487]

The 17-ship convoy sailed at night, portholes closed and covered, running lights off. No cigarette smoking allowed on deck as lit matches create light visible for miles on clear nights. Three short blasts on the ship's horn meant an emergency, all hands on deck and don't stop for anything.[488] The slowest ship determined sailing speed. A destroyer, one or two miles in front, led the convoy. Other destroyers circled. The ships sailed in offset parallel rows about five hundred yards apart.

At night with no running lights and no modern radar, ships' crews had to carefully handle the ships to avoid collision. Lookouts posted fore and aft.[489] Keep things quiet, no laughter, shouting, whistling or banging of metal. The only sound was propellers slashing the water and the beating of anxious hearts. Meeting the convoy, the passenger liner *Carpathia* of the British Cunard Line, took its place in the sailing formation. The *Carpathia* had earned a reputation in sailing history six years before when it rescued survivors of the sinking of the *Titanic*. The convoy cleared the lower New York Bay sailing past Montauk on Long Island, then past Nantucket Island, across the Georges Bank, past

Nova Scotia and St. John's, Newfoundland, and out to the open North Atlantic. In the far distance off the Irish coast, a U-boat, its captain and crew, waited patiently: torpedoes at the ready.

Lucy Walters and Grace Gibson had been at Camp Lewis, Washington, for about six months. They had arrived at Camp Lewis in November 1917 and began caring for the thousands of basic training troops at the camp hospital. The hospital never had enough nurses, and their heavy workload never slowed. When Walters and Gibson enrolled in the ARC, they accepted assignment category 1: meaning they would go where the need was greatest. By spring 1918 the need was in France. In May 1918 the Army told Walters and Gibson they were going to France. On May 18, 1918, Walters and Gibson boarded the train, probably in Tacoma or Seattle, and headed east twenty-five hundred miles to the nurses' embarkation station in New York City. The shortest and fasted route from the Pacific Northwest to points east would be the Great Northern Railway's Oriental Limited. When troops rode the train, federal government wartime rules required them to take the shortest route to the troops' destination.[490] The same train Walters rode west to Camp Lewis would probably be taking her and Gibson east.

The eastbound Oriental crossed Washington to Spokane, then across northern Idaho and into the large valley around Kalispell, Montana. East of Kalispell the Oriental crossed Marias Pass. In May snow would still cover the pass. Heading east coming off the Continental Divide, the Oriental picked up speed east of Shelby, Montana. Refueling at Havre with a full load of water and coal, the Oriental sped east to Malta and Glasgow.

The Oriental stopped at Glasgow, but not for long. What Walters thought while the train stopped at Glasgow [most likely she and Gibson were on the train] is lost to history. Speculation does no service. That day at the Glasgow train station, when the eastbound Oriental pulled in briefly, a small but profound sentence in the chronology of Montana history was lost forever when a war nurse, looking out the train window at the adopted home she knew, kept it all in her heart. Walters and Gibson continued east to Minneapolis-St. Paul, where they changed trains to Chicago. At Chicago they changed trains again and continued east. How long their journey took, and what their thoughts were looking through the train windows at an America they never saw before, are lost to history.

Virginia Flanagan was enjoying her nursing assignment at Letterman Army Hospital, San Francisco, California. Flanagan had enrolled in the ANC in June 1918, and her six months of stateside duty were over in December. On December 13 the Army reassigned Flanagan to Camp Kearney, California: near San Diego. She was to leave the next day. Flanagan wrote: "I had no time to say good-bye to all the dear places we had grown so fond of, and which had come to seem almost like a part of our possessions." Flanagan faced increased challenges at Kearney, she wrote:

> Frolli [Agnes Frolli, San Francisco, California] and I were so cold and homesick, we put out beds together, and that [is] how they stayed during out stay at Kearney…We were very discouraged with the present ward arrangement…Our trunks did not arrive, so three of us could not go on duty for two days. I was glad as I was very tired as well as discouraged and glad to have some time to get adjusted to the change. When our things arrived, I was assigned to [the] surgical ward, and given charge of this ward. There are 50 beds in each ward…except some things are quite primitive, such as homemade desks, no trays, spreads, or curtains, and often no linen.

On May 16, 1918, Flanagan transferred again. She wrote:

> …When I returned [to the nurses' quarters] I heard quite a commotion, much talking, and the place was all lit up. When I went into the room…someone thrust a glass into my hand, at the same time telling me that the word had come that some of the nurses were to be sent overseas. But, I was told I was not one of the lucky ones [going overseas]. I was awfully excited and drank down the contents of the glass without even knowing it was some very good wine someone had smuggled in…I could not sleep that night thinking about being left behind as I was one

of the first to come in the service [from Montana]. My best friend's [Frolli] name was among those to go. I was in the office of my ward the next morning when I was told that my name was on the list [to go overseas]...O! [*sic*] the joy and sorrow of it, I did want to go, but hated to leave the dear old place, and most of all my patients.

Flanagan apparently wanted to "see the elephant." She wrote: "But to go overseas was the height of my dreams, so I did want to go." Flanagan and the other nurses at Camp Kearney slated to go overseas quickly packed. For operational security the Army told the nurses not to talk about their destination and assignment. The Camp Kearney nurses and doctors held a dinner for the departing nurses the night before Flanagan and the others departed. On May 17, 1918, Flanagan and three others set out from San Diego by train for New York City. Flanagan would travel the farthest of any Montana nurse: San Diego to New York City. Of her traveling companions, Flanagan wrote:

> ...Very well pleased with our small party of four; Miss Brake, tall dark, and distinguished looking; Mrs. Brinkerhoff, pretty and very stylish, and she had a beautiful voice; Miss Frolli who had beautiful red hair, and hails from sunny California, and yours truly, Miss Montana, whom you know for better and for worse.

Flanagan and the others needed five days to reach New York City. They traveled through Chicago and Detroit. She wrote of missing connections in Chicago but seeing Niagara Falls in the early morning light. Flanagan and the others arrived in New York City, May 22, 1918. She wrote: "[We]...were four tired soldiers. Had we known that our real hard work was just beginning, we might have been pretty discouraged, but that was to come, and only our fervent duty to our country kept out spirits from lagging."[491]

At Fort Riley, Kansas, May 18, 1918, Effie Louise Fowler, Harriet Marie O'Day, Elizabeth "Sandy" Sandelius, and Harriet Vineyard, received orders to proceed to New York City and prepare to go across.

Going Across 151

Their average age was twenty-seven: Fowler the oldest, age 28; Sandelius, the youngest, age 25. They didn't write their thoughts, emotions, fears, excitement, or anxieties when they received notification to go. After six months at crowded, improvised, and many times diseased Fort Riley/Camp Funston, perhaps the women welcomed a change: good, bad, or indifferent. They were going to France, the land of distant romance; to Paris, the city of lights: an adventure of a lifetime. For "Sandy" and Harriet, however, France would not be the land of romance, France would turn unimaginably cruel.

Across America, Montana's nurses slated to go overseas, began the steady and purposeful railroad march to New York City. From Camp Lewis, Camp Kearney, Fort Riley, Camp Dodge, and others scattered across America, Montana nurses converged on the eastern seaboard, mostly at New York City, and ready themselves to "go across." In the beginning of the war this wasn't easy. America's rails weren't supporting the war effort, and change was needed.

America's government has never solely owned, or in peacetime solely operated, the railroads operating within its borders. At the beginning of World War I almost 200 major private railroad companies and corporations existed in America. These railroad businesses employed 1.7 million workers operating over 200,000 miles of track.[492] America's businesses, economy, and war effort, could not operate without railroads. These many railroad companies and corporations wielded political power over the Interstate Commerce Commission. Railroad owners weren't investing in better tracks, rolling stock, and other improvements in the national rail system. Railroad strikes occurred, many railroads went bankrupt. National railroads were not functioning as an efficient network to support war.[493]

In 1916 the Army Appropriations Act gave the President authority to take control of [but not nationalize] America's railroads in war. To meet the war effort immediately after America entered the war, heads of the nation's railroads met in Washington D.C. They planned to coordinate national railroad support. Part of the effort was coordinating and sharing rail assets. However, the overall poor condition of America's rail infrastructure and operations could not be quickly overcome. President Wilson needed immediate results, and in December 1917 Congress passed legislation giving Wilson operational control over America's railroads. Railroad ownership remained in private hands, but with the passage of the Federal Control Act of March 1918, the federal government controlled the operation of the railroads through the United States Railroad Administration [USRA]. To keep the nation's railroads solvent, the federal government would pay rent to the railroads based on the railroads' net income for the past three years. With the Federal Control Act the federal government bypassed the Interstate Commerce Commission, state regulatory bodies, and anti-trust laws.

The federal government could also set rail transport priorities. Part of the government rail objectives was setting rail transportation via the shortest routes regardless of who owned the rails. Because of this, troops [or nurses] did not have to ride trains in circuitous routes to their destinations. Government freight and troop shipments had the right-of-way on America's railroads.[494] The USRA ensured wartime rules and operations did not leave towns without rail service, and transcontinental routes, such as the Oriental Limited, were kept operational.[495]

The USRA achieved what it was supposed to do in wartime. It wasn't a perfect solution, especially with wages for railroad workers, but overall railroad support improved for the war effort while providing for the civilian population. The USRA would continue to 1920 when its legislative authority ended.[496]

Trains took the nurses east. Most likely the nurses arrived at New York City's Grand Central Station or Penn Station: both in midtown Manhattan. These elegant and ornate transportation palaces paled the small rail structures along Montana's vast routes on the high line or along the Yellowstone River in southern Montana. Instead of looking upward to the sky, nurses looked upward to the high arched ceilings crowned with glass panes and wrought iron supports. A sight in New York City it must have been.

In June 1917 the Army had established a nurses' mobilization station on Ellis Island in New York harbor. Since 1914 Ellis Island [actually three islands connected with foot bridges] had three large buildings used as immigrant hospitals. The administration offices were on island number one. The hospital was on island number three. Ellis Island had a ferry boat dock for the nurses to get to shore.[497] When the number of immigrant arrivals declined, the U.S. Immigration Department turned over Ellis Island to the Army. The Army designated

Going Across   153

a chief nurse to manage Ellis Island and began work to transform the buildings into a receiving station for nurses heading to France. Ellis Island originally handled all ARC base hospitals heading overseas. The nurses of one hospital, Base Hospital 28 [BH 28] from Kansas City, arrived in New York and prepared to go overseas. The nurses were scheduled to sail on the *Megantic* on or about Jun 11/12 with the hospital's doctors and men. However, scheduling got fouled and the nurses had to wait for another ship. The *Mauretania* would sail about two weeks later. One BH 28 nurse had to adjust quickly; history would record this nurse from Missoula, Montana, as capable and efficient.

Eula Bernice Butzerin was born July 22, 1891, in Lacrosse, Wisconsin, to Albert J. and Margaret Butzerin.[498] [499] Albert and Margaret had four children: Roy, Arthur, Anna Hazel ["Hazel"], and Eula.[500] In 1902 Albert moved his family to Missoula. A railroad engineer for the Northern Pacific railroad, in 1911 voters elected him for one term as Montana state senator.[501] In 1913 Eula's mother, Margaret, was a precinct chair of the Women's Equal Suffrage League in Missoula.[502] A train wreck killed Albert, January 26, 1918, near St. Regis, Montana. His family buried him in Missoula.[503]

Educated in Missoula, Eula graduated with honors from Missoula High School, class of 1909.[504] She enrolled in the University of Montana in 1910.[505] In 1911 she left the university and began nursing training at St. Patrick's hospital, Missoula. She finished her degree at Presbyterian Hospital School of Nursing in Chicago.[506] [507] By 1918 she was teaching home nursing in the domestic sciences part of Kansas State Agricultural College [present Kansas State University], Manhattan, Kansas. Eula was also attached to the Christian Church unit of the American Red Cross, Kansas City, Missouri.[508] Eula never married.

In early 1918 the Kansas City Red Cross Nurses Association selected Eula and nine other nurses to form Kansas City Nurses Unit number 1. These ten nurses readied for war service with Eula as chief nurse.[509] When WWI began, BH 28 formed in Kansas City with staff from the Christian Church hospital.[510] This large hospital [after WWI a veterans hospital] opened 1916. On May 28, 1918, Kansas State Agricultural College gave Eula a leave of absence to join BH 28 as the hospital readied to depart for France.[511] In June 1918, BH 28, with fifty officers, 150 enlisted men, and 150 nurses, readied to depart for France on the *Megantic*. Eula's two brothers, Roy and Arthur, both graduates of Missoula high school, enlisted together in the Army at Camp George Wright; Spokane, Washington, May 18, 1917. Arthur served in the infantry, Roy in the engineers. In May 1918 Arthur accepted a commission as an officer and served in Vladivostok, Siberia. Roy would stay in the engineers and serve in France.[512] On June 30, 1918, the *Mauretania*, with Eula Butzerin and about 150 nurses of BH 28, sailed to Liverpool, England, from New York City.[513]

As the nurses arrived at New York City train stations, hospital corpsmen detailed to Ellis Island, met the nurses and brought them to Ellis Island. Men with Army trucks gathered the nurses' baggage and brought the baggage to the Island by boat. In single file the nurses processed through the arriving station at Ellis showing their papers and documents. Daily at 9:00 a.m. Ellis Island had roll call for nurses; shore leave would be granted for the nurses if they hadn't received orders to sail. On shore at Hoboken, New Jersey, the nurses received identity cards and passports. As the nurses sat before large cameras with glaring lights, companions tried getting the nurse to smile, laugh, and look less-than serious. Developing the photograph took seven minutes.[514]

For passports a problem came when nurses arrived with no birth certificates, or documentation as to where and when they were born. By 1918 the government no longer required passports for Army and Navy nurses. In lieu of passports, the War Department issued War Department identifications called "Certificates of Identity."[515] These papers had a photograph and a fingerprint of the nurse's right index finger. The Army then stamped and issued the nurse a round circular metal disk commonly called a "dog tag." Nurses hung the 1¼ inch diameter disk around their neck like an unadorned necklace. The number stamped in the metal disk was the nurse's ARC registration number.[516]

With world war beginning in 1914, the U.S. government began the Bureau of War Risk Insurance. This comprehensive legislation included granting insurance to military members, men and women. On October 6, 1917, Congress expanded the law by creating the Division of Military and Naval Insurance.[517] Terms of insurance applied to men and women: including the Army and Navy nurse corps. The legislation specifically named female nurses as being eligible for the insurance. The government had massive challenges with processing insurance applications for almost two million Army and 200,000 Navy personnel. The government created War Risk offices in America and overseas to ensure military personnel had opportunities to complete insurance paperwork.[518]

The government issued insurance for amounts from $1,000 to $10,000 per person. The government deducted premiums from the insured person's monthly pay. Monthly premiums ranged from $5.75 for a $1,000 policy to a maximum of $57.50 for a $10,000 policy. The policy included death or disability and would be granted without a medical examination. If the military person qualified in death or disability, the government paid the beneficiary 240 monthly installment payments for the amount of the insurance policy. The beneficiary had to be an immediate family member or the insured herself. If the insured person died, the government paid the beneficiary the balance of the policy. The policy included reasonable governmental medical, surgical, and hospital services for those military disabled in the line-of-duty. The law also contemplated future legislation for re-education and vocational training for disabled military. Within five years after the war ended, the insured could convert the insurance to a peacetime policy with premiums adjusted for age.[519] When processing into Ellis Island or later in other mobilization offices, nurses were briefed on the insurance and had to decide if they wanted the insurance and how much.

More nurses arriving at Ellis Island overwhelmed the Island's ability to process and house the nurses. In December 1917 Mrs. Genevieve Walsh, Supreme Regent of the [Catholic] Daughters of Isabella, offered the [old] Colony Club building in New York City as a mobilization station. The Colony Club was a women-only private club at 120 Madison Avenue. The club had moved to a new building in 1916.[520] The Army accepted Walsh's offer as the old building could house 120 nurses. The delay in moving the nurses from Ellis Island, or anywhere on the eastern seaboard, was due to shipping priorities. Troops and equipment to France had priority; nurses went when ships had room.[521]

In late spring 1918 the War Department converted Ellis Island into a hospital. The nurses' embarkation station had to relocate. The War Department contracted to the Knott chain of hotels in New York City for ten hotels. The War Department selected these hotels due to their easy access to steamship piers on Manhattan's west side. Some hotels had already been designated as replacement stations.[522] These hotels then became the Army and nurses' mobilization stations. [David H. Knott owned the hotels, he would later run for sheriff of New York City, and be a bank president.][523] Mary C. Jorgensen was chief nurse of the New York mobilization station. She wrote: "Soon the daily reports showed nearly one thousand nurses housed in twenty different hotels, stretching from Washington Square to Seventy-Second Street. There, in America's largest city, it was no easy task to keep an eye on them [nurses] all..."[524]

In May 1918 many Montana nurses were traveling by train to New York City and preparing to sail to France. Arriving in New York City these nurses found themselves in a massive foul-up. Over 550 nurses going overseas as "casuals," [not going with a unit but as individual replacements], began arriving at the same time. Nobody in New York City knew these 550 nurses were coming. Jorgensen wrote: "They seemed to be in a chaotic state of disorganization." Jorgensen began assembling these 550 nurses in a local armory and sorting the confusion.[525]

Virginian Flanagan wrote of her arrival in New York City:

> ...My first impressions of New York City were formed under the most trying circumstances...it was extremely hot, and wherever we went there were hundreds standing in line waiting to be vaccinated, to get their pay, to have pictures taken, and to be fitted with overseas shoes, clothes, hats, etc. One finally gets the feeling that the Army has no feeling for [people]... since we were being banded like so many cattle.
>
> We were first sent to the Holley Hotel, but there was no room for us, so next we went to the Bristol Hotel, and were most unwelcome there. The four of us were put into a very ugly back room, one on a cot, one had a single bed, and the other two in a double bed. We scarcely had room to walk around the beds, and there was a mysterious bath in the wall with a door that was always swinging open most expectantly and kept us awake. And, to make matters worse, we had to drill for a couple of hours each day in an

entirely different part of the city. We had a very strict although nice [male] captain. If I hadn't been so tired, I could have enjoyed it.

We were in New York about three weeks and were moved from the Bristol [hotel] to the Jensen Hotel, which was in Washington Square…One day, we were sent to Wanamaker's to have our pictures taken for our passports…The passports, by the way, would scare any Hun if he ever sees them…Next, we went to Coward Shoe Company's wholesale for shoes. We were fitted with one pair of black "Cowards," and a pair of gumboots [overboots] also given polish, a polisher brush, and rubber heals…You think the shoes are too big, but they are really wonderful fit by the time you get two or three pair of socks on our scuffers…

And, thus we were shod, hatted, and dressed, and ordered to send home our last personal articles, so from then on, we had no individuality and became a small atom of what was later to be known as the AEF.[526]

Glenna L. Bigelow, nurse, ANC, wrote of the irony of having a Coward brand of shoe: "Is it not rather terrible that the American nurses must go to war with "Coward" imprinted on their soles? But Flanders' mud may transform them and thank goodness, anyway, for paradoxes."[527] [528] In the early days of the war the ARC gave a personalized box to the nurses arriving in New York City. The box had the nurse's uniforms and other items. Chief Nurse, Julia Katherine Stimson, BH 21, St. Louis, wrote:

> It took not much over an hour and a half before each nurse had received all her things and was free to go. Each one was given caps and armbands, a lovely soft cape lined with bright red flannel; a soft dark blue felt hat, with hat pins, a heavy dark brown blanket, a long heavy double-breasted dark blue military coat and a dark blue serge dress. The whole equipment is

excellent and extremely good in quality and fit was fine considering measurements had to be sent [in advance]. There was a box addressed to every single nurse, each one containing a dress and a coat. The dresses are very good looking....The effect of the whole outfit is very shipshape, though a little somber.[529]

Flanagan and the nurses also had to sign a statement reading they did not have cameras.[530] Flanagan and other nurses had time to walk about in New York City, but not far from their mobilization station hotels. Flanagan wrote of attending church services at St. Patrick's cathedral, and having lunch at the Ritz Hotel. She continued with her observations of New York City: "I found the nights in New York stifling, and suggested one night that we go out-of-doors for more air, but found it just as stifling there, not like good old Montana. I'm afraid I couldn't live in New York."[531]

One day in early June, Flanagan and the others received a well-disguised alert. Flanagan wrote when she and the other nurses returned to their hotel rooms a rolled knapsack with a rose attached was on each of their beds. This signaled the nurses they would be sailing soon. On Monday, June 10, 1918, the chief nurse at the Jensen Hotel, took Flanagan and the nurses upstairs, closed the door and told them they would be sailing the next day. The chief nurse told them they were not to tell anyone, or the offending nurse, lacking in operational security, would be left behind. Dora E. Thompson, superintendent of the ANC, had issued instructions to all Army nurses:

> Nurses are...cautioned to avoid giving out any information in regard to dates of sailing to Europe and the names of the boats upon which they expect to sail...Giving this information...jeopardizes the life of every person on the vessel. Letters to friends announcing departure should be left with the chief nurse at the mobilization place, with instructions not to mail them until fully two weeks after the departure of the nurse.[532]

Flanagan wrote:

Going Across

It was a strange feeling knowing that at last we were chosen to go over, after we had waited so long. And, we were a very solemn and subdued group of girls as we descended the stairs the next morning. Saying good-bye to this dear land of ours, and maybe never to return, or to see our loved ones again, was a sobering thought. But this is what we had joined the Army Nurse Corps for, and certainly didn't want to back out.[533]

The nurses could take a small steamer trunk and a suitcase. Experience from others showed the Army nurses what was needed for the duration of the war. Excess baggage was left behind or mailed home.[534]

Flanagan and her "faithful four" friends from military hospitals in California, had to overcome the sudden reality that war mobilization was not a game or a fanciful dance in the grand ballroom of the human experience. Working in crowded military hospitals in America demanded the most able, committed, and strong nurse. But at day's end, the nurse was still in America: the great land of freedom and security. The land where family, friends, and colleagues remained for support. Where mail arrived regularly, packages received relatively undamaged, and at night the only sounds heard were buzzing insects, soft breezes, and distant whistles of steam trains fading into the night. A quick weekend trip to town could get you toilet paper, soap, lotion, maybe a newspaper. You had a roof over your head, a decent bed to sleep in, a porcelain toilet to sit on, and you were dry with clean clothes; showers and baths nearby. In America you weren't facing bullets or bombs. Flashing lights and muted rolling thunder on the horizon meant distant rain storms and nothing else. You get lonely, you hide your tears, but fear hasn't arrived. A fear unlike anything you've felt or imagined. Cultures invent words, but no word exists to tell of the fear of a soldier in battle, or a sailor in the bowels of a ship: a ship taking on water and sinking fast. The only sounds you hear are screams from the deepest depths of a soul in battle torment, and the laughing of a thousand demons welcoming you to hell.

Adhering to orders, Flanagan and the others ate a hurried lunch and walked from the Jensen Hotel. They tried not to show in their faces that one of the most important events in their lives was about to happen. What they felt that moment they kept in their hearts. The chief nurse told all the nurses to break into small groups, don't attract attention, and go by separate routes to pier number 1 on Manhattan's west side. The nurses didn't carry any baggage: a nondescript truck, leaving from the hotel's rear entrance, took the nurses' baggage to the pier.[535] The walk from the Jensen Hotel near New York City's 9-acre Washington Square to the pier along Manhattan's west bank, was less than a mile through midtown Manhattan. How Flanagan and the others walked to Pier 1, purposely fast or nervously slow, is lost to history. You don't want your friends see you shake from fear. That's where courage comes from—not wanting your friends to think you're scared. You're afraid and they are afraid, you see it in their eyes, they see it in yours. You both refuse to shake from fear. Regardless of the pace, the nurses walked to the pier that June day. The only Cowards that afternoon were the shoes they wore, and they resolutely ground that name into the pavement.

At pier 1 the nurses saw the passenger line the *Megantic*. Named after Lake Megantic in Quebec, the ship was fifteen thousand tons, 550 feet long, almost seventy feet wide at its beam with three decks. Having one tall smokestack amidships, its twin four-cylinder steam piston engines driving twin screws, could make almost seventeen knots.[536] Flanagan and the others met at pier 1, and in two columns quietly boarded the *Megantic*. Flanagan and the "faithful four" wanted to stay together. The ship assigned berths by names in alphabetical order, Flanagan and Frolli, and Brake and Brinkerhoff, stayed together. Flanagan would later write that men of the 308th Field Signal Battalion were on the ship going across.[537] That night the *Megantic* stayed in port and prepared to sail with the tide the next morning. Flanagan wrote:

> ...We found [ourselves] in a not too bad state room with all port holes sealed so the bad Bosch would see no lights. We slept fairly well the first night, and during the early morning, drifted slowly and quietly out to sea in light fog. We could barely see a faint outline of the Statue [of Liberty] through the mist; the Statue, which was a reminder of the reason for all this sacrifice. What sacrifice was in store for us, we did not know, but were willing and even anxious to make

the supreme sacrifice if necessary. And why shouldn't we be willing, when on all sides of us were examples of the dear young boys going to what they knew to be certain death for many, but with a smile on their dear young faces, and a laugh ever ready on their lips, lips not yet old enough to show their manhood.[538]

These troop ships could be dreadfully crowded with conditions bordering on deplorable. Sometimes not enough berths or bunks were available; people had to sleep in shifts—if they could sleep at all. Sea sickness was common. Toilets overflowing, vomit throughout. With thousands of humans on board, many sick, the ship stunk. In heavy North Atlantic seas few could eat. Ship's food wasn't fine dining, basic rations quickly cooked were the rule. The only relief would be a trip outside to the deck.

For defense the merchant ships had deck guns to fire at U-boats. The deck guns could be lethal in ways not expected. To practice gunnery when the liners reached open sea, crewmen would throw overboard a floating barrel and use the barrel for target practice. This seemed to break the monotony of the voyage and provide macabre exciting entertainment to passengers. The SS *Mongolia*, a passenger liner fitted with three deck guns firing 6-inch diameter explosive projectiles, sailed from New York, May 19, 1917. On board were members of Army BH 21 from Northwestern Medical School, Chicago, and nurse Stella Judy from Deer Lodge, Montana. The next day the *Mongolia's* crew prepared for gunnery practice.[539]

The *Mongolia's* crew were using naval ammunition made before year 1900. Three basic pieces comprised the ammunition. A powder charge was in a cylindrical brass container. A press-fitted brass cup served as a moisture barrier and sealant on the brass container. Finally, an explosive projectile was press-fitted on the container having the powder charge. When the gun crew fired the gun, the explosive projectile could travel thousands of yards. The brass powder cup moisture seal behind the projectile also flew from the gun barrel: intact or in pieces, generally the latter. Few people ever see large caliber guns fire. Belching smoke, fire, and with ear-splitting noise, it's proper entertainment: like 4th of July but bigger and louder. Passengers that day, May 20, perhaps without command authorization from the ship, crowded on the *Mongolia's* deck to watch the big guns fire. The passengers included nurses from the base hospital sailing to France. The ship's gun crew began firing for practice.

The *Mongolia* fired three times. Immediately after firing a deck gun, three nurses on deck, Edith Ayres, Emma Matzen, and Helen Wood, collapsed on deck, bleeding. Ayers and Wood were killed outright and Matzen was wounded. The ship turned and immediately returned to New York City. Two theories surfaced as to what caused the nurse casualties: the brass cup moisture seal had ricocheted from the water and struck the nurses [not likely], or as a matter of the ammunition's dynamics when fired, brass fragments from the brass powder cup seal flew from the gun's muzzle [more likely]. Post mortem examinations showed brass fragments struck the nurses.[540] With deadly random chance and astonishingly bad luck, two Army nurses died watching the shipboard fireworks.[541] If Stella Judy witnessed the deadly accident she left no record.[542] The Navy's subsequent investigation laid no blame for the lethal accident and would in time replace the ammunition's brass ignitor cup moisture seal with wood or fiber substitutes.[543] With full military honors and great ceremony, Ayres was buried in Ohio; Wood in Chicago. They wouldn't be the last nurses to die.

Submarines weren't the sole hazard to ships. Crowded seaports brought collision hazards. On July 30, 1917, about 1,200 passengers, with nurses from Army BH 8, boarded the Army's transport ship the *Saratoga* at Hoboken, New Jersey. They were to sail soon. At about 1:30 p.m. the *Saratoga*, still at anchor, was rammed by the SS *City of Panama*. The collision tore a hole in the *Saratoga* and it began listing. *Saratoga*'s captain sounded the abandon ship signal. The nurses in various states of undress due to the heat of the day, manned the lifeboats and evacuated the ship. The *Saratoga* sank in less than twenty minutes. The nurses in lifeboats were rowed to Ellis Island. Their only possessions were the meager clothes they had on and what coats and capes their rescuers provided to shield the nurses from the blaring sun. For immediate resupply the ARC Council appropriated $14,000, roughly $200 per nurse, to outfit the now destitute nurses.[544] The Navy would buy the wrecked *Saratoga*, salvage it, convert it to a hospital ship and rename it the *USS Mercy*. The *Mercy* would be among the first Navy hospital ships to have female nurses on board for temporary duty[545].

U-boats didn't attack the SS *Great Northern:* a British ship did. On October 3, 1918, the British ship *Brinkburn*, slammed into the *Great Northern* about 500 miles off the coast of France. The collision killed seven Army passengers and wounded about fifteen others. Both ships remained afloat and the wounded were tended to.[546]

On June 11/12, the 17-ship convoy assembled in and around New York harbor.[547] Camouflage paint patterns tried to disguise the ship's appearance from periscopes of enemy submarines. The *Carpathia* sailing with the convoy had been painted in camouflage color schemes resembling giant teeth.[548] The USS San Diego was part of the destroyer escort for the convoy sailing to Liverpool, England. The convoy had lifeboat drills, and sometimes false alarms. Flanagan wrote of one alarm and a nurse's priority:

> …The Officer in Charge…said when we heard three short blasts from the horn at any time, we were to put on our coats and come on deck beside our life boats, and not to stop for anything. I had been sleeping with my coat pocket filled with what I thought I would need, enough to have sunk me had I had fallen overboard, and one night we were awakened by…blasts from the [ship's] horn. We all jumped out of our beds, put on our life belts and coats with our long hair streaming down our backs. Agnes [Frolli] couldn't find her stocking and refused to go on deck without her stockings. The other two said they could wait no longer, and I told Agnes that I thought I'd better go…Soon it got very quiet and before we found the lost stocking the others came back, Mary [Brinkerhoff] was furious because she had gone on deck looking the way she did. It was a false alarm, but had the ship been sinking, Agnes and I would have gone down with [the ship] all because of a lost stocking.[549]

Not all whistles were false alarms. The *Carpathia* had witnessed remarkable chapters in maritime history and survived. The ship had braved iceberg-choked waters to rescue *Titanic* survivors, and now served as a troop ship on the North Atlantic in the Great War. But the *Carpathia's* luck was running out. Somewhere on the North Atlantic, nurse Lucy Walters was on deck of the *Megantic*. The *Carpathia* sailing nearby in the seventeen-ship convoy. The convoy had departed New York, June 12, sailing to Liverpool. During daylight Walters was sitting on a deck chair breathing fresh sea air. Walters had a good view of the ship's crow's nest; the ship's signalman was high in the crow's nest. Suddenly the signalman began wig-wagging a flag message. The decoded message read: "Carpathia struck by submarine [deck gun] shell which [damaged] engines. Battleship standby. All other ships [begin] zig-zag in circles..."[550] The *Megantic's* captain ordered hard over on the helm, and the ship turned to begin evasive maneuvers avoiding U-boat gunfire. The hard turn rolled the deck to a steep incline. Walters wrote: "...I realized my [deck] chair was slipping...I found myself...in a corner of the deck where I knew a lower rail was missing. The chair was half off the edge of the ship! Screaming, I was clinging to the upper rail." Two doctors sailing on the ship grabbed Walters, she held on with an iron grip. The doctors lifted her to safety. Walters looked down to see the boiling waters behind the ship where she certainly would have been had the doctors not rescued her.[551]

Convoys normally took between ten to twelve days to cross the Atlantic to Liverpool. Because of U-boat activity, the convoy having the Montana nurses detoured to the north of Ireland. They sailed into the Irish Sea from the north rather than running the U-Boat gauntlet and entering the Irish Sea through St. George's Channel along the southeast coast of Ireland. Flanagan wrote: "It took two weeks to cross as we had to change course so often on account of submarines. I did not prove to be a good sailor...The only meal I ever really enjoyed was tea, and that was served on deck."[552]

In the convoy bringing the nurses to England, three ships in time would not survive. U-boat UB 87, commanded by Karl Petri, with ten sunk ships to his credit, would sink the *Missanbie* on September 9, 1918, off the southern coast of Ireland. Forty-five of *Missanabie's* crew died.[553] The morning of July 17, 1918, U-boat UB 55, commanded by Wilhem Werner, sank the *Carpathia* southwest of Ireland. Five crewmen of the *Carpathia* died.[554] On July 19, 1918, the cruiser USS *San Diego* entered New York harbor to meet a new convoy sailing to England. An explosion tore open the ship's port side [ship's left side facing forward].

Of the ship's officers and crew, six died; the rest reached safety. What caused the explosion, a torpedo or sea mine, is still debated.[555]

Flanagan's memoirs about "going across," ended with a cryptic, "We arrived in Liverpool on [Monday] June 24th, 1918 and went from there by train to Southampton." What she and the other Montana nurses saw, thought, and felt, when seeing the coast of Ireland, or the docks at Liverpool, is lost to history. She didn't write of having wobbly legs when getting off a ship's deck when stepping on land, or finally being able to breathe in deep breaths rather than with shallow pants of fear, or the sense of getting away from the shipboard stench. For a few days the nurses would rest. England would give them a safe respite— for a while. With a rolled knapsack and a rose, they had safely "gone across." Their long journey to war almost complete.

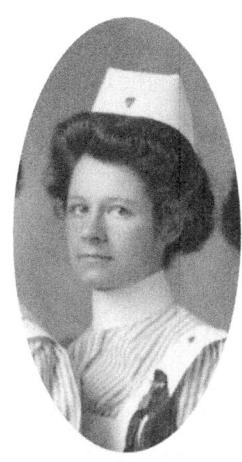

(*Left*) Virginia Flanagan
Courtesy The History Museum
Great Falls, MT

(*Below*) Army nurses receive gas mask training at Camp Kearney, (San Diego), CA. Courtesy National Archives and Records Administration.

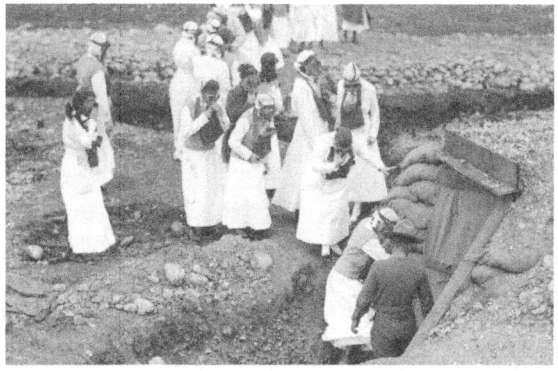

Chapter 11
OVER THERE

"War becomes real"

KING GEORGE V, AGE FIFTY-TWO, HAD BEEN KING OF ENGLAND since May 1910. The grandson of Queen Victoria and Prince Albert, some called George V an uninspiring fellow who would rather have lived a simpler quieter life. Ironically German Kaiser Wilhelm II was George V's first cousin and sworn enemy.[556] George V was now a war king, leading his people in a desperate struggle for survival. George V greeted American soldiers arriving in the kingdom. His printed greeting was folded in an envelope with "A Message to You from His Majesty King George" printed on the envelope. The greeting under the emblem of the royal Windsor Castle read:

> Soldiers of the United States, the people of the British Isles welcome you on your way to take your stand beside the Armies of many Nations now fighting in the Old World the great battle for human freedom.
> The Allies will gain new heart & spirit in your company. I wish that I could shake the hand of each one of you & bid you God speed on your mission.
> (signed) George R.I. April 1918.[557]

American nurses received their welcome from George V and dutifully noted it. Prior to departing America, soldiers and nurses could write their families about their pending sailing. The Army or the ARC would not mail the letter until two weeks after the soldiers and nurses sailed. This was for security to guard the ship's sailing date and name. It was also insurance in case German torpedoes ["tin fishes"] sank the ship. If the ship sank, the ARC had time to notify families without explaining why the family received a letter reading "all is well," when, in fact, the family's loved one was dead.[558]

America's slow mobilization for war disappointed and exasperated European allies. When America entered the war, European armies had been slaughtering each other with unrestrained carnage and ferocity for over two and a half years. To forever destroy the French army,

Germany began the war by attacking through Belgium in August 1914 with over one million men. During the opening days of the war during the Battle of the Frontiers, the French Army attacked with seventy infantry divisions, or about 1,250,000 men. French casualties during the battle exceeded 140,000 men: twice the number of the entire British Expeditionary Force in France at that time.[559] With luck, grit, and unimagined doggedness, exhausted French troops stopped the German advance at the first Battle of the Marne River in September 1914. Both sides dug in, and in time a 500-mile trench line extended from the English Channel to Switzerland. Artillery and machine guns turned the space between the opposing trenches into a grisly "no man's land." The carnage continued with little to show for it.

The Battle of Verdun in northeast France, from February 1916 to December 1916, was probably the longest sustained battle in history. Almost three-quarters of the French army were drawn to that human cauldron. Along a fifteen-mile front, Verdun has the wretched and hellish distinction of having the highest density of dead per square yard ever known in battle. An estimated 700,000 men fell, but no one knows for sure.[560] Explosive shells detonating near, or on, humans turn flesh and bone into pink mist: forever atomizing and erasing anything resembling an intact body. The human body simply disappears with nothing remaining to count. Heavy caliber artillery exploding in soft ground, forms a crater and throws dirt and mud skyward. The falling dirt and mud could bury forever a wounded or dead soldier falling in or thrown in the crater. Verdun was a grim battle; more than a century later, military historians still shudder at the name. The area around Verdun remains a pockmarked geological wreckage. After the battle France wouldn't be the same, Britain would now carry the fight.[561]

While Verdun flamed, roared, and slaughtered, combined British and French forces attacked the Germans along the upper reaches of the Somme River northeast of Paris. The battle took place from July 1 to November 18, 1916. The Somme is remembered as "...the greatest slaughter ever suffered by people who speak English."[562] In the first days almost sixty thousand British were casualties in the vainglorious Victorian notion of charging headlong to glory and honor and being instantly cut down by machine guns like sharp scythes on ripened wheat."[563] A small number of trained soldiers in fixed fortifications, manned with modern-for-their-day weapons, could stop a massed infantry assault. Defensive use of artillery and machine guns dominated World War I battles. At the Somme opposing armies fired almost two million artillery shells. Combined British losses were about 420,000; German losses more than 450,000. Mass slaughter for little gain.

Modern warfare had arrived and the British failed to adjust. Their officers, indifferent or ignorant, refused to acknowledge their centuries-old methods and tactics of warfare had wretchedly failed. A year later the British would fight another "imperial fiasco" at Passchendaele with similar terrible results. And always the mud, the dastardly damnable mud: exasperating soldiers and slowing the pace of war since French knights faltered against the English at the Battle of Agincourt in the fifteenth century.[564]

In 1917 the situation surrounding the French army became utterly perilous. French soldiers began protesting about stupidity of leadership, recklessness of decision, incompetence of officers, and overall lack of care for the common soldier. French soldiers mutinied and refused to move. The personal efforts of fabled French general Philippe Pétain calmed the situation. A closely guarded secret, the Germans never discovered the massive unrest in the French army. Few know of the French army mutiny even today.[565]

U.S. forces entered the war with an assortment of obsolete firearms, second-rate equipment, uniforms and helmets; but most glaringly, untrained soldiers. America relied on its allies to provide armaments, artillery, airplanes, and whatever the Allies could spare. An American infantry division of that time had between fifteen thousand to eighteen thousand men and about 4,500 horses.[566] Between two to five divisions create a corps. A corps is a lower-echelon tactical unit created to coordinate the fighting of its assigned divisions. Routinely a corps operates as part of a field army. A field army may consist of three to four corps.

America's First and Second Infantry Divisions were the first American fighting units to arrive in France. The Army formed the First Expeditionary Division [later the First Infantry Division] in late spring 1917. Few divisions were ever at full strength. Untrained and poorly equipped draftees and volunteers filled the ranks. Pershing called the recruits, "sturdy rookies."[567] The "Big Red One," the moniker of the First Infantry Division, wouldn't fire a shot in anger in France until October 1917.[568] The Army formed the Second Infantry Division in

September 1917. The Second Infantry Division would not see action until June 1918 at the fierce Battle of Belleau Wood.[569] The first National Guard units arriving in France were the Twenty-Sixth and Forty-Seconded Infantry Divisions. These divisions wouldn't be ready for combat until early 1918. Both divisions, no longer in active service, would remained fabled in American military history.

American soldiers were slow in coming, but six preconfigured American base hospitals with doctors, nurses, and medical equipment, had arrived in France less than eight weeks after America entered the war. On May 19, 1917, Montana nurse Alice Ralston sailed on the *St. Paul* as a member of BH 10 formed in Philadelphia. BH 10 would soon gain the distinction as having some of the highest decorated nurses in battle in American history to date. BH 21, formed from personnel of the Barnes Hospital, Washington University, St. Louis, Missouri, sailed with BH 10 on the *St. Paul.*

Clara Noyes, head of the ARC Department of Nursing, tried to be in New York City when any group of nurses sailed. Noyes would write of the nurses going to France:

> It is an inspiring picture to see the nursing personnel of a base hospital ready to embark. The dignified uniform of dark blue cloth, the scarlet lining of the cape, the caduceus and the letters "U. S." on the collar...are significant and impressive. Complete understanding of the nature of the mission is expressed on their faces. There is no laughing or joking, yet there are no tears. Courage is written on each countenance and service wherever required is their purpose.[570]

The first two base hospitals sailed so quickly the nurses traveled in civilian clothes. Nurses of the other base hospitals received uniforms and equipment at New York City.[571] After receiving uniforms and equipment, BH 10 and BH 21 sailed without destroyer escort for protection against U-boats. The *St. Paul* had deck guns for defense. On May 26 U.S. destroyers, based in Queenstown, Ireland, met the *St. Paul* off the Irish coast and escorted the ship to Liverpool. The *St. Paul* entered the Mersey River estuary and docked at Liverpool early evening, May 27. Owing to weather, the base hospitals did not disembark until morning, May 28. The nurses stayed at Liverpool's Adelphi Hotel. The next day they departed for London. In London they stayed at the Waldorf Hotel for nearly a month getting oriented for duty in France.

In England BH 10 saw the British Women's Voluntary Aid Detachment, or the V.A.D. The V.A.D. had women of all classes doing work supporting the hospitals, even driving ambulances. The V.A.D. didn't have nurses but had trained help. In London BH 10 learned the British custom of calling nurses, "sister."[572]

The U.S. State Department in England insisted that arriving medical staff, doctors and nurses, have U.S. passports. The U.S. consulate in London began issuing emergency passports to members of BH 10 and BH 21. Alice Ralston posed for her passport photograph in a nurse's outdoor dark blue uniform, appearing black in her photograph. Her chin is down, but focused eyes looked up in resolve. She doesn't wear glasses. Ralston's dark short hair parted down the middle.[573] The State Department hadn't grasped the full reality of the coming war. Requiring passports was impossible for hundreds of thousands of Americans coming through England. The State Department agreed to accept War Department issued Certificates of Identity.

Helen Fairchild, Jane Isabelle Stambaugh, and Helen Grace McClelland were Ralston's colleagues at BH 10.[574] Fairchild joined BH 10 and, like Ralston, volunteered to go overseas in May 1917. Fairchild wrote extensively to her family in America. She wrote of nurses' uniforms:

> "…We were in uniforms all the time, and our street uniforms are heavy dark blue serge, made very military, one piece, with big broad pleats over the shoulders with rows of big, black buttons down both sides, and swirls, with panels front and back, made quite short little white bands around the collar and sleeves and short blue hats. At first we didn't like the idea of having to wear uniforms all the time, but we have learned the wisdom of it now, for it gives protection [from the weather]…[575]

On June 28 Ralston and BH 10 departed for France from London.

Taking a train to the port of Southampton on a pleasant spring day, they boarded an English hospital ship escorted by destroyers. Arriving at the port of Le Havre, France, the next morning at 4 a.m., the medical personnel quickly disembarked, but for twelve hours found no support available. They didn't eat for almost a day until a resourceful American military officer bought food and drink from a nearby French village.[576] A British V.A.D. arrived with ambulances to take the Americans to their destination at Le Treport on the English Channel northeast of Le Havre. Driving through mud and rain, the Americans finally arrived at British General Hospital 16 [GH 16] Le Treport. GH 16 was located in one of the most forward points of the British Zone near the front battle lines.[577] GH 16 was constructed entirely of huts and tents arranged in a half-circle. BH 10 staff soon noted the hospital was depressing and had few creature comforts.[578] Margaret A. Dunlop, chief nurse at BH 10, wrote of the nurses' quarters:

> …Little huts were added so that by winter the nurses were entirely housed in huts instead of tents. The little huts were one-story wooded structures partitioned into small rooms holding two nurses [per room.] Each room had for equipment a small stove holding about ten pieces of coal. Other equipment the nurses provided themselves. The little stove proved our greatest friend. With the ten pieces of coal per week per ration, we leave it to the imagination how we secured sufficient warmth and hot water. For bureau or wash stands we used Red Cross packing cases, begged, borrowed or stolen, which we cover with [a heavy cotton fabric]. A small triangular board nailed in the corner of the room made a closet. A collapsible canvas basin, or in the case of the more fortunate ones, a while enamel basis and pitcher were the toilet articles. The beds were canvas cots, the mattresses squares of cotton pads known as "biscuits." Later we [pooled] our [money] and bought from the British Red Cross chairs and [cotton fabric] for curtain.[579]

Ralston and BH 10 would have to make do with what they had.

Resourcefulness, initiative, grit, and determination would be needed and soon.

Two days behind the *St. Paul*, General Pershing and staff sailed on the SS *Baltic*, May 28. They were to travel incognito, but, in the words of President John F. Kennedy during the Cuban Missile Crisis, "There's always some [SOB] who doesn't get the word." Many of Pershing's staff arrived in full uniform with luggage plainly marked "General Pershing's Headquarters," effectively trouncing any secrecy of travel. Added to the failed attempt at concealment, gun batteries on Governor's Island gave Pershing and the *Baltic* a full and loud ceremonial salute.[580]

After ten days at sea, Pershing and staff docked at Liverpool. The final destination was secret, but cable traffic from newspaper reporters revealed Pershing's whereabouts.[581] Arriving by train in London, joyous crowds met him. He began attending obligatory briefings, meetings, hand-shaking events, teas, and church services. Pershing didn't stay long in London. On June 13 he and his staff crossed the English Channel to France, where again, joyous crowds hailed his arrival. Pershing brought a token force with him. Waving the flag was all they could do for the moment. Pershing spent the first few days in Paris attending social engagements. A handsome man and widower at aged fifty-seven, who spoke French, Pershing soon became close to a French woman selected to paint Pershing's official portrait.[582]

By June 16 Pershing toured the battle lines, staying beyond gun fire. Looking at enemy battle positions through binoculars, Pershing made no comment as to disposition of forces or proposed battle plans.[583] He began resisting, diplomatically but firmly, French and British insistence that American troops be placed immediately under French or British command. Prior to sailing for France, Pershing met with U.S. secretary of war Newton Baker. President Wilson, through Baker, gave Pershing orders that "In military operations against the Imperial German Government you [Pershing] are directed to cooperate with the forces of the other countries employed against the enemy; but in doing so…the forces of the United States are [to be kept] separate and distinct…the identity of which must be preserved."[584] Wilson and Baker also knew the American people would not stand for European generals commanding American soldiers. Generals who had repeatedly shown utter disregard for the lives and well-being of their soldiers.

Pershing had little regard for trench warfare: the grinding death-by-attrition method of war prevalent among French, British, and Germans. He also had little use for the way France trained troops. Pershing would train American soldiers in the art of maneuver warfare: draw the enemy into the open from entrenched positions, and destroy the enemy in open battle.[585] One of Pershing's generals, Major General Robert L. Bullard said of French battle tactics: "A French soldier never rests until he had dug a hole, and after that he never rests anywhere but in the hole."[586] However compelling their common cause in war, it was exceedingly difficult for allies to combine their forces, and to suppress their national rivalries and pride under the authority of a single commander not of their nation and character.[587]

Pershing departed Paris and made his headquarters at Chaumont: about 140 miles east-southeast of Paris at the confluence of the Marne and Suize Rivers. With his staff he began forming the combat forces of the AEF. This would take time. Pershing's staff began working the millions of details to prepare an army for war. This meant having reliable communications. An old American army saying is a piece of paper makes a man a general, but communications makes him a commander. Wireless radios were in their infancy in the early twentieth century, but the French had telephones.

In World War I telephones meant survival. Among the many challenges facing Pershing and his staff in organizing for war, was using the French telephone system. This wasn't a matter of convenience, Pershing needed dependable communications to relay military orders, adjust artillery fire, direct resupply, and care for wounded soldiers. Laying lightweight telephone wires from command posts to forward units and artillery guns was terribly dangerous, but it could be done rapidly with wire spools on horse-drawn wagons or trucks. Switchboards could be wagon-mounted and follow the battle. Erecting telephone wires back to major command centers was challenging but not impossible given technology, soldier initiative, skill, and courage.

France had few telephone lines, and the French/English language challenge became an impediment when using French telephones. Army Signal Corps captain Robert B. Owens had an idea. A highly educated man of letters, he was quick to solve technical problems. He recommended bringing French/English speaking American [mostly women] telephone operators to France. Owens' idea worked its way up the chain of command. The Army Signal Corps decided on using women telephone operators in France. The Army's reasons were, first, the "unquestioned superiority of women as telephone switchboard operators," and second "the desire to release for service in the more dangerous telephone centrals at the front, the male operators…in the larger offices at Army headquarters and in the [major supply depots]".[588]

By November 1917 Pershing decided against having Army male telephone operators to continue using the French telephone system. Army colonel Parker Hitt, chief signal officer, First Army said: "Our experience in Paris with the untrained and undisciplined English-speaking French women operators…with willing but untrained [American] men operators was almost disastrous."[589] On November 8, 1917, Pershing sent a message to America reading: "On account of the great difficulty of obtaining properly qualified men, request organization and dispatch to France…women telephone operators all speaking French and English equally well.[590] Pershing's detailed request included three chief telephone operators at a salary of $125 a month, nine supervising operators at $72 a month, twenty-four long distance operators at $60 a month, fifty-four operators at $60 a month, and ten substitute operators at $50 a month. These salaries were comparable to what operators earned in America. AEF operators would have the same allowances as Army and Navy nurses and wear uniforms.[591]

The Army gave Captain E.J. Wesson, Civilian Personnel Section of the Signal Corps, the mission of recruiting American bilingual telephone operators. Officially these operators formed the Women's Telephone Unit of the American Signal Corps, (WTU). Colloquially America and history would call them the "Hello Girls." The Signal Corps said it needed about 500 operators. One hundred would go immediately to France and the rest would stay in America as reserves. Wesson first recruited in newspapers in Montreal, Canada, and creole-speaking areas of Louisiana. Three hundred to 400 women applied, but the Army found only twenty-five qualified in language and telephone switchboard operating skills.[592]

The Army had other requirements. The women had to be between twenty-three and thirty-five years old, pass a physical and psychological exam similar to that given an officer, and also have her background checked by Army security. The applicant had to submit an affidavit from her previous employer as to the woman's character and ability. The Army did not restrict the job to single women. Erroneous information surfaced that the Army would allow wives of officers and enlisted men in Europe to apply for operators' positions. The Army quickly said no to that.[593] Lacking qualified recruits, Wesson began recruiting nationwide in trade magazines, journals, and newspapers. The Army asked cooperation from the Bell Telephone System, and the Independent Telephone System. In December 1917 Montana newspapers began printing the first Army national recruiting advertisements for women telephone operators. The *Butte* [MT] *Daily Post*, December 5, 1917, printed a short national notice from the Army chief signal officer. The notice read:

> A unit of 150 telephone operators, able to speak both French and English, for immediate service in France, will be formed under the direction of the army signal corps…
>
> The operators, enlisted for the duration of the war, will be given allowances of quarters and rations accorded American nurses, in addition to their pay, and also will wear the same uniform.
>
> In seeking recruits for the new service, the announcement of the chief signal officer says: "Young ladies, physically fit, with command of the French and English languages, desirous of obtaining these positions, should apply by mail to room 826, Mills Building annex, Washington."

In time the Army received 7,600 applications for about 500 positions.[594] Wesson soon concluded: "It would be impossible to [command and control] American troops without these girls. They are going to astound the people over there by the efficiency of their work. In Paris it takes from 40 to 60 seconds to complete one call. Our girls are equipped to handle 300 calls an hour."[595] The recruiting drive reached Montana. Montana's switchboard operators, on occasion, already had their hands and their headsets full.

The University of Montana, in the scenic and quiet western Montana city of Missoula, lies at the base of a small mountain on Missoula's east side. The city changes as students arrive or depart when school begins or is let out. In 1917 Missoula's telephone operators either breathed relief or braced for the increased phone traffic when school let out or began. "Missoula 83" was a number the operators mumbled in their sleep for nine months during school. The women's dormitory at the university had one telephone in the lobby, the number? "Missoula 83." Every young man at the school with courting on his mind, soon knew the number by heart. Every Missoula telephone operator would soon scorn the number and the operator's repeated answer of "83 is busy."[596]

At the turn of the twentieth century about 80 percent of telephone operators were women. Most men in the wire communications business were telegraphers.[597] In 1917 Missoula had its own private branch exchange, or PBX. This was a self-contained telephone system, mostly for local calls. A user could ask for a long-distance line, but this required special handling from the local operator. Telephone users did not dial a number. The user would lift a hand-held receiver from its carrying hook on a telephone, this completed a circuit to the main switchboard where an operator would see a small light come on. The operator would take a male electrical plug, insert it into a hole on the switchboard connecting the circuit. The operator would ask: "Number please?" When given the number, [hopefully not "Missoula 83"] the operator would insert a connecting plug into another numbered hole. She would then turn a crank that rang the other phone. When the other person answered, this completed the call. Periodically the operator would listen in on the call to see if the call was completed. With the many wire plugs going every which way on the switchboard, the board could look like a spider web.

The operator had to manage this spider web of connections. She also had to memorize the connecting holes on the switchboard. With great nimbleness of fingers working the many circuit connecting plugs, the operator had to keep up with the "plug count."[598] The plug count was the required number of make and break telephone connections in a given time. She had to track the plug count at her station by writing down the number of calls. This showed if the operator was working hard or not. A low plug count on a high-volume telephone time-of-day meant the individual operator wasn't keeping up and could be fired.[599]

University students had departed for summer break. Fourth of July festivities were coming soon. Missoula telephone operators were getting hot under the collar and not because of summer heat. Long hours, increased telephone usage, insufficient pay, and rising calls for unionization among telephone operators had reached a decision point. On Tuesday, July 3, 1917, eighteen Missoula telephone operators suddenly took off their headsets, unplugged their switchboards, got up and walked out of the Mountain States Telephone Company office. Missoula went dead. Men of the Brotherhood of Electrical Workers, Local No. 408, supporting the Missoula women operators, also walked off the job in a no-notice wildcat strike. When leaving the telephone office, the women said they wanted better wages than $40 a month. They also wanted recognition for their switchboard operators' union and closed shop [union only] hiring. The Mountain States Telephone Company could not do anything without conferring with the main office in Denver.[600] The Missoula telephone operator's strike lasted three days. The telephone company met all the women's demands. Their pay scale increased to $65 a month with no wage ceiling for longevity. They had their union and closed shop hiring. However, this labor agreement applied to Missoula and nowhere else.[601]

Missoula operators weren't alone in their efforts. Telephone operators nationwide were doing much the same in 1917: strikes, labor organizing, and demands for better pay. Leaders of six thousand west coast telephone operators threatened a general strike if Pacific Telephone and Telegraph didn't meet the operators' demands of better pay and benefits. The telephone operators, affiliated with the International Brotherhood of Electrical Workers, said: "We want to be regarded as human beings instead of machines." Pacific Telephone and Telegraph met all their demands.[602]

In March 1918 Mary E. Vannier was working as a saleswoman for the Sanden and Ferguson Company in Helena. A Canadian by birth, she came with her family to Deer Lodge in western Montana. A capable woman, she was a women's delegate at the 1909 Montana Federation of Labor convention at the Carpenter's Union Hall in Butte.[603] Vannier learned of the Army's recruiting for bilingual telephone operators. She spoke fluent French, and had worked as a telephone operator for the Mountain States Telephone and Telegraph Company in Butte. When she took the WTU qualifying examination, she was the only applicant to pass in Montana and Wyoming.

For training on switchboards, the Army established six training sites in large telephone offices in America. The sites were, New York

City; Chicago; Lancaster, Pennsylvania; San Francisco; Jersey City; New Jersey; Atlantic City, and Philadelphia.[604] The Army gave Vannier orders to report to Jersey City, New Jersey, for training. Part of the American Telephone and Telegraph Company training would be in downtown Manhattan, where operators worked at a busy telephone exchange.[605] Vannier would also receive military specific training. Military switchboards didn't use numbers, they used call signs. The telephone to the commanding general of the First Infantry Division might be "Big Red Six." Calling the Marine Corps, an operator might have to know "Leather Necks," or other perplexing telephone codes like "skeezer," or "narndull." Animal names of all sorts might be used for switchboard locations. For security these code names changed often. Operators then had to memorize another list of perplexing names for Army switchboard centers supporting on-going battles.

On June 28, 1918, Vannnier sailed for France on the SS *Lapland* with Signal Corps Unit No. 4. Built by Harland and Wolff of Belfast for the Red Star Line, the *Lapland* was a newer ship.[606] Signal Corps Unit 4 was the fourth group of WTU operators to France. This unit had sixty-two operators on board.[607] Vannier would serve almost three years overseas. Before sailing to France, Vannier had her photograph taken in New York City. In the photograph she sits while wearing the Army Signal Corps uniform. Vannier wore the wide brimmed hat with the Army Signal Corps colored cords around the hat. She was wearing the high-necked military coat with the WTU organizational position icon on the white brassard on her left coat sleeve. Looking over her left shoulder to the camera, the handsome young Montana woman smiles confidently.

The Army did send operators to military cantonment areas and training bases in America. Here operators received training on military-related words, ranks, and procedures. Army training bases grew in size and number. These bases needed telephone operators. This meant women working in Army bases and the Army didn't like that. Telephone traffic to these training bases demanded experienced operators. Regardless of the Army's reluctance to have women on bases, the Army had no choice. The Army began preparations for civilian women on base.

When small town America found its younger women were going to military bases alongside thousands of young men, the age-old issue of "the boy-girl thing," raised its head. Mothers didn't want "scarlet women," around their sons, and fathers didn't want their daughters around young soldiers looking for one last hurrah before going to war.[608] These concerns were real. The Army surgeon general in his 1919 annual report to the president reported the Army was treating over two thousand cases of venereal disease *every day Army-wide* [italics added]. Next to the 1918 influenza epidemic, venereal disease prostrated more American soldiers in American and France than anything in World War I.[609] The Army and the YMCA began an extensive campaign to offer soldiers relaxing activities in training camps, other than partaking of the world's oldest profession.

Lena Anderson-Roy lived in Bozeman, Montana, and worked at the Willson and Company mercantile establishment. She had never operated a telephone switchboard, but she was fluent in French. Pershing first wanted operators fluent in French; in time the Army found comparatively few women were expert in both. The Army decided it could train women to operate a switchboard faster than teaching them French. The Army soon publicly said: "Knowledge of switchboard is also necessary, but if you do not have this knowledge and if all the operators needed are not obtained…you may be accepted without previous experience and given the necessary training by some telephone company."[610] If the woman spoke French, that was the major hurdle. Anderson-Roy fit the bill and applied to for the WTU.

She applied through the Bozeman Telephone Company. The Army accepted her application. The enthusiastic [and perhaps naive] Anderson-Roy said: "…You know I am going to wear a uniform, and while the work is going to be hard, just think of the thrills we switchboard operators are going to have in active service."[611]

The women of the WTU would indeed wear an Army Signal Corps uniform designed by the Army War College. The uniform consisted of a coat and skirt of navy blue serge, tailored shirtwaist [blouse constructed as a shirt] of navy blue cloth or similar material, with a straight-brimmed hat of blue felt. The hat had the official orange and white cord of the Signal Corps. The women didn't wear official military rank insignia, such as stripes worn by enlisted men or sergeants. A white brassard was worn on the left sleeve of the women's coat. The brassard had embroidered icons indicating the *organizational position* [italics added] of the wearer.[612] Anderson-Roy described the insignia as: "…The different ranks are distinguished by the different insignia on the white brassard worn on the left arm. Operators will wear a [blue outline of a telephone mouthpiece], supervisors [wear] a gilt laurel wreath beneath the [mouthpiece symbol], and chief operators wear the two symbols with lightning bolts used by the Signal Corps.

Anderson-Roy continued:

> General Pershing told us in a communication sent out by the War Department that this is to be a task of a nature and size that would appeal only to brave and patriotic women, and I am going to try and be brave. I am sure I am patriotic. When we applied we were told that the signal corps wanted only level-headed women who were resourceful, able to exercise good judgment in emergencies and even endure hardships if necessary. I only hope that I shall live up to all these requirements.

Because Anderson-Roy didn't know how to operate a telephone switchboard, the Army told her to report for intensive training at the Helena branch of the Mountain States Telephone Company. There Anderson-Roy would be trained by Montana's best, Merle Egan.

In 1913 the Mountain States Telephone Company, Helena, Montana, expanded its operations in Lewistown, Montana. The telephone company invested much money and built a new exchange building in Lewistown. The building had concrete floors, with modern batteries and a ten-horsepower back-up generator. The building had its own heating plant. Electrical engineers installed the latest telephone circuit boards and distributing panels. The telephone exchange could handle 1,600 lines with a maximum capacity of eight thousand lines. The chief operator's desk monitored operations. The exchange had three long-distance switchboards switchable to local calls at night. The building had rest rooms adjoining the switchboard room. The rest rooms had women's lockers and wash basins. An outside iron stair exit, easily reached by operators, ensured fast egress in emergencies. Fourteen girls and three back-ups operated the exchange.

Mountain States Telephone brought an experienced team to switch over to the new building. The district manager in Helena brought the plant supervisor, and traffic superintendent. He also brought chief operator, Merle Egan.[613] Egan had been the chief operator at Helena for many years. Egan knew the latest switchboard technology, and apparently was a very good instructor. When war came, Helena saw Egan as an energetic supporter of the war effort. Egan didn't speak French. She didn't apply for the WTU as she knew the Army first required French-speaking operators. Egan was an excellent writer and editor as she was the associate editor of the *Mountain States Monitor*: the Mountain States Telephone Company's magazine. Egan edited the information about the company's northern district.[614]

On September 20, 1918, the Army dropped the French-speaking requirement for its operators as the AEF had grown and had installed over 1,500 miles of its own telephone wires. When Pershing and his staff first sailed to France in May 1917 the cargo hold of the SS *Baltic*, carried material and equipment, and telephone poles, to install and operate one local battery telephone system in France.[615] The AEF soon conducted its business between American offices and didn't need French operators.[616] Egan and other operators who didn't speak French, saw their chance and applied for the WTU. The Army accepted their applications. Egan raised her right hand and swore the loyalty oath before the adjutant general of Montana.[617] Egan was on her way to France.

Montana had other experienced chief operators willing to serve. Celia Ann Grimmeke was chief operator in Butte. Born in Calumet, Michigan, October 11, 1886, to Bernard and Charlotte Grimmeke, she graduated from high school in Calumet. She made her way to Montana with her family, and in 1910 began working for the Mountain States Telephone Company in Butte. Promoted to chief operator, she gained a reputation as having tact with customers and ability to soothe angry telephone users.

Grimmeke didn't speak French, but when the Army had relaxed the French language requirement, Grimmeke applied for the WTU. The Army accepted Grimmeke in August 1918. The Army didn't give her much time to report for training in New York City. She quickly went to the Butte Army recruiting office and got travel orders to the American Telephone and Telegraph Company training station in New York City.[618] The Butte telephone operators gave Grimmeke a farewell ceremony. The operators wanted to give her a commemorative watch as a going away present, but Grimmeke's travel orders came too fast. The operators gave her a cash gift at the Butte train station.[619] Grimmeke received her signal corps uniform: probably in New York City. A photograph shows her in profile in smartly-attired Signal Corps uniform with a soft-sided smooth hat, not the wide-brimmed hat with Signal Corps cords. Signal Corps crossed-flags insignia is pinned to her hat. Her expression is one of pride, resolve, and determination.[620] Grimmeke sailed for France on September 11, 1918.[621]

Little is known of Montana's Marie Paul Adams. A daughter of Louis Paul from St. Ignatius, Montana, she may have grown to womanhood around Arlee, Montana: north of Missoula.[622] She apparently entered the WTU from Butte. The *Montana Standard*, November 11, 1929, quotes Adams as saying she was stationed at Souilly, France. Some Montana women departed for war with great fanfare; others quietly, almost anonymously.

Thirty-three American telephone operators, with chief operator Grace Banker, sailed from New York City to Liverpool, March 6, 1918.[623] They arrived in Liverpool and traveled to Paris, where they received three days intensive training. The March 29, 1918, edition of the *Stars and Stripes* newspaper had a page 1 article titled: "Hello Girls Here in Real Army Duds." The article trumpets the women wore "real Army costumes," and the women showed real originality by substituting skirts for the more conventional olive drab colored breeches common soldiers wear. The *Stars and Stripes* article seemed to make levity of the women and their mission. In summary the newspaper reads the women were "capable plus."

Soon 233 operators arrived in France. The Army assigned operators to the Paris office, to Pershing's headquarters at Chaumont, and to the Signal Corps headquarters at Tours, France. A few operators were kept in reserve to go where the need was greatest. The AEF assigned its best operators to large offices and toll centers. In September 1917 American AEF operators each day handled 200 long-distance calls and four thousand local calls. By March 1918 local calls exceeded seventeen thousand a day. The AEF would soon assign operators to the headquarters of each numbered Army in the AEF.[624] On March 19, 1918, the office of the AEF chief signal officer, along with the signal personnel division and signal supply, moved to Tours, France: about 130 miles southwest of Paris on the Loire River. Tours was safely behind the battle lines and intermittent German shelling of Paris. Of the cathedral city of Tours, Anderson-Roy wrote:

> Here in constantly increasing numbers we have American and British women in uniform composed of Y.W.C.A. girls, Yankee telephone girls, Red Cross workers, and English women war workers of all kinds....
>
> Again, how many travel worn nurses have landed here between meal hours, enroute for a new post having been in many cases 10 and 12 hours without food! What would they have done without the hurriedly prepared bread and jam and tea, sometimes served to a group of 30 or 40.
>
> When plans were finally matured and it was decided to send telephone girls from the United States to Tours, there was scurrying about to get lodging for [the girls] in this congested city. The Y.W.C.A. people after a distracting hunt for suitable quarters succeeded in leasing a small hotel. [It was a] dirty hole. To see it now, clean and quaintly pretty in its new dress, it would take an equal imagination to picture it as it was.
>
> The telephone girls are a light-hearted lot...and although they are more or less under army discipline, that is a feature they laud instead of bewail. Their [food] is taken at the barracks where they work...[625]

Anderson-Roy would also write of the inauguration of the American Signal Corps Women's club and the Foyer des Allies: a club in Tours for French, British, and American women.[626]

The Navy also began preparing for war and established naval hospitals in Europe. The Navy had fewer nurses than the Army. At the end of 1918 the Navy had slightly over one thousand nurses.[627] The Navy reluctantly reported it had fewer assignment opportunities than the Army. Nurses signed up for the Army for the chance to go more places.[628] Alice Canon, age twenty-eight, Lewistown, Montana, enrolled in the Navy Nurse Corps, September 14, 1917. Canon received her graduate nurses training in Los Angeles, California, 1914. After graduating, Canon stayed in Los Angeles.[629] Canon became part of Navy Base Hospital 3, [BH 3] formed in Philadelphia, Pennsylvania, on December 10, 1917.[630]

The Navy sent BH 3 to Leith, [Edinburgh] Scotland, on July 29, 1918. The hospital was a tenant of the British Army and took over buildings of the Leith Parish Poorhouse at Seafield. After frustrating negotiations with local authorities, America spent over $40,000 improving the buildings. When the Americans arrived, fifty British patients were in the buildings. After improvements the hospital had over one thousand beds.[631] In Leith the American nurses stayed in local hotels and three houses.[632] The Navy established another hospital in Strathpeffer, Scotland, near Inverness.

In 1917 forming advanced medical support wasn't an AEF priority. The Army had sent available American doctors and nurses first to stateside military training bases. What few American nurses in France in 1917 were helping the British. By February 1918 five Montana nurses were in France: Alice Ralston and Sally Connor from Butte; and Genevieve Larson, Gertrude Sloane, and Martha Daigle from Missoula. Ralston, Daigle, and Larson, were sent to the British Expeditionary Force. Ralston was with BH 10 that took over a British general hospital near the front battle lines.

In war much is made of "firsts." For Montana women in World War I, Ralston has three distinctive firsts: She would be the first female from Montana to officially enroll in the military as a nurse; the first recognized female military veteran from Montana, and the first Montana female to be under fire in World War I.[633] Ralston and BH 10 would soon see firsthand the horrors and death at an earthly hell called Passchendaele.[634]

Chapter 12
UNDER FIRE

"Into the cauldron"

BRITISH SOLDIERS CALLED THE TOWN "WIPERS." For non-French speakers, pronouncing the Belgium town, *Ypres*, [EE-pur or EE-prah] as "wipers" seems practical. In World War I British soldiers near Ypres published a humorous and satirical trench magazine call "The Wiper's Times." Ypres, an ancient city in the flat Flanders region of west Belgium, is about twenty miles east of the English Channel: almost straddling the French border. In history ancient and modern armies have fought brutal battles around Ypres. In World War I Ypres occupied important ground directly in the path of the planned German army advance on Paris. Five savage battles from autumn 1914 to autumn 1918 largely obliterated Ypres. Hundreds of thousands of Allied and German soldiers fell there. Canadian physician Lieutenant-Colonel John McCrae's immortal poem, "In Flanders Fields," is a memorial to a friend who died in the Second Battle of Ypres, May 1915.[635]

In 1917 the war had entered its third year: largely a stalemate of trench warfare. Year 1916 exhausted Allied and Germany armies at Verdun and the Somme. The war strained Britain. On December 16 the British parliament formed a new government with a new prime minister, David Lloyd George. On the eastern front by year's end 1916, Russia had lost almost five million men: killed, wounded, captured, or missing.[636] Russia collapsed in the 1917 revolution. This collapse released German soldiers fighting on the eastern front to come west reinforcing the German army along the French and Belgium borders. France and Britain faced a common battlefield enemy, but the two allied countries squabbled. In spring 1917 the French formed a new government. French and British high command changed their high-level troop leaders. And America remained far in the distance.

In 1917 the Allies planned more attacks on German battle lines. French general Robert Georges Nivelle, age sixty, looked battle-weary, old, distant, portly, and uninspiring. But he was a charming and forceful speaker. He spoke fluent English and persuaded French and British leaders to agree with his war plans. Nivelle convinced French and British leaders he could win. With that, Nivelle replaced the French commander-in-chief General Joseph Joffre. Joffre, age sixty-four, lost his job as he failed in appallingly costly battles.

In spring 1917 Nivelle wanted to attack German lines near the Belgium border north of Paris. Nivelle's plan was the British, commanded by British field marshall Douglas Haig, would support the attack. Haig wanted to attack farther north near Ypres. His strategic plan was to advance along the Belgium coast and capture German U-boat bases. Haig wanted to capture Belgium sea ports: Antwerp among them. French and British military leaders quarreled as to who would command the effort and for how long. Haig, adhering to his long-held notion he was an ally and not a French subordinate, finally and reluctantly agreed to be under French command during the spring offensive.[637]

A massive artillery barrage on German lines opened Nivelle's six-week spring offensive on the cold and snowy morning of April 16. The offensive lasted until mid-May with mixed results at high cost. The British achieved limited success near Arras south of Ypres. The French achieved some gains, but with tremendous casualties. The German army held. In Nivelle's offensive the French army had reached the limits of its endurance. In one week beginning April 16 the French army lost thirty thousand killed, 100,000 wounded, and four thousand missing. Mass mutinies began in the French army and Nivelle was sacked.[638] Britain would take the military initiative until the end of 1917.

British naval command wanted German U-boat attacks stopped. The British navy's concern was U-boat attacks would restrict shipping from the United States. British naval command pressured Haig to attack north near Ypres and seize German U-boat bases along the Belgium coast. In June 1917 Haig attacked. He was successful in the Battle of Messines: six miles south of Ypres. With this success the British government approved Haig's continued offensive drive north beyond Ypres.[639] Haig and his staff would badly miscalculate on one thing no general can control—the weather.

European cities can be farther north on the globe when compared to cities in North America. Paris, France, is nearly on the same latitude line as the U.S.-Canadian border west of Minnesota. London, England, is as far north as Calgary, Alberta, Canada. Ypres, Belgium, where Haig wanted to attack, is also about as far north as Calgary. Western Europe has seacoast weather: cloudy, cold, mist, and fog. Relentless drenching rains could come with prolonged penetrating cold weather. Mud, unimaginable deep black goo, vexed the most ardent of European souls and soldiers in the field.[640] Haig and his staff thoroughly checked historical weather records for Flanders before scheduling an offensive near Ypres. They knew rain would come but decided it would be acceptable for maneuver warfare across open ground. The Third Battle of Ypres, and Passchendaele Ridge, was on for July 1917.

On Tuesday, June 12, 1917, BH 10 with Montana nurse Alice Ralston, began operations at Le Treport, France: about eighty miles west-southwest of Ypres. BH 10's officer's, nurses, and staff, immediately saw the immense effort facing them. BH 10 was equipped for 500 beds, but faced over two thousand patients. BH 10 could not treat that many and called for immediate medical reinforcements. Reinforcements, thirty doctors and nurses from America, would not come until September 22.[641] BH 10's war report read: "Few of [the staff] had ever come in contact with sickness and suffering on a large scale before." The British Women's Motor Ambulance Convoy No. 10, with about thirty-five to forty well-maintained ambulances all driven by women, supported the hospital. The women ambulance drivers stayed in a large garage with the ambulances near a Le Treport hotel. BH 10 reported the British women drivers were, "Always willing, cheerful, and obliging, never driving fast or carelessly, so as to spare the patient every unnecessary jolt, they won the universal admiration of everyone who saw them..."[642] Le Treport had a train station. At the station the wounded were transferred to the trains for movement south.

Shortly after arriving in Le Treport, horrors of war bathed BH 10. A mustard gas attack along the front sixty miles east of BH 10 brought about 600 gas casualties to BH 10 in less than forty-eight hours. BH 10 chief nurse Margaret A. Dunlop wrote:

> The first hard experience in nursing came...when an exceedingly large convoy of patients, overwhelmed by mustard gas, was received. These patients were horribly gassed and were pictures of misery and intense suffering...The nurses worked hard and faithfully during this short period, but the awfulness and immensity of suffering and cruel barbarity of

war...were a soul-harrowing experience...It was a tremendous strain on mind, heart and body, being untrained to the handling of such large numbers, and not [experienced] to the immensity of the work.[643]

Dunlop wrote that with experience, the American nurses learned to manage mass and grisly casualties, and "the fear of not being equal to the task gradually disappeared."[644]

The British offensive at Ypres began with a massive artillery bombardment. When heard from distant miles, artillery barrages seem as indistinct thunder: a continual rumbling unlike anything yet heard. A person struggles to conclude what the sound is and what it means. The ominous rumble seems to foreshadow something dark and sinister. At night muted flashes from explosions light the horizon. It seems the rain of brimstone on biblical Sodom. Battle-hardened soldiers look with disbelief and wonder who could survive such hellish baptism?[645]

The infantry assault at Ypres began July 31, so did the rain. Rain fell for twenty-eight days in August. The artillery bombardment destroyed the earth's natural ability to drain water. Explosives destroyed river banks and canals. The area around Ypres turned into a sea of unimaginable mud: sucking down wheels, horses, artillery, and wounded and dying men.[646] The British suffered heavy casualties at Passchendaele Ridge near Ypres. Cold weather and vast mud eventually stopped the Third Battle of Ypres in November 1917. Historians dispute casualties, but 250,000 British and 217,000 German casualties seems the butcher's bill. In his memoirs, Lloyd George wrote, "Passchendaele was indeed one of the greatest disasters of the war...No soldier of any intelligence now defends this senseless campaign..."[647]

Ralston and the American nurses at BH 10, were fast learning combat medicine. The long line of medical care for wounded soldiers began with combat medics. Triage, or assessing the severity of wounds and what to do next, began with the medics on the front line. The general theory of procedure began with medics doing what their training and available equipment and bandages allowed. Stretcher bearers carried the wounded through bombardment, mud, and gunfire to the nearest first aid dressing station. Dressing stations were as near the front as reasonable: mostly in make-shift shelters. After treatment in the dressing station, transport carried the wounded to the nearest casualty clearing station. Transport might be stretcher bearers, horse-drawn wagons, or motor ambulances. The AEF estimated four stretcher bearers needed one hour to transport a wounded man one thousand yards and return an empty litter to the starting point.[648] An ever-changing muddy crater-filled battlefield extended the time. The fluid battlefield situation demanded initiative and courage to get the wounded to help. Each station rearward from the front lines in the line-of-care for the wounded, had increased ability, training, personnel, and equipment, to medically treat the casualty.

The British established casualty clearing stations [CCS] behind the front trenches and beyond range of enemy artillery. This meant about four to ten miles behind the first line of trenches. The CCS were clusters of tents with surgical teams generally having two surgeons, an anesthetist, two nurses, and two corpsmen. The CCS personnel were volunteers from nearby base hospitals. At the CCS when casualties arrived, surgeons triaged the patient. If immediate life-saving procedures weren't required, surgeons would stabilize the patient and send the patient to the nearest base hospital. If immediate life-saving aid was needed, surgeons performed operations at the CCS. Attending nurses were surgical nurses. In many battles, where critically wounded soldiers overwhelmed available doctors, surgical nurses triaged arriving wounded and performed minor surgical procedures.

Trench warfare changed war surgery and battlefield medical treatment. Tetanus, lock-jaw, contaminated wounds, war gas wounds, and gas gangrene were in such massive volumes that front-line doctors, nurses, and corpsman had to improvise treatment and learn fast.[649] From the CCS, ambulances or hospital trains carried the wounded to the nearest base hospital: generally sixty to one hundred miles distant. For rail transport, ammunition trains had priority over hospital trains.[650]

On July 22, 1917, BH 10 received its first call for volunteers for two CCS operating teams. Each team would have two doctors, one nurse, and one corpsman. Ralston's colleagues, Helen G. McClelland, and Helen Fairchild, volunteered for a CCS operating team.[651] They were chosen for their ability, experience, and reputation. McClelland was at CCS No. 61 from July 22 to October 6. Fairchild was at CCS No. 4 from July 22, to August 18. At each CCS they lived in tents, and during bombardments worked in make-shift dugouts. They worked twelve to sixteen hours a day.[652] For her heroism under fire at CCS No. 61, Helen Grace McClelland, nurse, ANC, would receive the Army's Distinguished Service Cross: second only to the Medal of Honor. Nurse Helen Fairchild never survived the war. While in France she became seriously ill in December 1917. She died three days after emergency surgery. Fairchild is buried in France.

Rouen, a medieval city on the Seine River about forty-five miles south-southwest of BH 10, is the capital of the region of Normandy. In World War I Rouen was the clearing center for eleven British hospitals. American BH 21 and BH 10 had sailed together to France. BH 21 took over British General Hospital 12 [GH 12] at Rouen.[653] Arriving in Rouen about the same time as BH 10 arrived in Le Treport, BH 21 chief nurse, Julia Stimson, wrote many letters home describing conditions. Stimson began writing of the quaintness of the countryside, the churches, trees, and available cuisine. When war's reality came, her letters became less a tourist, and more a war nurse. Of the weather she wrote on June 30: "It is a cold, rainy day and you'd be surprised to know how really cold it is. At night the night nurses are already wearing all their heavy underwear and their sweaters and their capes. I don't quite see how they are going to manage when real winter comes. We had just two warm days..."[654] In July when the Third Battle of Ypres began, BH 21 began receiving many casualties, the same at other base hospitals. Stimson wrote:

> The other night at midnight I went to the [casualty] receiving tent to see [an incoming] convoy...Doctors worked with [flashlights] with two feeble electric lights. The ambulances arrived at the back door and our stretcher bearers were all there ready to receive [patients]...The stretchers were brought in and laid on the dirt floor as close together as possible... Nurses get the infected and dirty clothes [off] and to the fumigator...unless the patient is in very bad condition...That night sixty-four men, most of them stretcher cases were brought in...and taken to their wards in twenty-five minutes, which you can see is pretty speedy work.
>
> The men have very little to say when they first

come in. They are tired out and forlorn and often in pain and dazed…Most are "G.S.W." [gunshot wound]. Some are unbelievably awful, whole [body] parts blown away…all flesh across the shoulders or between the thighs, where a shell tore right through from behind. I cannot see how some of them live, and live so bravely and cheerfully.[655]

Nursing is an intimate and personal profession. Doctors see the patient for a much shorter time than nurses: especially in combat. Doctors assess the patient from the moment the patient arrives to departure. The assessment isn't a constant doctor-observed minute-by-minute progression. The doctor relies on nurses' observations, and initiative to manage the medical situation within the nurses' ability, training, and common sense. Olive Dent, a British member of the V.A.D. served as a nurse assistant in one of the frontline British war hospitals for two years beginning 1914. An American base hospital unit would later take over the British hospital she worked at. Dent's diary gives a personal and innermost look at combat nursing on the front lines. She wrote: "Active-service nursing…is intensively fascinating, interesting and [rewarding]. The men come practically straight from the trenches, and are deeply grateful for, and appreciative of, the cosy [sic] beds, the cooked food, the absence of vermin…and our [nurses'] attempt to make them comfortable and happy. They have not grown irritable with the tediousness of nursing or wearisome convalescence." Dent gave a veiled warning: "Active-service nursing is distinctly chequered [sic], here today, and there tomorrow, wherever the work is heaviest, and with unexpected happenings…The time-table person who doesn't like to be disturbed from the even tenor of her ways would find little joy in it."[656]

Dent wrote of getting acquainted with the wounded men through day-to-day chit-chat and cheering them with humorous nicknames befitting their situation. She tended the men, cleaned them, fed them, and kept up their spirits in spite of their terrible wounds. And many men died in front of her as she held their hand. At the military cemetery near her hospital, Dent wrote:

> ...Long lines of smooth graves, each headed with a little wooden cross, it is a picture of majestic simplicity, of infinite pathos, nothing tawdry, nothing trivial, nothing but the grandeur of simplicity...Those are the dead who won our freedom. May we cheat time, and ever retain the thought. May it compel us to greater patience, greater fortitude, greater forbearance in the work that is to come."[657]

Winter came and fighting subsided at the end of 1917. The European winter of 1917/18 was the harshest in memory. Persistent penetrating rain, relentless cold, snow, and mud vexed military and medical efforts for months. As the AEF grew with more troops arriving in early 1918, the AEF medical command estimated it needed 171 base hospitals and sixty-eight evacuation hospitals. With many competing priorities and limited number of transport ships, the Army decided infantry and machine gun units had absolute priority.[658] Since U.S. forces had not been seriously engaged in fighting, medical units and nurses had to wait for transportation to France.

In March 1918 Germany launched an offensive against the British left flank at Arras northeast of BH 10. At Arras the British would slow the German advance with heavy losses. The Germans regrouped and launched another furious attack. The Germans gained little.[659] BH 10 was caught in the attack. On March 21 the British called for another CCS from BH 10. Jane Isabelle Stambaugh, nurse, ANC, volunteered. BH 10, the CCS, and Stambaugh, faced crushing odds. During the British retreat, the CCS had to move fast among battlefield locations. During one bombing raid on Amiens thirty-five miles east of BH 10, Stambaugh was wounded by hostile fire and evacuated to England. In 1932, for heroism under fire, nurse Jane Isabel Stambaugh, ANC, would receive the Silver Star Medal retroactive to World War I.[660]

The German advance threatened to cut off and isolate BH 10. BH 10, with Alice Ralston still present for duty, was ordered to evacuate all patients south to Rouen and BH 21. BH 10 chief nurse, Margaret Dunlop, wrote of the evacuation:

> This meant the evacuation of over 10,000 men in two or three days. As many of the patients had but small

chance of living under the best conditions, it [the evacuation] seemed a heart-breaking thing to do...An order came at ten one morning that forty-five nurses should be ready, bag, bedding, and baggage [in two hours] to be sent out of the area. [Thirty nurses were sent] to Rouen; fifteen [sent] to Etreat.

...The remainder of the nurses were ordered to be pack up ready to evacuate with [whatever they could pack]. Anxiety was in every heart but we made little outward show. Time went on and the Germans were held. After two weeks' suspense, more patients came and we were told to carry on without equipment... The tide was [eventually] turned.[661]

On receiving the evacuated wounded from BH 10, Stimson wrote:

We were all so hard pushed physically that [our commander] wired for help and we received a mobile unit from the AEF. The fifteen nurses [from the mobile unit] were soon lost in the shuffle. They were all young, inexperienced, little things from Kentucky, who had not seen a patient since they had landed [in Europe]. Some of them were only twenty-one years old, fresh from small hospitals. It seemed heart-breaking to thrust them into this unbelievable hell of a hospital...Such a baptism of fire they got that first afternoon. The poor little dears, they will never forget [this].[662]

After the German offensive in spring 1918, Pershing began realizing he was making a serious mistake common to generals: he was neglecting his supply and service support. Generals wage war by looking at maps, and with broad sweeping waving of hands, show where troops are to move and attack. Professional logisticians, with their ledger books, spreadsheets, and reams of inventory paperwork, remain a general's frustrating reality and infuriating nightmare. As the general trumpets his masterful attack plan, the supply officer quietly shakes his head, and leaning toward the general whispers, "We don't have the ammunition, transport, fuel, food, or medicine to do that." Monuments and grand memorials, with upright generals on noble mounted steeds, exist in abundance throughout the world. Generals honored forever when history anointed them with eternal grandeur and remembrance from thankful citizens. Honor exists in infantry charges up the enemy-held hill, and generals holding victory flags. No monument or battlefield glory exists for the supply officer who moves tons of bacon, beans, bullets, and bandages, to keep an army moving to fight another day.

In World War I the AEF faced unprecedented logistical demands. AEF soldiers would consume 165,000 *tons* of meat, 250,000 *tons* of flour, 57,000 *tons* of bacon, 49,000 *tons* of sugar, 20,000 *tons* of evaporated milk, and *two billion* cigarettes. Chewing tobacco was not included in the cigarette count. The AEF also brought thousands of horses. Horses need forage, America would ship 427,000 *tons* of feed for the horses. [Italics added.] For medical supplies ARC volunteers in 3,870 chapters throughout America and Montana, rolled over *two hundred fifty million surgical bandages*, and sewed almost *twenty-three million hospital* garments [italics added].[663] The Army's supply chain had three main problems: lack of trained personnel, lack of a centralized logistics command, and many uncoordinated actions and functions.

Pershing began realizing another frustrating fact of modern war: the so-called "tooth to tail" ratio. Generals want many frontline combat riflemen to fight the enemy. However, for every combat rifleman about seven support soldiers exist somewhere immediately behind the rifleman to provide fire support, ammunition, transport, food, signal, medical help, and clerks typing paperwork. In World War II the ratio was as high as one combat soldier to fifteen support soldiers.[664] Combat infantry platoons are supposed to have about forty soldiers. Due to casualties, lack of replacements, sickness, authorized absence, desertion or jail, platoons rarely have all its soldiers. In World War I, the AEF never had its full complement of required doctors and nurses.

Secretary of War Newton Baker soon learned of Pershing's supply and support problem. Baker wanted to send the number-two man on the general staff, General George W. Goethals, acting quartermaster general of the Army, to the AEF and take control of the supply and support mission. Goethals, an engineer by trade and capable man, had built the Panama Canal. By April 1918 Goethals was assistant chief of staff of the Army, and director of the Army's Purchase, Storage, and Traffic Division.[665] Pershing learned Baker wanted Goethals to control AEF's supply. Pershing didn't want the number-two man in the Army in Pershing's sphere of operations. Pershing told Baker he [Pershing] wanted the AEF supply and services to remain under one head—Pershing. Pershing appointed his chief of staff, General James G. Harbord, as overall in charge of AEF supply and transportation.[666] Harbord continued a systematic buildup and laying a foundation for AEF's logistical support. The AEF built large shipping docks, miles of new railroads, storage depots, and training areas. Until the AEF built this support foundation, Pershing couldn't fight a sustained battle. Without medical the AEF would bleed to death.

From December 1917 to spring 1918, America sent less than 900 nurses overseas. Most were individual replacements to fill various vacancies. All but two Montana nurses in World War I [Ralston and Butzerin] went overseas as individual replacements. The AEF first established its office of the chief surgeon in Paris. By January 1918 the office had moved to Tours: the main AEF supply base about 125 miles southwest of Paris, well behind the front lines. Headquarters of the AEF Army Nurse Corps was also in Tours. Arriving Army nurses were staged in Blois: about thirty miles from Tours on the north bank of the Loire River midway between Tours and Orleans.[667] When nurses of the ANC arrived in France, they immediately came under the command and control of the office of the chief surgeon, AEF. Nurses asked a basic question, "Who's in charge?"

In France the greatest administrative difficulty facing arriving nurses was the AEF did not have a chief nurse with authority to get things done. Pershing's overall supply problem extended to nurses. No person with authority was coordinating all the nurses' supply and personnel needs with uniforms, equipment, assignments, transfers, and resignations. The AEF surgeon general admitted the AEF did not have accurate records on, and did not know for certain, where its doctors and nurses were stationed.[668] To begin working these matters, the surgeon general of the AEF appointed nurse Bessie S. Bell, ANC, to the surgeon general's staff. Bell was capable, competent, and efficient, but lacked the needed dynamics, forcefulness, and support to sufficiently advocate needs of the nurses. Given that, the chief nurses of the American base hospitals had to rely on their initiative, and resourcefulness to meet the nursing requirements they faced. The AEF would not get a capable chief nurse until November 1918 when the AEF appointed Julia Stimson, former chief nurse, BH 21, as chief nurse, AEF. After the war, for her leadership and abilities, Stimson would receive the Army's Distinguished Service Medal.

Montana nurses began arriving in the AEF in late spring 1918. Harriet O'Day, Margaret MacCauley, Elizabeth Sandelius, Virginia Flanagan, and Harriet Vineyard reported to Blois, France, in June 1918. The AEF assigned them to BH 43 at Blois. BH 43 became operational in early July 1918. The hospital occupied seven buildings in Blois. BH 43 required more people as each building began operating as a separate hospital. BH 43 had one thousand beds, but soon expanded to 2,300 beds. For a time, BH 43 received and processed all incoming nurses to the AEF[669]

Other Montana nurses arrived in June: Effie Fowler, Grace Gibson, Lucy Walters, and Mary Hall. The Army assigned Fowler, Gibson, Walters, and Hall to other hospitals throughout France. Walters, the indomitable nurse from Glasgow, was sent to the largest AEF hospital complex in France: BH 8 at Savenay on the west coast of France. The AEF tried to establish specialty hospitals based on type of wound. BH 8 began as maxillofacial wound hospital but soon accepted all casualties.

History doesn't say if these few Montana nurses from mining camps, railroad stops and cities, became acquainted, friends, buddies, or tent mates. They traveled together across the ocean, braved submarine menace for almost two weeks at sea, went by rail to London, crossed the channel to France, and were sent to Blois. The AEF assigned five Montana nurses to BH 43. It's hard to think these women didn't meet.

What few restful hours people have in war, especially on the front lines, they talk of and think of everything: mostly sleep and food. One person is generally the tent cook. Regardless of gender, someone has an inherent ability to take canned food or stale rations, however sour and unpalatable, and create a feast. They laugh in exhaustion-induced humor. They create a world, however small, that they can survive in. At day's end they talk and think of home. They're careful not to cry or show emotion. Leaders have to be strong, they cannot break under pressure. If so, it becomes a cancer and shakes the unit irreparably. Unit members rely on each other, for at times that's all they have. Frontline soldiers facing bullets, bombs, shrapnel and death every day, have earned the right to be critical of those who haven't. By some force of will gathered from a spirit borne of Montana hardship and dogged independence, these women were rising to a call of service previously unknown.

Thousands of American troops poured into France. In August 1917 over eighteen thousand had landed. By June 1918 well over a quarter million had arrived, with more coming. America shouldered a greater share of combat. French marshal Ferdinand Foch, became, at least on paper, the supreme commander-in-chief of the Allied armies. Pershing refused to give up command to Foch and insisted the AEF remain an independent army. Pershing, mindful of his instructions from Wilson, refused any suggestion to permanently break up the AEF and give his soldiers piecemeal to French or British armies. In his workings with Foch and other Allied commanders, Pershing was regarded as one of the most successful military diplomats of the war. In negotiations he never unintentionally lost his temper and had great personal charm.[670]

On May 27 the Germans began their hardest drive of the spring. They caught the Allies off guard and pierced the French lines. Pershing sent three divisions, the First, Second, and Third Infantry Divisions to reinforce the French. Among the Americans was the Fourth Marine Brigade composed of the Fifth and Sixth Marine Regiments. On the afternoon of June 3, the Germans attacked the Marines with fixed bayonets. The Marines cut them down with expert rifle fire. On June 6 the Marines were ordered to take a hill overlooking the French forces. To take the hill the Marines' charge across the fields of red poppies at Belleau Wood remains storied in American military history. The Marines suffered severe casualties, it was one of the costliest battles in Marine Corps history. The battle would last until June 26 when the Marines finally cleared Belleau Wood in one of the bloodiest and ferocious battles America fought in World War I.[671]

The Third Infantry Division, protecting Paris from German advance, would face the Germans on the bend of the Marne River near Chateau-Thierry. The Third Division refused to withdraw under intensive German attack, earning the division their famous moniker, "The Rock of the Marne." No German unit breached the lines of the Third Division.[672] American casualties were coming fast. American medical units, wherever they were and whatever their size, faced a torrent of wounded men.

The evacuation hospital ["evacs"] was an American invention to serve battlefield wounded. These hospitals had 500 beds, each division had two evacs. Evacs were mobile units designed with essential medical equipment to follow an infantry division in battle. The hospitals were set beyond enemy artillery range about ten to twelve miles from the front lines. Ideally the hospital would have ten operating teams, each with two doctors, a nurse, a corpsman, and anesthetist or nurse-anesthetist. The evacs were to be located near rail lines to quickly move the wounded farther to the rear.

When American troops were fully engaged in battle, the AEF still did not have enough nurses to meet the increased demand of caring for the wounded. Front line evacs needed nurses. The AEF began stripping base hospitals of available nurses and sending the nurses to evacs. The ARC war journal reads: …"Base hospitals have been stripped of every available officer and nurse for the purpose of forming surgical teams [supporting the troops]…The situation was saved only by the self-sacrificing spirit of the officers, nurses, and men…It was not at all uncommon for nurses to work fourteen to eighteen hours a day for weeks at a time…"[673]

Montana nurses served in the evacs. Mary Hall was born in England in 1879 and immigrated to America. She was trained a nurse in Los Angeles. She came to Montana and nursed in Missoula.[674] Hall entered the ANC at Missoula in January 1918. The Army first sent her to Camp Pike, Arkansas, and then to France in June 1918. The AEF assigned her to BH 18 at Bazoilles-sur-Meuse, northeast of AEF headquarters at Chaumont. During the German offensive in summer 1918, AEF needed nurses wherever found. Hall was reassigned to Evac 6 the third week of July. Evac 6 arrived at Meaux, on the Marne River northeast of Paris, July 20. Evac 6 was designed as a 350-bed hospital, but during the first hours of the Second Battle of the Marne, the hospital was receiving 200 patients *every hour* [italics added.] Immediately before the wounded came, Evac 6 received thirty nurses as reinforcements. Hall probably was among the thirty.[675] Daisie P. Beyea, a reserve nurse, wrote of conditions at Evac 6:

> In an open wheat field, with an ammunition dump on one side and artillery on the other, while the boys were throwing a pontoon bridge across the Marne

in front of us, we began to [prepare to move]…Oh, the flies, the dead horses, and the dead Germans! At three a.m. the [artillery] barrage started. The then word came down the line: 'The boys go over the top at five!'. A flash of light, the roar of the guns and then the very earth rocking under our feet as we fumbled with our helmets and gas masks. Crash after crash followed all day long until five, when the ambulances began pouring in. The tents were overflowing, but still the ambulances line the roads. Darkness came, lit every few seconds with an exploding shell…Nurses and doctors were working faster and faster. The strain grew intense.[676]

The battle front rapidly advanced and Evac 6 had to move forward. On July 28 all patients were relocated and the hospital prepared to move. As Allied troops moved forward, the evacs moved with them keeping several miles to the rear. By August 25 Evac 6 had largely finished supporting the Second Battle of the Marne. The hospital would move to Souilly: a few miles south of Verdun. By August 27 the hospital was receiving more patients. Evac 6 would have little time to rest. The Meuse-Argonne offensive would begin in September: the last great offensive of the war.[677] Hall would stay with Evac 6 for the remainder of the war. Three of her cousins fighting in the British army would die in the war.[678] [679]

In war, soldiers size up each other fast. Can you put your life in the hands of the person next to you? Is their judgment sound? Will they break under fire? Even in combat, war has an ironic respectability born within the human experience that people nurture. Sometimes a unit has a person, a kind courteous person that in the realm of simple decency, the Army should have said, "You're too nice, you stay home." Maybe Ann should have stayed home. She didn't, and she saw war few Montana women did.

Ann Emelia Dobias was born December 17, 1891, in Sleepy Eye, Minnesota:, the daughter of Joseph and Mary (Peterka) Dobias. She finished her schooling in Angus, Minnesota. Ann entered the Warren Hospital Nurse's School in Warren, Minnesota. In 1913 she graduated with honors.[680] She followed the railroad and nursed in Glasgow,

Montana. When war came Ann entered the ANC at Glasgow in January 1918.[681] The Army assigned her first to Camp Pike, Arkansas: near Little Rock. Ann had a photograph taken of her in full ANC uniform wearing a wide-brimmed nurse's hat. With her wire spectacles over compassionate eyes and with a slightly rounded face, Ann looked pleasant and ready. But sometimes soldiers have to work hard to convince themselves they are indeed ready: if that is possible in war. In August 1918 Ann sailed from New York City to France. She arrived when the Allies and Germans were locked in the last desperate furious battles of World War I. Originally assigned to BH 15, Ann either volunteered or was sent to the front battle lines to Evac 5.[682]

Evac 5 was assigned to the First and Second Infantry Divisions. The divisions were in heavy fighting. Evac 5 moved to Crepy near Paris to receive wounded and gassed soldiers. At the end of August, Evac hospitals 5 and 6 were at Chateau-Thierry. The wounded were sent first to field hospitals, and those not needing immediate life-saving treatment were sent to the evacs. Evac 5 had five large tents erected in line from admission to surgery to receiving wards.[683] Dobias was a nurse anesthetist. She worked surgeries. Several evacs and field hospitals served in and around the thundering battlefields near Chateau-Thierry. In late August these evacs and field hospitals combined, treated almost six thousand patients, performed over 700 surgeries, and recorded 133 patient deaths.[684]

Of the challenges at Evac 5, Dobias wrote:

> ...Have been on a surgical team giving ether, and moved often, following the American drives. Have traveled over some very interesting ground since leaving America, old and new battlefields, ruins, shell holes and everything else...
> We are living in tents and oh boy it gets cold! We have to pinch ourselves in the morning to see if we are all there, break the ice in our drinking cups, wash our faces, then beat it for our mess line...pass our outdoor kitchen cooks, throw everything together in our kits, and stand in the mud and water to eat. Wonderful life! Like living on a [Montana homestead] claim. We sit on the ground, woodpile or tomato cans. Food is

good, black coffee, oatmeal, dry bread and dirt...we seem to be happy through all this roughing. It does not seem to hurt us.[685]

In another letter Dobias wrote:

It is perfectly wonderful to see the smile break over the stern, sober faces of our boys returning from the front...when they hear our American voices as they call it...Most the time we are here, we wear our grey uniforms, rain coats and rubber boots, and sweaters, oceans of them, if you happen to have more than one, for its [sic] cold, beastly cold, wet and muddy. A white uniform is a thing of the past, and trench coats and caps have taken their place. Must close [now], its [sic] getting too dark for me to see and we don't have lights.[686]

Dobias stayed with Evac 5 through the battles near Ypres, the Meuse-Argonne and the Oise-Aisne offensives. She stayed with Evac 5 after the armistice. When war ended, because of her qualifications as nurse anesthetist, the AEF assigned her to several hospitals in France. Ann would not return to America for another year.[687]

Gertrude Sloane, from Missoula, entered the ANC late in 1917. As one of the first Montana nurses to arrive in France, Sloane first reported for duty at the ARC military hospital in Paris. The ARC established the hospital and operated it jointly with the AEF: hence the title "Red Cross Military Hospital." At times the hospital accepted American, Allied, and civilian wounded. ARC Military Hospital 1 was a hybrid hospital operating to help French civilians and Allied wounded under rules established by the Army judge advocate.[688]

Sloane served in Paris until January 1918 when the Army assigned her to BH 15 at AEF headquarters, Chaumont. During the Second Battle of the Marne, the AEF established Mobile Hospitals 1 and 3. A mobile hospital was intended to be smaller and quicker to move than an evac, but could still treat seriously wounded nearer the battle line. One Army corps had two mobile hospitals.[689] When the Second Battle of the Marne got perilously close to Paris, the AEF needed medical reinforcements. The AEF war report read: "The work referred to was done at the most critical period of the war, when Paris...was almost in the grasp of the enemy and when everyone was working under the great pressure, both physically and mentally."[690] The AEF assigned Sloane to Mobile Hospital 1 [MH 1] in July 1918. In June MH 1 treated two thousand patients. On July 29 MH 1 and Sloane moved about two miles east of Chateau-Thierry and was attached to Evac 6 where Mary Hall worked. Combined, the two hospitals performed 1,711 operations from July 29 to August 20. After the Second Battle of the Marne, Sloane returned to ARC Military Hospital 1.[691] [692]

American Base Hospital 57 [BH 57] opened in Paris, September 19, 1918. BH 57 occupied a large municipal school: "a very handsome stone building with two large courtyards, a small paved garden, and a glass-enclosed sun parlor."[693] The hospital had eighteen hundred beds for Allied soldiers. The Kingdom of Siam was one of twenty-nine countries that had declared war on Germany and the Central Powers. The King of Siam sent twelve hundred men to France to fight.[694] The king's men needed medical care and many were admitted to BH 57. Nurse Cora Viola Craig, from Glasgow, Montana, arrived in France after serving six months at the Fort Riley, Kansas, hospital. The AEF assigned her to BH 57.[695] [696]

Craig never married and had no children. She wanted to be a missionary among the Siamese. When war came she became a nurse and entered the ANC. At BH 57 she asked to be assigned to the ward treating Siamese wounded and sick soldiers. To her pleasure she was assigned to treat the Siamese. The King of Siam noticed her care and commitment to his soldiers. He awarded Craig an engraved silver medal in appreciation of services rendered to Siamese officers and men while on the western front. The medal had an engraved portrait of the king and an inscription reading, "In appreciation of services rendered the Siamese volunteers." Craig is probably the only woman in Montana or maybe in the United States decorated by the King of Siam.[697]

Nurse Virginia Flanagan and her three friends were sent from Paris to Blois: the nurses' staging base. By some mix-up the Army sent them back to Paris. They were stationed at the Red Cross Hospital in Paris at Neuilly. During the Second Battle of the Marne, wounded from Chateau-Thierry overflowed the hospital and Flanagan wrote "there was a general air of depression." She could hear and see the artillery fire and wrote many civilians had left Paris. The courage of the wounded soldiers made a lasting impression on her. She wrote:

> …I have never seen such cheerful and courageous patients as our soldier boys, and it was hard to understand. I recall asking a boy with a far-away look in his eyes what he was thinking about, and he replied, "About my buddies out there in the rain and the cold, and here I am in comfort." My thought was…[he had] wounds that might never heal, and if they did, would leave terrific scars which he would have always.[698]

Along the battle lines the AEF was getting desperate in finding nurses. A pretty and ever-smiling twenty-five-year-old nurse from a gritty Montana mining town volunteered.

Elizabeth Dorothy "Sandy" Sandelius was born April 10, 1893, in Cokedale, Montana. Her parents, Peter and Christina [Ek] Sandelius, were Swedish immigrants among many immigrants who came to Montana's mining towns. Townsfolk accurately named Cokedale due to the 122 brick coke ovens lining the narrow valley on the north side of Miner Creek beneath Canyon Mountain. From nearby mines, miners brought coal to the coke ovens where controlled burning removed water, coal-gas, coal-tar and other impurities from the coal. A fuel remained with few impurities and high carbon content. Coke ovens poisoned the landscape. Smoke and gas came from the ovens leaving a cheerless place where breathing became an effort and green vegetation a rarity under fine ash.

Sandy grew to womanhood in this narrow valley beneath tall pine covered mountains bordering the north region of the Yellowstone. By 1914 she had graduated from the Training School for Nurses at St. John's Hospital, in Helena. In June 1914 she became the 265th registered nurse in Montana.[699] In 1916 she was the superintendent of the Stillwater Hospital in the small railroad town of Columbus, Montana. Columbus, county seat of Stillwater County, was sixty miles east of Cokedale at the confluence of the scenic Stillwater and Yellowstone Rivers. Mineral deposits existed southwest of Columbus. Thomas C. Benbow began a chromium mine in the Beartooth

Mountains near Columbus. He was also a gadgeteer and eccentric. He enjoyed designing airships using torpedo-looking balloons. Benbow seemed good at it as he won a $50,000 prize in the 1904 St. Louis World's Fair for the longest distance flown by an airship he designed.[700]

Cebron Benbow, Thomas' son, met Sandy in Columbus. Cebe ["Seeb"] and Sandy fell in love. War clouds loomed. The Army needed nurses, and Cebe was interested in entering Army aviation. Duty called both. Wanting to finalize their lasting devotion to each other, Cebe and Sandy quietly married in Columbus, October 6, 1917: Cebe's twenty-fourth birthday. Two weeks later on October 20, Sandy took the loyalty oath at Columbus, Montana, and entered the ANC.

Early in World War I the Army prohibited married nurses from enrolling in the ANC. Sandy never told the Army she was married. In her official War Department documents, she gave her name as "Elizabeth D. Sandelius." At five feet five inches tall, 140 pounds, with brown hair and brown eyes, Sandy looked progressive for the times. She had a pleasant face, engaging eyes, and playful girlish smile. She wore her hair short and combed back over an open neck light-colored blouse for her official War Department certificate of identification. She was twenty-five when she went to war.[701] The Army assigned her husband, Cebe, to an Army aviation training base at Mather Field, California. Cebe and Sandy never served together in war.

After serving a six-month tour-of-duty at the military hospital in Fort Riley, Kansas, Sandelius sailed to France in June 1918. The Army issued her the round "dog tags" common to soldiers. Her tags read, "Elizabeth D. Sandelius, AEF 12660." The number was Sandelius' Red Cross registration number. The Army assigned her to BH 15 at AEF headquarters. The Army established BH 15 in the French artillery base at Chaumont. Sandelius could not take a camera, but she collected tourist postcards of Chaumont and the French base.[702]

The Second Battle of the Marne saw the AEF in desperate fighting along the trench lines north of Chaumont and along the Marne River. The Twenty-Eighth Infantry Division met the German army at the Battle of Chateau-Thierry, July 18. Fighting continued through the summer. The AEF with the Twenty-Eighth Division needed immediate medical help. The Twenty-Eighth Division had four field hospitals [FH]: FH 109, FH 110, FH 111, and FH 112. A field hospital is smaller than an evac and quicker to move, but it can still do surgeries.

Sandelius volunteered for FH 112. FH 112 set up at Chateau-Thierry in the ruined buildings of a local hotel. Field hospitals intentionally tried not to use tents. Clusters of tents meant soldiers were there, and enemy artillery fire followed. The hospital operated in a triple capacity: divisional triage, treating seriously wounded, and acting as a divisional evac. From July 25 to August 9, FH 112 received almost five thousand patients and performed over 200 surgical operations.[703] After August 9, FH 112 moved to Cohan, France. Cohan was a rural crossroads village with few undamaged buildings. FH 112 set up tents near the roads at Cohan.

The battle sector near Chateau-Thierry required more medical help. FH 112 needed reinforcements. Navy Operating Team No. 1, [Navy 1] from Navy Base Hospital 1, Brest, France, was called forward to help the Marines fighting on the front lines at Belleau Wood. Navy nurses Mary Elderkins and Katherine McCarthy were surgical nurses in Navy 1.[704] On August 11 Navy 1 had to find FH 112 somewhere along the blazing, exploding, and dangerous front lines. FH 112 had moved again closer to the fast advancing front lines. The Navy had to do the best they could, move fast under fire, and find FH 112. Elderkins wrote:

> ...An officer [from FH 112] said he feared it would not be possible for any of us to go on that night, as the [Germans] were shelling the roads and [firing many] gas shells in the vicinity of [FH 112]. Nevertheless, [I and the other nurses] started up. We were provided with helmets and gas masks.
>
> That was a wild ride. We passed through village after village where not a house had been spared, and the only signs of life were the military...Ammunition trucks were racing in both directions, and ...no lights were allowed...About a half hour before we reached [FH 112] we were stopped and told that all masks were to be [at the ready.] We had no more than adjusted them when the real gas alarm came...We arrived at [FH 112] in pitch darkness...Gas alarms sounded continuously.
>
> In the morning, we found ourselves in a little

town called Cohan. [FH 112] was at the foot of the hill; from the top you could get a good idea where the fighting was…At night it seemed like the battle was being fought just outside our tents.

…The days were intensely hot and the nights bitterly cold. The flies were unbearable. We had air raids night after night with no opposition for there were no anti-aircraft [guns] nearby and seemingly few French or American airplanes.

When we were not operating at night, we spent the time from darkness to dawn in a cellar twenty feet underground. It just held seven cots and thirteen nurses were supposed to sleep there. It we sat erect on the cot our heads struck the rough stone above. Water dripped on us all night long. Huge black bugs crawled about and after we quieted down we could hear the rats. We, ourselves, felt like rats in some trap, for in case of a direct hit our chances of getting out were slim.

On the morning of [August 10] the Germans had found our range. They opened fire on us, or rather on their objectives about us. With shells falling all about us, we went back that night three miles.[705]

Nurse Gertrude Bowling, ANC, would also write of FH12 and the difficulty in getting a gas mask on unconscious patients.[706] She wrote of the shelling and treachery of people thought friends:

…One morning we heard…a new sound, the long, shrill whistle of the Hun's Big Bertha [artillery] followed in a few seconds by the crash of explosion… All my life I have read of the whistle and whine of shells. The vacuum left over our heads as the shells seemed to pass lower and lower, was so vivid in our minds, we thought we could reach up and touch it with our hands…Many bombs exploded near us… Two proved to be duds. Had they exploded quite a few of us [would have been killed]. Later we learned a woman spy had signaled the [German] planes with a flashlight from the top of a hillside on which our tents were placed. She was a middle-aged French woman and pretended to speak no English, until her condemnation was [revealed].[707]

FH 112 operated at Cohan for about a month under frequent shelling and bombing. The Army nurses did not withdraw to safety but stayed with the wounded. On August 12 a German aerial bomb dropped within fifteen feet of a hospital tent but did not explode.[708] On September 11 the Twenty-Eighth Division closed FH 112, and the hospital moved by truck and train to Moussy, northeast of Paris. Major General Charles H. Muir, commanding general of the U.S. Twenty-Eighth Infantry Division, would cite Elizabeth Sandelius, ANC, for heroism under fire. The citation reads:

> For eight consecutive days in August 1918, [Elizabeth Sandelius] was on duty with Field Hospital Company 112 operating north of Cohan, France. Notwithstanding nightly air raids upon the town, harassing shell fire during the daytime, she repeatedly refused to retire to the rear and continued to administer to the needs of the wounded, exhibiting at all times a splendid spirit of self-sacrifice, courage, and devotion to duty which largely contributed to the welfare and rapid convalescence of the wounded officers and soldiers entrusted to her care.[709]

After the Second Battle of the Marne, Sandelius returned to BH 15. She later transferred to BH 90, also at AEF headquarters, for the duration of the war and months beyond.

With no letup the battle lines heaved, thundered, and bled through summer and into autumn. Pershing was ready to occupy a large section of the Allied battle line. His plan was to attack a German bulge in the Allied line, called a "salient", at St. Mihiel. On the Meuse River, St, Mihiel was about twenty miles south of the slaughter-hole of Verdun and sixty miles northeast of Pershing's AEF headquarters. Pershing expertly planned the attack. Due to his lack of foresight in getting support troops, engineers, medical, and transportation support from America during the AEF buildup, Pershing relied heavily on Allied support.[710] The attack on the St. Mihiel salient began September 12. The attack was the AEF's first battlefield victory.

Pershing cleared the Germans from St. Mihiel and began shifting American forces to take part in a battle along the entire western front called the Meuse-Argonne Offensive. Pershing would attack on a twenty-mile front in northeast France in the Argonne region. The wooded hilly Argonne region of northeast France is about forty miles long and ten miles wide. It has deep valleys and watersheds. It would be a hard place to fight in the attack. The Germans were not expecting Pershing to attack soon.

On September 21 Pershing moved his battle headquarters to Souilly: about ten miles southwest of Verdun. Telephone operators of the WTU went with his headquarters. Montana's Mary Vinnier and Marie Paul Adams, went to Souilly. They began serving in direct combat communications. Few records exist of the hours worked, the calls connected, the artillery fire commands relayed, and the desperate calls for help, that Pershing's WTU telephone operators handled during the last final and desperate attack in the Meuse-Argonne. Pershing would cite Vannier for meritorious service in his combat communications center at Souilly.[711] Pershing could be a dashing fellow, and after the war on February 2, 1919, at a tea party, Vannier, then a chief operator, had the honor of dancing the first dance with him.[712] [713]

On September 26 Pershing attacked north after a tremendous artillery barrage on the Germans.[714] Many of his soldiers that day served America years later in higher authority: Colonel George C. Marshall, Lieutenant Colonel George S. Patton, Jr, and an artillery captain from Missouri, Harry S. Truman. Patton was severely wounded in the attack.[715] As the attack began, casualties mounted and medical support was thin. Help needed and fast. BH 15 would be called upon again for medical help. Evac 4 arrived in France in June and went into action almost immediately during the Second Battle of the Marne. Evac 4 now faced another even greater Allied offensive. Many doctors and nurses already assigned to BH 15 reinforced Evac 4. Harriet Marie O'Day, nurse, ANC, BH 15, went to Evac 4 to help. On the bloody fields of France near Verdun, she was a long way from her home in Billings, Montana.

O'Day was born February 16, 1890, in Sumner, Bremer County, Iowa, near where Iowa, Minnesota, and Wisconsin meet. She was the second child of William and Elizabeth [Daly] O'Day. As a child she moved with her parents to St. Paul, Minnesota, and then in 1906 to Billings. Elizabeth worked as a nurse in the Billings Northern hospital.[716] By early 1907 William had abandoned Elizabeth, Harriet, [called "Hattie"] and William Jr. The court granted Elizabeth a decree of divorce in Billings in 1907.[717] Harriet went to school in Billings. In 1910 Elizabeth married a Fergus County, Montana, rancher and had moved near Lewistown. Harriet went with her mother. Elizabeth' second marriage failed three years later. Harriet enrolled in nursing school at St. Joseph's Hospital in St. Paul, Minnesota. After graduating, Harriet returned to Billings and worked as an ARC registered nurse. When war came Harriet entered the ANC, November 14, 1917, at Billings. After serving at Fort Riley, Kansas, O'Day went to France in June 1918 with several Montana nurses. She worked at BH 43 until the Allied offensives in spring 1918. In July 1918 the AEF reassigned her to BH 15.

It isn't known if the AEF asked for nurse volunteers, or assigned the nurses regardless of the nurses' wishes, to the desperately short-handed evacs on the front lines. O'Day departed BH 15 mid-July and began treating wounded at Evac 4 near Chateau-Thierry during the Second Battle of the Marne, and later during Pershing's Meuse-Argonne Offensive.[718] In mid-July Evac 4 had set up operations in a wheat field at Ecury-sur-Coole, on the Marne River at Champagne about forty miles west of Verdun. Nurse Sigrid M. Jorgensen, ANC, arrived with O'Day at Evac 4. Jorgensen wrote:

> On July 14 our troops were making the first big offensive by themselves. We were dumped off in the middle of a wheat field outside a small town called Ecury. [Evac 4] consisted of ten [large] tents, a dozen large khaki tents and numerous smaller one. This whole hospital was just twenty-four hours old when we arrived...A dozen tired but cheerful nurses greeted us.
>
> Our operating room...had four tables arranged down each side [of the tent]. The night teams relieved

the day teams. There was no stopping for explanations. The faces of the wounded all around us on the ground and on the tables, everywhere we looked seemed to say: "When will my turn come?"[719]

By July 17 heavy casualties were overwhelming Evac 4. The hospital received about 1,200 patients in forty-eight hours. During the onrush of patients, practically the entire hospital had no sleep for seventy-two hours. The hospital moved with the offensive and passed through Chateau-Thierry on August 6. On passing through Chateau-Thierry, Jorgensen wrote:

> ...Everywhere along the road we saw ruins, torn trees, dead horses, [and] shelled roads...
> Our entrance to Chateau-Thierry was five days after the Germans left. The city must have been very beautiful before the attack...Now almost every house was shelled to pieces...no civilian inhabitants remained.[720]

On midnight August 24 a German airplane bombed the hospital, the bomb hit the ground but did not explode. The bomb was a "dud." The end of September saw Evac 4 in the Meuse-Argonne Offensive. When the offensive began, Evac 4 reported the horizon was "a blaze of light and sleep was impossible." The AEF was taking heavy casualties and ordered Evac 4 to increase its capacity to 900 beds. Many American wounded were not found for over three days.[721]

On October 29 the first detachment of Evac 4 left for Fromerville on the Meuse River: a deserted village about three miles west of Verdun. Jorgensen wrote:

> Our last camp at Fromerville will never be forgotten by any member of our little hospital. It was hardship, sacrifice and toil from the day we came there. Something seemed to tell us that this was the last fight, and that it was going to be to the bitter end.[722]

Winter weather began in late October and early November. Drenching cold rains came. Jorgenson wrote:

> The mud and cold will always be associated with our stay at Fromerville. Our uniforms had at this time been considerably changed. Instead of uniforms with such trimmings as white collars and caps, we were then wearing high rubber boots, trench coats, and rain hats, not to speak of sweaters and underwear. They were on in several layers. The mud was so deep we could hardly get about, and the work was piling in on us.[723]

Fromerville was well within German artillery range. Verdun never ceased being a place of human misery, death, and utter destruction. Nearing the final hours of war both sides were hemorrhaging artillery and gunfire. Anything resembling military was a target. Collections of tents in the open were never safe. The Germans had 8-inch artillery and were using it expertly. Jorgensen wrote:

> The tents were pitched on the top of a hill overlooking the ruins of the village. Verdun was only about four kilometers from us. At this time the Germans were shelling Verdun very heavily, but we never dreamt for a minute that they were after out little camp, when one morning [November 3] they got our range and threw over thirteen shells. Headquarters was shelled down completely; some shells struck the tents, and the shrapnel flew in every direction. The details cannot be explained; it all happened so quickly. The concussion of the air when these huge shells burst was terrible. No one knew where the next one would fall, but I am glad to say there was not one coward among our nurses.[724]

Cassie White, from New York, was chief nurse at Evac 4. She gave the order for all nurses to lend immediate assistance to evacuate the wounded to the top of a nearby hill away from the artillery fire. One explosion knocked her down. She got up and kept going. Jorgenson continued in her report:

> All who were able to do so helped the boys. Some carried stretchers, others went about with bandages and dressings, and still others did their best to cover the boys up. As usual it was raining, and it was cold. We lost two of our best sergeants, and one officer and twelve boys were wounded…[725]

O'Day wrote three letters home to Montana to assure her mother, Elizabeth, that Harriet was safe. Weeks later, Harriet found the AEF hadn't mailed any of Harriet's letters. She hurriedly sent a cable to Elizabeth reading Harriet was alive and reasonably well. O'Day wrote her mother about Fromerville and a Montana wounded soldier:

> We were in Fromerville [near] Verdun on Sept. 30 and were…shelled on Nov 1. Three of the men on night duty were killed…I was terribly upset about Hobensack, a prince of a fellow from Montana who lived four hours after having a horrible piece of shrapnel tear through his abdomen.[726]

After the artillery barrage ceased, Evac 4 moved all patients to Souilly. Evac 4 would finally be released from duty on February 18, 1919. For heroism under fire at Fromerville the nurses at Evac 4 and Harriet M. O'Day, were cited in dispatch by Pershing.[727] Nurse Sylvene Nye, Evac 4, would receive the French Croix de Guerre with gilt star.[728]

From the field hospitals and evacuation hospitals, available transportation took the wounded arrived to the many base hospitals in the AEF. Langres, south of Chaumont, was a large AEF training base and home to the AEF officer command school. The ancient city on the Marne River was built on a fortified limestone outcropping of the same name about 300 feet above the surrounding fields. Langres had two base hospitals: BH 88 and BH 53. The AEF built both hospitals at the base of the promontory on Langres' east side. On September 16 BH 53 began receiving American wounded. BH 88 would become operational on October 7. Being south of Pershing's headquarters at Chaumont but near the battle lines, both hospitals received many wounded: largely by rail. Five Montana nurses served at BH 53: Eunice Collins, Susie Welborn, Elizabeth Sterling, Clara Ruff, and Florence Biddles: soon to call Billings her home. Maude Osborne from Laurel, Montana, served at BH 88.

The official report of BH 53 largely followed the challenges of other hospitals: lack of supplies, lack of proper food for patients, no coal stoves for heat or hot water, and always the incessant rain and mud. BH 53's unit report read:

> Shortage of blankets, the non-arrival of coal stoves, the lack of oil for lanterns and small cooking stoves in the wards all combined to make the cold weather in October a very unpleasant experience. The patients lay wakeful and shivering while the night nurses and corpsmen put on all available sweaters.. [and other clothes]…and tried hard to work with frost bitten fingers or sat by candle light thinking of all that might be done for the patients in the way of hot drinks, hot water bottles, etc, if only there were oil for the stoves.[729]

A military force cannot expect its people to continue without rest. Rest does not imply laziness or being a "slacker." Rest is needed for the human body and the human mind to regain strength and resolve. Soldiers don't need much other than a good cup of hot coffee, a decent meal, and an hour or two away from danger and distress to recuperate: so did the nurses of the AEF and BH 53 and 88. Even in the stress of tending battle wounded, the nurses of BH 53, and other places throughout the AEF looked to recreation of their making. BH 53 nurses scheduled dances with any band they could find. The ARC had reading rooms and rest areas for the nurses. The YMCA and ARC huts were the nurses' principal means to relax: if for a few minutes from the duties of tending the terribly wounded and gassed.

For their outstanding service in war and to the City of Langres, the mayor of Langres, in ceremony assembled, on March 9, 1919, awarded the soldiers, doctors, and nurses of BH 53, the coat of arms of the City of Langres. The mayor said:

> All generations who have lived upon this promontory from which springs our Marne [river], glorious in a two-fold victory, all our ancestors unite with us in paying homage of the appreciation and admiration for the whole people of America. It is with joyful pride that we attach this coat-of-arms to your colors and place them as insignia upon the uniform of your personnel.[730]

The AEF would not allow members of BH 53 to wear the Langres coat-of-arms on the left shoulder of their uniforms. To mollify BH 53 soldiers, the AEF designed a less ornate shoulder patch having interlocking numbers "5" and "3." Nurse Florence Mary Marvel Biddles, was born in Newton, England, and after the war would became an American citizen. A trained nurse from the Royal Salop Hospital in Shrewsbury, England, she would soon live in Montana. She served as a nurse at BH 53, and proudly sewed the original Langres coat-of-arms to the left shoulder of her formal ANC uniform. In the one photograph taken of her in her full uniform with the Langres coat-of-arms, the diminutive and handsome Biddles has a look of dignity, firmness, and resolve. History dares to remove the Langres coat-of-arms she and the other nurses rightfully and forever earned.

In war, rumors abound: rumors of weather, attacks, troop movements, promotions, card games, home-made booze, and surrender. Beginning November 1918 rumors of an impending armistice went up and down the battle lines. Rumors reached Evac 4 and its nurses, but this time the rumors were fact. The Armistice was signed, the guns went silent. Jorgensen wrote:

> It was difficult for us to realize that the end was so near. We will never forget November 11th when the news reached us that the Armistice had been signed. To think that once again we were to have peace.
>
> Even though our wounded continued to come in for twelve hours after the Armistice, the change was felt everywhere. In the profound stillness after the barrage ceased, we all had our own little way in which we may our joy known. Now that it is all over…we

look back on the days of hardships, but strangely enough, it is not the discomforts we think of, because they were small compared to the joy it was to have been permitted to be up with our boys at the time when they needed us most, and I do not believe but that if the time came again when we were needed, every one of us who went to the front would ask to go again.[731]

Going home was no longer a short-lived dream in the muddy blood-soaked fields of France.

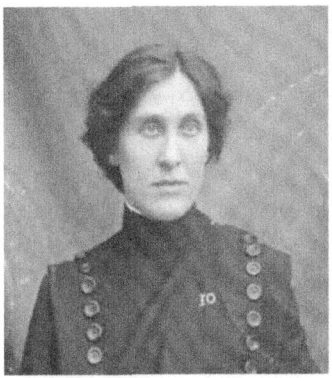

(*Left*) Alice H. Ralston. The embroidered "10" on her uniform designates Base Hospital 10. Courtesy National Archives and Records Administration

(*Below*) Base Hospital 10, Le Treport, France. Courtesy National Library of Medicine

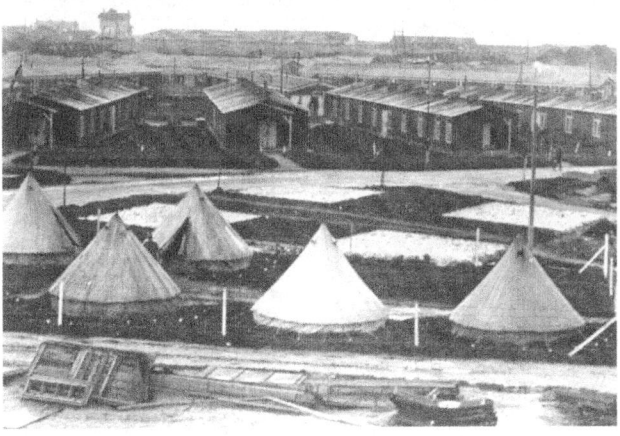

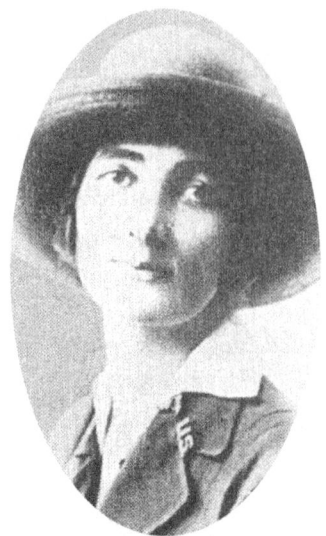

Harriet O'Day
(From Gail, W. W.)

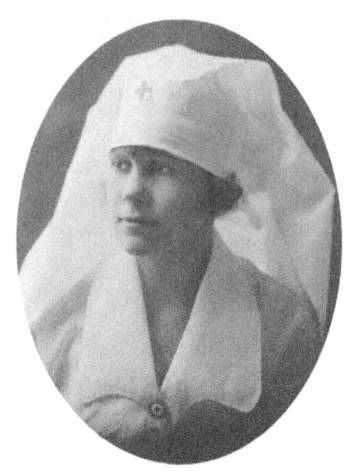

Elizabeth D. Sandelius
Nurse graduation
Courtesy James Benbow

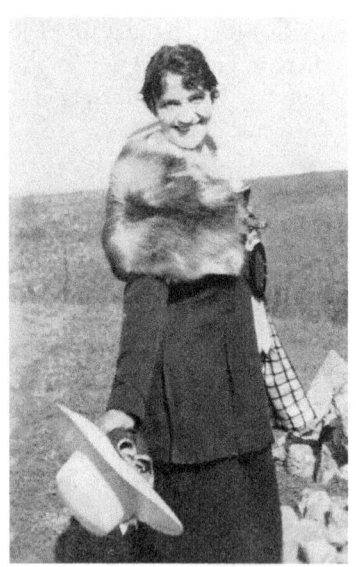

Elizabeth D. Sandelius
Courtesy James Benbow

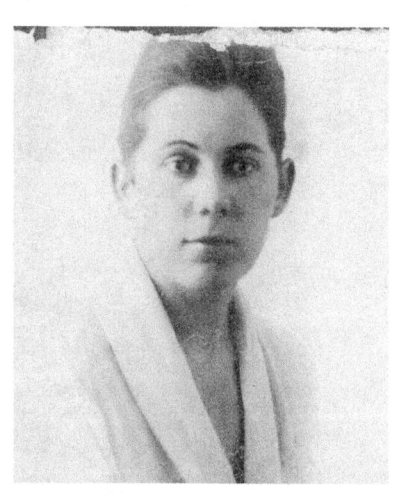

Elizabeth D. Sandelius
War Dept ID photo
Courtesy James Benbow

Elizabeth D. Sandelius
War Department, Certificate of Identification
Courtesy James Benbow

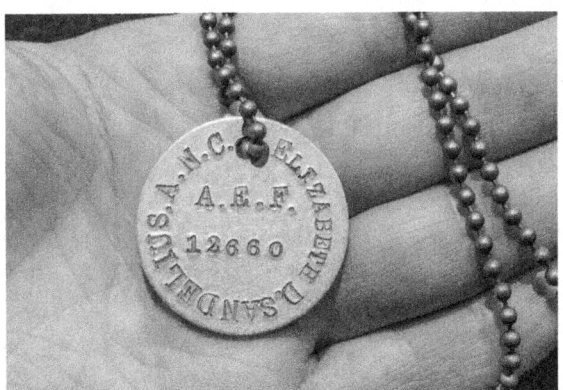

"Dog tags" of Elizabeth Sandelius, Army Nurse Corps, as held by the author. Sandelius' AEF ID number is her American Red Cross registration number.
Courtesy James Benbow, with photograph by the author.

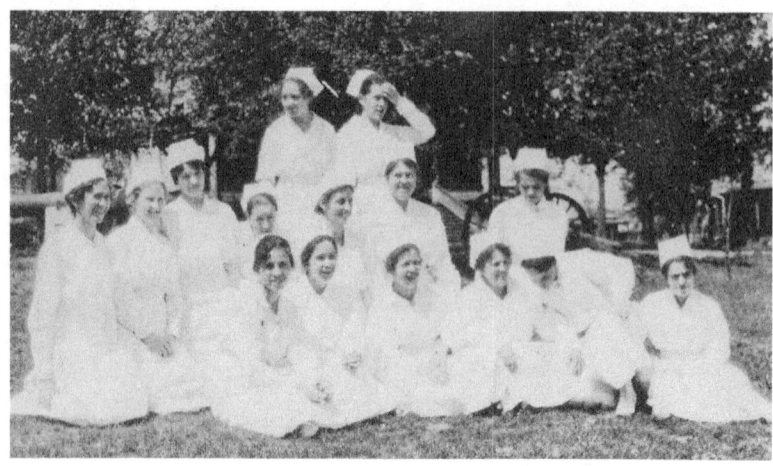

Nurses, Army Nurse Corps, Fort Riley, Kansas.
Elizabeth Sandelius is front row left.
Courtesy James Benbow.

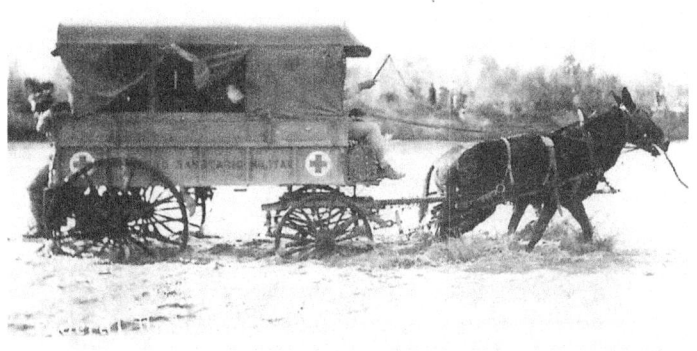

A WWI U.S. Army horse/mule-drawn ambulance crossing a rain swollen stream near the battle lines
Courtesy Bernice Welborn Hash

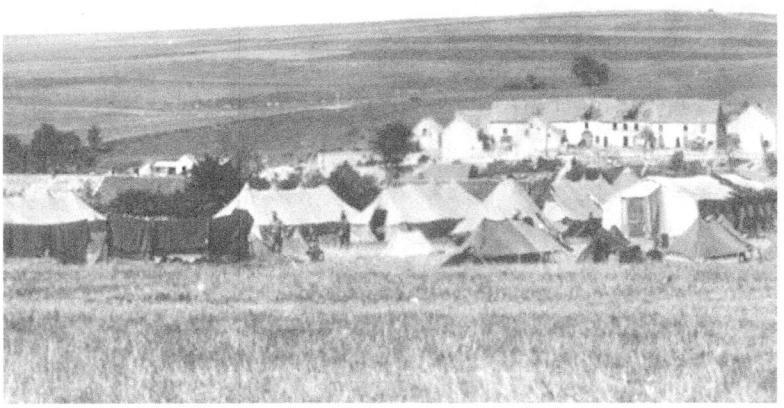

Field Hospital 112, Cohan, France
Courtesy National Library of Medicine

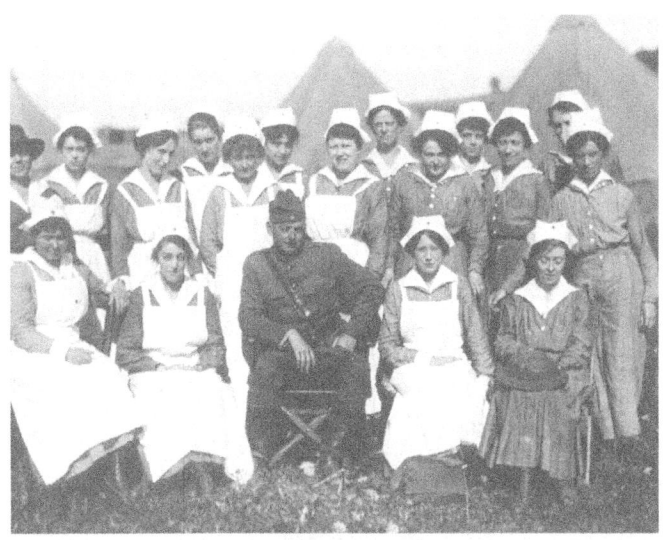

Field Hospital 112, Cohan, France. Nurses and commander.
Courtesy National Library of Medicine

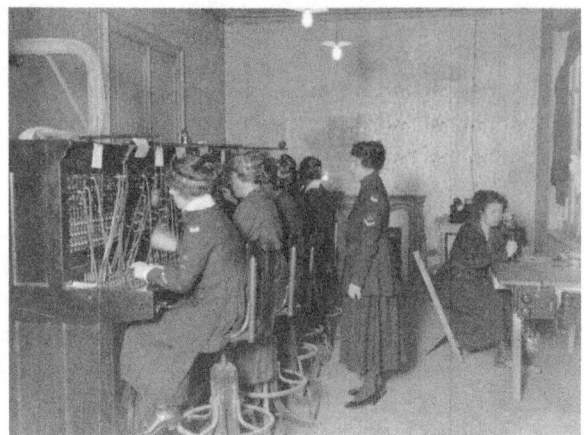

Telephone operators, U.S. Signal Corps, France
Courtesy National Archives and Records Administration

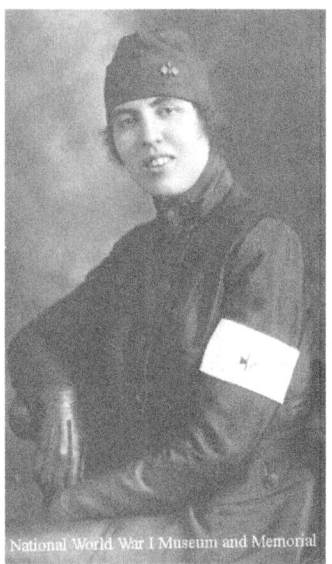

Merle Egan, Helena, Montana, U.S. Signal Corps.
Courtesy National World War I Museum and Memorial

Chapter 13
GOING HOME

"A veiled pride"

BATTLE HAD TORN THE EARTH TO PIECES. The earth was severely wounded. Rain fell, not from clouds but from divine tears. Humans had no tears left to shed. Shrapnel and blast shredded trees into unrecognizable upright flayed sticks. Birds flew away long ago and hadn't returned—if they could return and find anything to perch upon. Country animals, rabbits, quail, and deer were gone: killed or stampeded. Death everywhere: flies, maggots, bloated animals, and what remained of human bodies not buried or hastily covered. Fetid water pooled. Stench lingered and impaled itself in clothes, noses, and memory.

Sleep, ironically, didn't come; everything was too quiet. Almost a mystical quiet. You wait for the guns to fire again, you're conditioned to the gunfire. Now the quiet; you cope with quiet. There's little cheering, just relief. Oddly, guilt and shame come: not in abundance, but they still come. Guilt because you walked away unharmed, and the other person next to you got killed. Angry hot shrapnel got him, not you. Shame comes from knowing that for the briefest time, you entered a realm you feared, a realm once thought beneath common and decent people. Battle removed you from the common and the decent. War is a wretched debasement of the human experience. You participated and you survived—at least physically. People mend from this, but they truly never heal. A veiled pride grows slowly: pride that you rose above the common and prevailed. You're alive and that matters.

The guns once roaring, were now silent. Wars would come again, but for now, the Great War was over. One-by-one, people began the long trek home. For two Montana women who saw war first hand, another journey began: a journey to find their brothers killed in battle somewhere on the torn and bleeding earth of France. Two women dedicated to say a last goodbye.

Eula Butzerin had entered the war with Base Hospital 28, Kansas City. BH 28 was established at Limoges, on the Vienne River about 220 miles south of Paris. BH 28 was a recovery hospital for severely wounded soldiers. On September 26, 1918, during the Second Battle of the Marne, Eula's brother, Roy, was killed-in-action near Chateau-Thierry. Margaret Butzerin, the mother of Eula, Arthur, and Roy, still lived in Missoula. The Army notified Margaret that Roy was dead.[732]

Somehow Eula learned of Roy's death and began the long search for him. In spring 1919 she traveled north to Paris from Limoges. The farther north she went, battle destruction grew outside any window she looked through. By persistence and initiative, she found Roy's military unit. A supply sergeant had Roy's personal effects and gave them to Eula. She learned American dead were buried in a cemetery near the battle area. The Army assigned a French guide to take Eula across the devastated war-torn battlefields to the Meuse-Argonne American Cemetery near the village of Romagne-sous-Montfaucon: about fifty miles northeast of Chateau-Thierry. In time the 130-acre cemetery would hold the honored remains of over fourteen thousand American military dead: the largest in Europe.[733]

History doesn't record Eula's thoughts as she and her French guide looked upon the thousands of makeshift grave markers of American dead. She kept looking and by determination, fortune, or divine favor, found an upright stick with Roy's round dog tags hanging from it.[734] Her final goodbyes to her brother she kept within. Arthur survived the war and came home to Missoula. Roy would never be brought home to Montana. He lies forever in the ground he fought to keep free.

By 1914 Ulysses Welborn had sold his ranch and farm in western Montana, and moved with his youngest son, Ulysses Marion Welborn, to west of Jordan, Montana, in remote Garfield County near Smoky Butte Creek.[735] War came and Ulysses' oldest children, Susie and Frank, were serving in the Army. After Susie's assignment to Camp Dodge, Iowa, the Army assigned her to BH 52 and BH 53 in France. During the Second Battle of the Marne, Frank was killed-in-action on August 3, 1918. The Army notified Frank's father, of Frank's death.[736] Susie was enroute to France then. How she learned of her brother's death isn't known.

After the Armistice, Susie, the resolute Montana girl who perhaps grew to womanhood too soon carrying for her four younger brothers and four younger sisters, struggled to find Frank's grave. When war ended, the Army canceled its restriction on soldiers taking photographs. Susie found that Frank was buried in the Oise-Aisne American

Cemetery. Susie kept photographs of the 36-acre Oise-Aisne American Cemetery about fourteen miles northeast of Chateau-Thierry. Over six thousand Americans would be buried there. Upright wooden crosses in precision rows originally marked American graves. Like Roy Butzerin, Frank was never brought home to Montana. How Susie said goodbye to her brother, Frank, buried among the thousands who died, she kept within.

At the outset of the war, America wanted to continue a policy of returning home its war dead. In past wars fought overseas, returning America's dead didn't pose insurmountable logistical or hygiene challenges. World War I changed that. No one in America could have imagined the battle deaths America faced in World War I. Hard reality struck. Tens of thousands of Americans fell in France: many hastily buried as best war conditions allowed. Upon investigation of how many war deaths and where buried, the War Department accepted reality. The War Department called upon the Army, Navy, and Marine Corps to agree to a new burial policy of America's war dead overseas.

The War Department convened a joint military council to determine what actions were needed regarding the bodies of men who should die at sea or abroad. The council also found France had a military law prohibiting the transportation of bodies in war. The joint council agreed all officers, enlisted men, and civilian employees of the Army, Navy, and Marine Corps, who had died or might hereafter die in France, *shall* [italics added] be buried in France. After the war, the remains shall be brought back to America for final interment. The remains of military or civilians who died on board ship, shall be embalmed and returned to the America.[737] The council determined most American families wanted their deceased loved one returned home for burial.

After the Armistice was signed, the French minister of war examined the subject of American war dead buried in France. The French War Ministry established a national commission to study the matter. France conferred with America on matters of French law and transportation of disinterred bodies. The War Department's policy remained that if American families wanted the body of a family member returned, the War Department would do so. If the family didn't want the body returned, then America coordinated with the French government for an appropriate grave marker and perpetual care of the grave.

France decided that repatriation of American, French, or other allied dead, would cause too many problems. France proposed a law in its national legislature reading that no deceased French, American, or allied military member killed-in-action during the war or having subsequently died beginning January 1, 1919 for the next three years, could be transported by rail or road in France. The American State Department, U.S. Senate, and the Committee of Foreign Relations, protested the proposed French law.[738]

General Pershing wanted order and honor for America's dead in World War I. The AEF Graves Registration Service, with offices in Paris, took on the task of recording the location of burial for American war dead in France. In 1923 Congress established the American Battle Monuments Commission [ABMC], an independent branch of the federal government. The ABMC establishes and maintains U.S. military memorials, monuments, and markers where American armed forces have served overseas since April 6, 1917. The ABMC designed, built, operates and maintains America's overseas commemorative cemeteries and memorials. For America's World War I dead, American presently has seven military cemeteries in France, one military cemetery in England, and one in Belgium. Almost 31,000 Americans are buried in these cemeteries.[739]

Beginning with the Spanish-American War, the Army authorized burial of American nurses in Arlington National Cemetery. If the nurse's family wished, the superintendent of Arlington National Cemetery would receive the nurse's remains with burial in the cemetery.[740] Section 21 of Arlington National Cemetery is informally called "the nurses' section." In 1938, a 10-foot white marble statue depicting a caped nurse was dedicated in section 21. The statue, called "The Spirit of Nursing," overlooks the area where many American military nurses are buried.

World War I ended, the dead buried, but the fight to save desperately wounded men didn't stop. Over ten thousand American nurses were overseas in France, waiting for transportation to France, or enroute to France. The total strength of the ANC worldwide was over 21,000. The Army never had enough nurses. At war's end 266 nurses had died from non-combat related causes: 164 in the United States and 102 overseas. No American nurse died from hostile fire.

Thousands of nurses remained in France in the many base hospitals to treat American wounded too badly hurt to immediately send home.[741] Patients selected as priority to return to the United States were those deemed permanently unsuited physically for any military duty, and those who would require at least six months of further treatment to return to active duty.[742] Hospitalization on a large scale was planned for Savenay: on France's west coast. Savenay became a barracks city with thousands of recovering wounded soldiers. Brest, St. Nazaire, and Bordeaux, were the three principal ports of embarkation to return to America. Savenay would become an AEF embarkation hospital. The AEF would transfer many Montana nurses to Savenay.[743]

At Savenay the AEF medical command established a treatment ward for "psychoneurosis." The Army struggled to diagnose, treat, and manage the mental state of soldiers who saw too many battlefield horrors, and mentally collapsed. "Shell shock," "1,000-yard-stare," "battle fatigue," are now called post-traumatic stress disorder. It didn't stay exclusively with soldiers. Two sisters from New York, Gladys and Dorothy Cromwell, served in the war as nurses. They may have spent a long time on the front lines. Friends said the two were exhausted. In January 1919 they sailed home on the French liner *Lorraine*. While heading to sea, the two sisters linked arms, jumped overboard and drowned. They left notes in their staterooms reading they wanted to "end it all."[744] Marcia Lucille Lange, born in Livingston, Wisconsin, entered the ANC at Havre, Montana. She went overseas and served in three separate hospitals in France. When Lange returned to America she wrote of the nineteen nurses she went overseas with, seventeen came back invalids.[745] Lange didn't elaborate on the nurses' disabilities.

BH 53 served also as a convalescent camp before the hospital moved to Savenay. A corpsman at BH 53, Private First-Class Bill Schira, wrote extensively about the hospital. Apparently he made a lasting impression on nurses: especially nurse Clara Ruff from Great Falls, Montana. In his journal, January 29, 1919, Schira wrote: "Miss Clara Ruff left at 7:30 p.m. for home. [She] got a discharge. Clara's sister died and left 3 small children [and Clara] must take care of them. She gave me her [ANC] pin…"[746]

The U.S. Navy Cruiser and Transport Force, Atlantic Fleet, had the responsibility to bring American military and American wounded home. The Navy had two hospital ships, the *Mercy* and the *Comfort*. Each had a 300-patient capacity. Their combined capacity and turn-around time could not exceed an average of 600 to 900 patients a month. The Army first expected the Navy hospital ships to carry America's war wounded. A joint Army-Navy medical conference soon decided civilian troop transport ships had to be used for medical transport. The transports would have a contingent of medical staff on board for care of the wounded in transit.[747]

The Navy ensured the ship transporting the wounded had needed infrastructure for the wounded. The ship had proper support, food, [even ice cream] bunks, and recreation. A Navy medical aid team at St. Nazaire, near Savenay, drafted and managed a system of patient loading on the transport ships. Each patient had one of five different colored tags attached to the front of the patient's garb showing what class [including psychiatric] of onboard medical ward the patient would be sent to. The card had the patient's name, rank, organization, and diagnosis would also be on the tag. The Army gave the Navy twenty-four-hour notice as to when the patients were ready to board. When patients boarded, the Navy had hot coffee and sandwiches immediately available. Onboard medical teams began any needed medical treatment and continued medical monitoring throughout sailing to America.[748]

Not all nurses went home soon, many stayed with the Allied army of occupation in Germany immediately after the war. Harriet O'Day, the Billings, Montana, nurse who survived German artillery and bombardment for weeks on the battle lines, went to Tuabach and Koblenz, Germany, after the Armistice. At Tuabach she would write of her observations and bitterness about war:

> It is very fine to come into Germany as victors, and the Americans have met little unpleasantness…and the people in this place are very nice and have turned the place over to us with good grace, but of course this country and the people have to respect Americans. They are a beaten nation and they know it and their faces show it, and they don't like us because we got into the war and drove them back when they were ready to win. France they have always hated, and the same with England. But it's mutual. They [France and England] have good reason for their hate…and so have we when we think of the hundreds of white

crosses in that devastated France.

France has a soul and her people have a spirit, but the moment you step into Germany it is machine-like and the people speak of brute force and it's so easy to see how impossible it was for [Germany] to win the war against a civilized world and the United States of America.

...I hope the peace terms are severely just [against Germany]. They should be made to pay and be crippled forever.[749]

As the wounded sailed home, the nurses slowly went home too. The nurses went home largely the same as they went over: mostly by themselves. The first units of the American medical department to return to America were the original six base hospitals that went to France. BH 10 and Montana's Alice Ralston were among the first to head home. This time no U-boat threats existed. Blackout conditions weren't needed on ship. Smoking, laughing, cheers rang across the waters when returning military and nurses saw the Statue of Liberty in New York Harbor.

The nurses had time to think about many things. They thought of their status in the military. They were professional women with credentials; they worked under hostile fire, and they saved lives. These women were not the hired help. The women worked in military units with doctors who had military rank and command authority to get things done: especially when battle jeopardized the lives of terribly wounded men. In a letter to a friend in Michigan, Montana nurse Ann Dobias wrote of her battlefield experiences. She said she worked with an Army colonel who said Ann's abilities ranked her as an Army captain. Ann said she did not have an officer's commission but had heard of talk to get nurses an officer's commission.[750] Nurses asked why didn't they have commissions as officers?

Military rank is always a position of service, and never a position of privilege or having more money. Rank has inherent authority to get things done. Overall, the nurses' position was they needed rank to direct the treatment of their patients. When wounded arrived, nurses needed authority to direct the medical treatment of suffering men. Nurses needed at least an authorized outward military rank insignia showing their position and authority. This would plainly show the nurse's position so soldiers wouldn't question her say-so about medical care of her patients.

In May 1917 the American Nurses' Association, in convention assembled in Philadelphia, passed a resolution reading proper military authorities should specifically define the status of nurses in military hospitals, and confer upon the nurses the authority necessary to control the situation and general welfare of patients. In summer 1917 the War Department said nurses in the ANC had authority pertaining to their professional duties in and around military hospitals, and at all times were to be obeyed accordingly and receive the respect due their position. This lacked details and was open to interpretation. The War Department said nothing about military rank for nurses.

In 1918 legislation was introduced in Congress for the general reorganization of the ANC. Legislation looked at the number of executive officers in the Nurse Corps, increased salaries and compensation, and consolidating all regulations concerning the Nurse Corps. Two congressman, Willfred W. Lufkin, R-Mass, and John E. Raker, D-Calif, introduced legislation giving nurses commissioned rank as officers with appropriate rates of pay. However, after conference with each other and with General William C. Gorgas, surgeon general of the Army, Lufkin and Raker abandoned their proposed legislation and supported the concept of "relative rank" for nurses.

The British, Australian, and Canadian armies had relative ranks for their nurses. Those armies ensured their nurses wore recognizable rank insignia on their nurses' uniforms. Relative rank was not commissioned rank. It didn't conveyed authority of command similar to a line-serving officer and did not have the same pay. Relative rank was quasi-rank, largely symbolic rank. It granted nurses authority to wear rank insignia and have authority to direct matters in and around military hospitals. After World War I the nurses had to struggle for the right to wear gold overseas service chevrons on the lower left sleeve of their nurses' uniform. A gold chevron shaped as the letter "V" point down indicated the nurse served at least six months overseas.[751]

Congress in 1919 passed legislation reorganizing the ANC. The legislation did not include rank for all nurses. Army leadership continued to oppose rank of any kind for nurses. Nurses in the Army did not have a champion similar to Secretary of the Navy Josephus

Daniels. Daniels ensured women entered the Navy as yeomen [F] and receive equal pay and allowances as men. Nationally women's nursing organizations continued lobbying Congress for relative rank for women nurses. Nurses testified on Capitol Hill for five weeks to ensure relative rank would pass. Nurses were successful. On June 4, 1920, President Wilson signed the Army Reorganization Bill that gave women nurses relative rank in the ANC. This ended a long legislative struggle for women's recognition in the ANC.[752] It was partial recognition, however. For women, Congress would not pass legislation authorizing military officer commissions with full pay, allowances, and status as the men, until 1947 and 1948.[753]

The guns of war went silent, but messages still crackled over AEF telephone wires. American women of the WTU continued connecting telephone calls at switchboards across France. The business of war ended; the business of peace earnestly began. Telephones had to work and work well. Montana's five WTU women stayed in France for some time after the war. After Mary Vannier's service in France, the Army transferred her to Italy, Belgium, and England. She would not return to her home in Helena, Montana, for over two years.[754]

Merle Egan, also from Helena, admirably showed her skills at the Signal Corps headquarters, Tours, France. When the Paris Peace Conference convened involving thirty-two countries and nationalities, the AEF chose Egan as the conference's chief telephone operator.[755] In June 1919 she returned to America thinking she and the other women WTU members were military veterans. Egan married Harold "Hal" Anderson when she came home. Anderson, an employee of Mountain States Telephone, wrote the Army requesting a World War I victory medal for Merle. The Army replied she was not eligible for a medal or an honorable discharge certificate as she had not served in the Army.[756] The Army told this to each WTU member seeking any manner of veteran benefits or recognition. This was baffling as the women had to take a loyalty oath, wear uniforms, and were subject to military orders, and the Army treated them as soldiers. The head telephone operator of the AEF, Grace Banker, would receive the Army's Distinguished Service Medal for her service in World War I, but even she was deemed not a veteran.[757]

This began an almost sixty-year struggle led by Egan-Anderson to gain veteran status for the women of the WTU. Many bills were introduced in congress to recognize these women as military veterans. None passed. The Army, the Veterans Administration, and the American Legion, all opposed veteran status for these women. It would take the veiled threat of a lawsuit in federal court to win veteran status for the women in 1977. In 1973 a federal lawsuit for veteran status was successful for the 350 U.S. civilian members of the World War I Russian Railway Service Corps in Siberia.[758] The WTU women probably would have used this lawsuit as precedent to gain veteran status. Egan-Anderson said: "If I do get a Victory Medal it should be for fighting the Army all these years.[759]

As thousands of American nurses sailed home, the president of the American Nurses Association, Clara Noyes, recommended an ARC Bureau of Information be established for returning nurses. The Bureau would serve as a clearing house for information, employment opportunities, and options for returning nurses. The Bureau of Information was established, but the ARC wasn't prepared for the physical, emotional, and mental state of many returning nurses. An ARC staff member, Laura Hartwell, wrote:

> The state of mind of some ex-members of the American Expeditionary Forces resembles somewhat [of] the forlorn desolation of a homeless cat. While this is true of both men and women, it applies especially to the returned overseas nurse…who live [their lives] in a trunk…and who make their homes wherever their hat happens to be…[760]

The ARC determined the returning nurses needed some process to return to civilian life. The Bureau of Information in time managed over two thousand nurses for job placement or future employment.[761] Many nurses entered the U.S. Public Health Service. But most wanted to go home.

When you return from war you're not sure where you belong. When you were home, you wanted to go "over there." When you were "over there" you wanted to be home. Now that you are home, you want to turn and go back. You think if one of your friends over there gets hurt or killed, maybe you could have saved them if only you'd have stayed and looked out for them. You exist in a different "no man's

Going Home   231

land." A no-man's-land that has no gunfire, but a sense of impermanent wandering.

The Army expedited discharging nurses from service. The Army decided when nurses arrived in New York City or eastern ports of debarkation, the respective port commander had authority to issue travel orders to the nurses returning them home for separation from duty.[762] Virginia Flanagan wrote about her arriving at New York:

> We sailed on July 6, 1919, from Savenay enroute to Brest [to sail] on the *Aquitania*, destination New York. We arrived in New York City on July 20, 1919 and reported to the Nurses Demobilization Center at Hotel Albert for future orders. I left this station on July 25th for home in Fort Benton, Montana. [At Fort Benton] I was relieved from active duty on September 11, 1919.[763]

Newspapers didn't trumpet the arrival of nurses at American ports of debarkation. No welcoming parades. New York City newspapers would print the ship's name, how many soldiers, and maybe how many nurses were arriving. That was all. Nurses then made their way to the nurses' demobilization center at the Hotel Albert in midtown Manhattan for out-processing. The Army would give the nurses a one-way passenger train ticket home. The nurses departed New York City. Physically the war was over for them. Yet the women would face an indifferent America, an America struggling with women's place in the national realm. America would not give women the right to vote in federal elections until the passage of the Nineteenth Amendment to the Constitution in 1920.

"Welcome home, Soldiers, Sailors, and Nurses." The *Great Falls Tribune* printed the large printed banner on page seven of the *Tribune's* July 4, 1919, edition. Great Falls welcomed home all veterans of the Great War, even nurses. Great Falls was determined to enthusiastically welcome home Cascade County's war veterans. The city planned "the greatest celebration in Montana history" for July 4, 1919. The Elks Club thought of the idea, and Great Falls business men backed it with donations of $12,000. The celebration would honor retuning service men with a big military parade, beautiful floats, decorated streets, sports carnivals, fireworks, street dancing, and speeches by dignitaries. A big barbecue was assured with four steers and whole pigs over a large fire. Ten thousand sandwiches were planned. The celebration would begin at 9:00 a.m. and would last all day with fireworks at night. The city said it would be the first opportunity to thank those who waged war against "the Hun." The parade was to have every soldier, sailor, and marine, and nurse in Cascade County who returned from the service. Organizers expected one thousand returning Cascade County military to lead the parade.

A special ceremony was planned for Gibson Park in Great Falls. The ceremony would be for Cascade County veterans returning from the Great War. The ceremony would present a war victory medal to returning Cascade County military veterans. The medal would have an eagle with wings spread suspended underneath a colored ribbon. The word "victory" embossed above the eagle. John E. Moran was the chairman of the Medal Committee. As well he should, for Moran was a Medal of Honor recipient from Great Falls. Born 1856 in Vermont, Moran had enlisted in the First Montana Volunteers to fight in the Philippine Insurrection. He received the Medal of Honor for action in the Philippines on September 17, 1900, when enemy forces attacked his patrol. Captain Moran led a counterattack against the enemy and saved Moran's men. Moran returned to Great Falls and dedicated his life to public service. He was a peace officer, undersheriff, and deputy county clerk before he was elected county clerk and recorded. Moran would die in 1930 and be buried in Highland Cemetery, Great Falls. An upright white marble veteran headstone marks his grave. Gold lettering on the headstone reads he was a Medal of Honor recipient.[764]

Moran wanted to ensure the women war nurses of Cascade County also received the victory medal in the ceremony. The nurses were instructed to meet at the prescribed time and place with the Army, Navy, and Marines, and march with the men, escorted by a band, to Gibson Park for the ceremony. Ladies of the ARC would present the medals and pin them on the recipients. Each recipient of the victory medal would have a small card to present to the ladies of the Red Cross attesting to their county residency and military service. It was suggested the nurses march with the medical corps veterans.[765] Cascade County reported sixteen nurses served in the Great War.[766] The *Great Falls Tribune* did not read which nurse, if any, received the victory medal.

Glasgow, Montana, didn't give Lucy Walters a parade when she returned by train in early April 1919. Seventeen months prior, Lucy left Montana for war without ceremony or fanfare; she returned the same way. Lucy had homesteaded west of Glasgow near Vandalia. Federal homestead law read homesteaders had to be on the homestead land for at least five years to "prove it up." Lucy and thousands of homesteaders went to war and had to leave their homesteads. Luckily the U.S. government knew war conditions affect things. A general act of June 1, 1898, provided that military service of a homesteader in the Army, Navy, or Marine Corps, during the Spanish-American War, or during "any other war in which the United States might be engaged," should be equivalent to a residence upon the homesteaded land for the same length of time. The homesteader's land entry was "protected against contest." Lucy Walters, Ann Dobias, and Cora V. Craig, World War I veterans and homesteaders in Valley County, Montana, would not lose their land and their homes due to war.[767]

Montana's women veterans of World War I returned and reentered life as best they could. Their war travels and service in America and overseas, gave them a perspective few had then, and now. As nurses with experience and professional credentials, they could relocate if they wanted. Many women moved away from Montana and didn't return.

Montana women who served in World War I didn't leave many written accounts of their time in war and their experiences and friendships they left behind. Virginia Flanagan wrote briefly of events she saw. She guardedly opened her heart. What Flanagan didn't write is how to say goodbye to friends you bonded with under fire and in hardships of war. Friends who shared adversities and privations never thought possible. Friends you shared more than day talk, but shared life, sorrows, hopes and innermost fears. Friends unlike you've ever had before or thought you would have. They held your soul. You gave them a lasting hug, or hearty handshake, held back tears, set your quivering jaw, and nodded a good-bye. You promised you would write, but in time you found the memories lost or too painful. You moved on and so did they. When sunset quieted the day and people settled into their reflections, you remembered the long ago and the people you walked with. You looked to the sunset and thought, "It was good."

234 KNAPSACKS AND ROSES

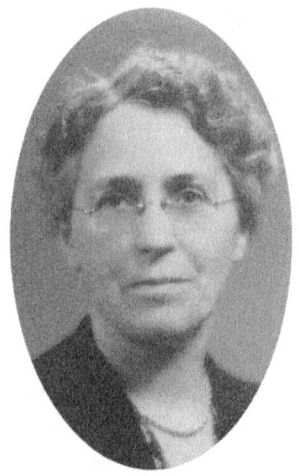

Eula B. Butzerin
Courtesy University of Chicago

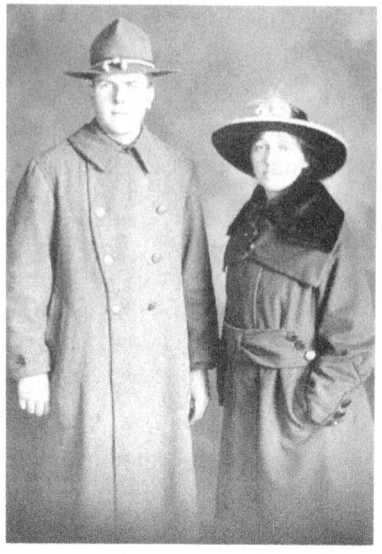

Siblings, Frank and Susie Welborn
Courtesy Bernice Welborn Hash

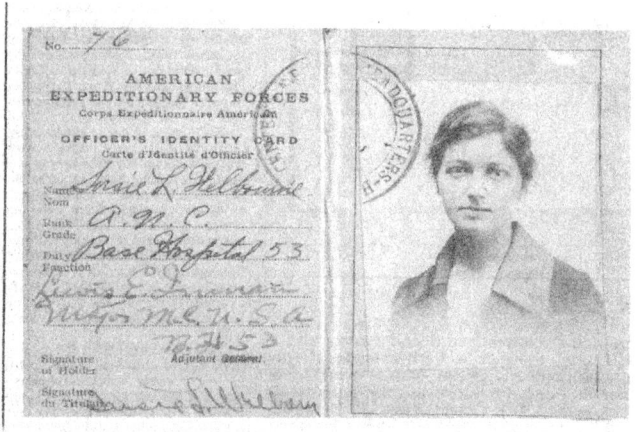

Susie Welborn's ID card at Base Hospital 53, Langres, France
Courtesy Bernice Welborn Hash

Going Home 235

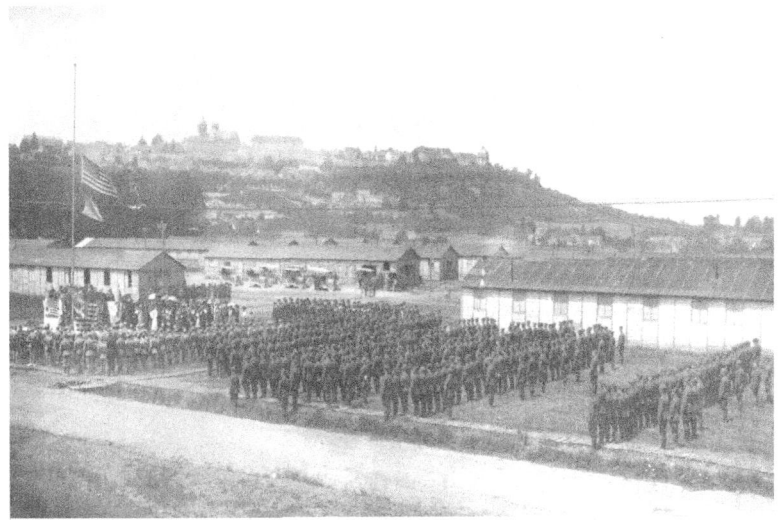

Memorial service, Base Hospital 53, Langres, France
Courtesy Bernice Welborn Hash

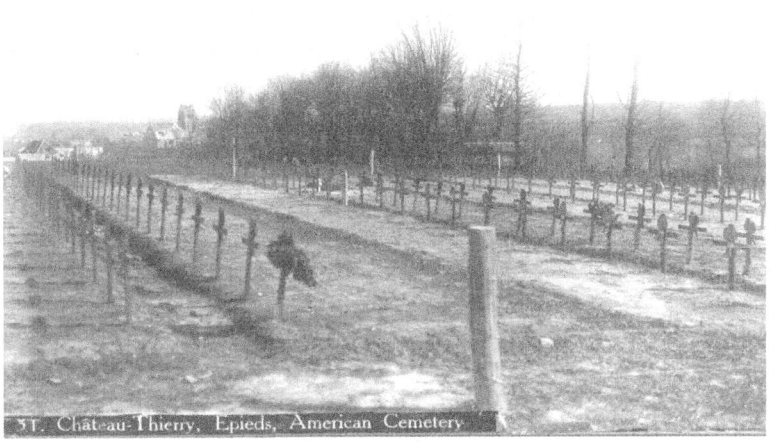

American military cemetery, Chateau-Thierry, France
Courtesy Bernice Welborn Hash

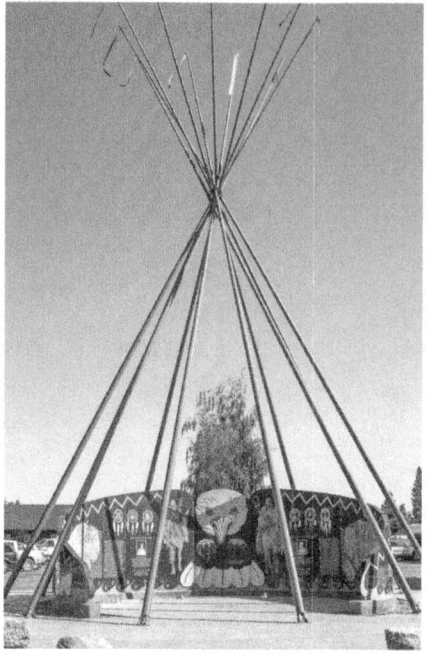

Eagle Circle Veterans Wall of Remembrance
Confederated Salish-Kootenai Tribes
Pablo, Montana
Courtesy of the author

Through the author's research, Regina McIntyre-Early, nurse, U.S. Army Nurse Corps, is the first known and proven female World War I veteran from a Montana American Indian tribe. McIntyre-Early was a member of the Confederated Salish-Kootenai Tribes (CSKT). Her name was entered on the CSKT *Eagle Circle Veterans Wall of Remembrance* in tribal ceremony, July 7, 2017. (*Above*) Her name as engraved on the black granite *Eagle Circle*. Courtesy of the author.

EPILOGUE

"Forgotten no more"

CROWDS GATHERED ON THE YELLOWSTONE COUNTY courthouse lawn, Billings, Montana, Thursday, April 6, 2017. One hundred years ago that day, America entered World War I. A century later in Montana, that April day began cold. Thankfully no snow fell. Drifts had melted, grass was greening, and tree leaves were wakening. Montana gambles with the weather in early April: a lovely sunny day can welcome spring, but a late blizzard could torment you one last time. Winter departed two weeks prior; citizens didn't mourn its leaving. On the courthouse lawn folding chairs faced an impressive, large, and heavy bronze plaque. Crowds gathered, the elderly sat. More people came and stood reverently, silently, thinking.

A decorative steel support, ebony in color, held the plaque. One side of the support had a medical caduceus, expertly cut in hardened steel as if from a skilled surgeon's knife. A silhouette of a dove holding an olive branch was on the other side of the support. The symbols represented healing and peace. A kind and quiet war veteran offered the thought for the symbols. He and others had seen hard war. The veteran recommended healing and peace to shoulder the heavy plaque.[768]

The plaque had twenty-three names. Names in precision vertical lines as if they were in military ranks for one last roll call. Their stories many, their service legion, and their names forgotten. Years of research found twenty-three women military veterans of World War I with ties to the county. They were born there, entered military service there, or were buried there. The plaque permanently honored them beneath a tall flag pole and majestic Colorado blue spruce trees. The women were previously unknown volunteers who went to war one hundred years ago: a war thought to end all wars but ended up frightening the Almighty Himself.

About 8:30 a.m., to the west of enormous spruce trees, seven well-past-middle-age men lined shoulder-to-shoulder as best they could.[769] Years and long-ago wars had taken their youth. A war veteran praised the women and said of a nation's belated resolve:

The greatest tragedy for America's servicemen and — women is not that they may die in war. The greatest tragedy is they may be forgotten: forgotten in life and forgotten in death by the very same nation and people they swore an oath to defend. Within the realm of human possibility and endurance, the armed forces of the United States leave no serviceman or —woman behind, in body, in memory, or in spirit...[770]

Remarks concluded, the men of the honor detail came to attention as best their once proud and now aging bodies allowed. The command, "ready-fire," given smartly. In unison the seven men pulled the triggers three times on their ceremonial rifles. The blank cartridges didn't fire bullets but spewed flame from rifle barrels. Tall buildings on three sides of the crowd echoed and magnified the sharp report from the rifles. The crowd flinched.

A lone bugler stood at precision attention near the rifle detail. The bugler held a battered bugle bought for ten dollars in a Missoula, Montana, pawn shop years before. Once thought useless and junk among the cast-off icons and remnants of people needing fast money, the bugler had carefully lifted the scarred and dented bugle from the wall in the shop. Small mounds of solder showed woeful tries at repairing damage the bugle had faced in its century-old service. The skilled bugler wasn't inspecting the bugle but honoring it. He breathed life into it and found it whole. The bugle resonated with timbre and respect. The bugler opened his wallet, paid the pawn shop ransom, and returned the instrument to honorable service.

Over a thousand times since found in Missoula, the scarred instrument in the hands of its master have sounded "Taps" as a final tribute across fields of veterans' graves and memorials from Montana to the terrible bloodied fields at Gettysburg, Pennsylvania. That April day the bugler smartly came to attention, the bugle crisply to his lips. "Taps" rose above the somber moan of Montana wind bending the pines near the memorial plaque. With final note sounded, the bugler ended the service.[771]

Two roses adorned the plaque: roses laid by a frail woman who saw war decades before, and in modern times, a veteran wounded in Afghanistan. Crowds gathered and gently touched, with reverent thanks, the names of the women on the plaque. Bringing devotion, compassion, skill, courage, humanity, and simple decency, America's and Montana's women blessed and upheld the calling of freedom a century ago. We are better for them. These women are forgotten no more.

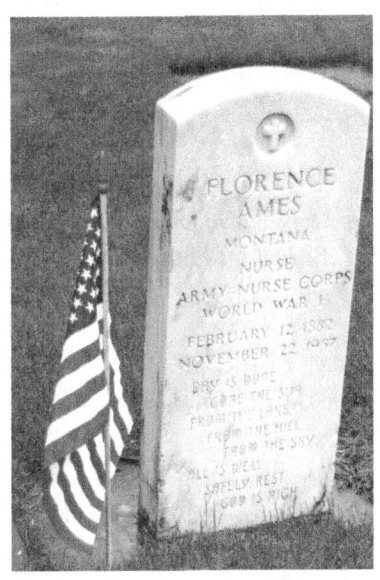

Grave of Florence Ames
(1882-1957)
Nurse, Army Nurse Corps
Montana
World War I
Mountview Cemetery, Billings, MT
Courtesy of the author.

"Day is done
Gone the sun
From the lake
From the hill
From the sky
All is well
Safely rest
God is nigh"

Lyrics to the bugle tune "Taps" engraved on the headstone of Florence Ames.

APPENDIX A

Available information follows on the post-war history of some of the women named herein. The women are listed alphabetically by maiden name. Information is from the author's research.

Mina Aasen. ANC, WWI, WWII. Prisoner of War, WWII. Angel of Bataan. Career Army officer. Bronze Star recipient. Retired 1947 in San Francisco with rank of captain. Never married. Died in Minot, ND, Apr 1974. Buried in Minot.

Florence Ames. ANC, WWI. After WWI, a career nurse in the U.S. Public Health Service. Never married, traveled widely. Retired 1953 in San Francisco. Died there Nov 1957. Buried in Mountview Cemetery, Billings, MT.

Lena [Anderson] Roy. Army Signal Corps, WWI. Returned to Montana. Never remarried. Died 1975 in Minnesota. Buried in Skibtvedt Cemetery, Battle Lake, MN.

Merle [Egan] Anderson. Army Signal Corps, WWI. Married Harold Anderson. Spent decades advocating for veteran status for women who served in the Women's Telephone Unit of the American Signal Corps. She is thought buried in Washington.

Alice Amelia Becklin. ANC, WWI, WWII. A career Army nurse. Served worldwide. Retired with rank of lieutenant colonel. Never married. Died Oct 1984 in Red Lodge, MT. Buried in Red Lodge.

Ruby Bohart. Navy Nurse Corps, WWI. Never married. Died May 1963. Buried in Bozeman, MT.

Bertha Becker. ANC, WWI. Believed died in Washington D.C. Burial location unknown.

Appendix A 241

Florence [Biddles] Myers. ANC, WWI. In 1922 married Neil Myers in Chicago. Moved to Fromberg, MT, and then Billings, MT. She died Mar 1976 in Billings. Buried in Mountview Cemetery, Billings.

Eula Butzerin. ANC, WWI. After the war she served as associate professor of nursing on faculty of the U. of Wisconsin and U. of Illinois. Graduate degree from Columbia University. Head of American Red Cross Nursing education. Retired to Washington. Never married. Died in Washington, Jul 1978. Cremated. Ashes scattered in the Redwood forests of northern California.

Sally [Connor] Chapman. ANC, WWI. Married William Chapman in Shanghai, China. He was later sentenced to federal prison for embezzlement of federal funds. Sally died Feb 1952 in Los Angeles and presumed buried there.

Emily [Covert] Heaton. ANC, WWI. While as a nurse, married Lieutenant Nathaniel D. Heaton in Allery, France. Divorced soon after. She returned to Montana and was head of the Montana State Association of Registered Nurses. Was superintendent of Good Samaritan Hospital, Portland, Oregon. She died Mar 1974 in Eugene, OR. Cremated. Ashes believed scattered at sea.

Cora Viola Craig. ANC, WWI. Returned to Montana and worked her homestead north of Glasgow. She never married. Craig retired to Kansas City, Missouri, to be near family. She died there Sept 1944 and is buried in Forest Hill Cemetery. The whereabouts of her silver medal from the King of Siam is unknown.

Artie [Cullop] Finch. Navy yeoman [F], WWI. After the war she returned to Montana and married Frank Finch. They later divorced. She died Apr 1974 and is buried in Willamette National Cemetery, Portland, OR.

Martha [Daigle] Graef. ANC, WWI. She went to Mexico City, Mexico, to serve in the American hospital. Married Luis Graef there. She died Dec 1967 in San Diego, CA, and is presumed buried there.

Ann E. [Dobias] Montgomery. ANC, WWI. Returned to Montana and homesteaded near Glasgow. She partnered with Lucy Walters to operate the small clinic/hospital in Malta, Montana. Married Mancie Montgomery and moved to Detroit, Michigan. They had no children. She died in Detroit from appendicitis in Sep 1922 and is buried in Detroit.

Vera Elder. Navy yeoman [F], WWI. Returned to Montana and is thought to have married Anthony McQuaig. She died Feb 1987 in Sacramento, CA. Her burial location unknown.

Virginia Flanagan. ANC, WWI. Returned to Great Falls, MT, and continued nursing. Never married. Died Aug 1962 in Great Falls and buried in Mount Olivet Cemetery, Great Falls.

Catherine [Flynn] Lauerman. ANC, WWI. Returned to Billings, Montana, and continued nursing. Married Albert Lauerman. She died Apr 1936 in Billings. She is buried with her husband in San Francisco National Cemetery, CA.

Florence [Ford] Hathaway. ANC, WWI. A widow prior to entering Word War I, she returned to Great Falls, MT, and married Rollin Hathaway. She died Nov 1940 in Great Falls and is buried in Highland Cemetery.

Lydia [Fousek] Boyle. ANC, WWI. Returned to Great Falls, MT, worked as a hospital librarian. Married Albert Boyle late in life. She died Aug 1972 in Great Falls and is buried in Mount Olivet Cemetery.

Effie [Fowler] Sparrow. ANC, WWI. Returned to Montana. Married Charles Sparrow. She died Feb 1930 in Deer Lodge, MT, and is buried in Hill Cemetery; Anaconda, MT.

Annabelle [Frye] Balle. ANC, WWI. Returned and married Charles Balle in Spokane, Washington. Widowed by 1940. Died Feb 1966. Burial location unknown, presumed in Washington.

Grace [Gibson] Sullivan. ANC, WWI. Returned to Montana and married [?] Sullivan in Lewistown. Died Jan 1943 in Portland, OR. Buried in Riverview Abbey Mausoleum, Portland.

Emeline [Gonczy] Stewart. ANC, WWI. Returned to Montana and became Public Health Service nurse in Great Falls. Married Lewis Stewart. She died Nov 1983 and is buried in Highland Cemetery, Great Falls.

Mary Gregory. ANC, WWI. Returned to Montana and nursed in Great Falls for an unknown time. Her date and death and burial location presently unknown.

Celia [Grimmeke] Berry. Army Signal Corps, WWI. Returned to Montana and married William Berry. They raised a family. She died Nov 1960 in Butte, MT, and is buried there.

Esther [Hervin] Crowther. Navy yeoman [F], WWI. Married Kriss Crowther. Died Nov 1963, Spokane, WA. Buried in Spokane.

Violet [Hoffman] Hodgson. ANC, WWI. Married Dr. Joseph Hodgson prior to entering WWI. Returned to Montana. Divorced. Died Nov 1950, Los Angeles, CA. Burial location unknown.

Ella [Hornke] Gruner. ANC, WWI. Married Charles V. Gruner. Died Aug 1960, Helena, Montana. Buried in Forestvale Cemetery, Helena.

Margaret Hughes. ARC, WWI. Montana Director of Red Cross Nursing Services. Married before WWI to "Reverend" Reginald Norris. She later found Norris to be a serial bigamist who left a trail of married women across the United States. The *Anaconda* [MT] *Standard*, Oct 16, 1899, reported "marriage was his pastime." She filed charges against him. A Montana jury found him guilty of bigamy. The presiding judge sentenced Norris to the Montana state penitentiary at Deer Lodge. Hughes later served as Director of Child Welfare Division in Montana, and the Minnesota Children's Bureau. Hughes retired to Oregon. Her date of death and burial location unknown.

Wilhelmina "Minnie" [Hume] Andrews. ANC, WWI. Returned to Montana and ranched along the Teton River. Married Charles Andrews. Died Aug 1975 and is buried in Golden Gate National Cemetery, San Bruno, CA.

Mary [Hutton] Hutson. ANC. Married Seba F. Hutson possibly in Iowa. She died Mar 1929 in Benton, IL, and is buried there.

Alice Johnson. Navy yeoman [F], WWI. Lost to history.

Stella Judy. ANC, WWI. Lost to history.

Louise [LaFornaise] Schneider. ANC, WWI. Returned to Montana and was a nurse in Havre. Entered the U.S. Public Health Service and moved to California. Survived spinal meningitis. Married Raymond Schneider. She died March 1984 and is buried in San Francisco National Cemetery, CA. Valley County, Montana, historical society has her WWI uniform.

Marcia Lange. ANC, WWI. A high school teacher in biology, she became a WWI nurse. After the war she moved to California to be near family. Died in Los Angeles May 1932 of an unspecified illness. Presumed buried in California.

Genevieve [Larson] Rose. ANC, WWI. Returned to Montana and married Stewart Rose. She died in Great Falls, Jan 1965, and is buried in Highland Cemetery, Great Falls.

Ethel [Lezie] Brown. Navy yeoman [F], WWI. After the war married James M. Brown in Lewistown. Moved to Minot, ND. Her date of death and burial location are presently unknown.

Louise Lindeberg. ANC, WWI. Returned to Montana. Never married. Died Jan 1952 in Custer County, Montana. Buried in the Lindeberg family plot, Custer County Cemetery, Miles City, MT.

Lucy Marshall. ANC, WWI. A Canadian citizen, after the war she did not return to Montana. Died Mar 1975 in Old Barns, Nova Scotia, Canada.

Regina [McIntyre] Early. ANC, WWI. Member of the Confederated Salish-Kootenai tribes. Married Joseph Early in Manhattan, New York City. Died Jan 1923 in New York City. Buried in Polson, MT.

Dora [Mecklenburg] Driscoll. ANC, WWI. Returned to Montana and elected chair of the Montana State Association of Registered Nurses. Married Michael Driscoll in Great Falls, MT. She died July 1941 and is buried in Highland Cemetery, Great Falls.

Elizabeth Valine Messner. ANC, WWI and WWII. Career Army nurse. Served for thirty years worldwide. Achieved rank of lieutenant colonel. Retired July 1947. Died June 1963 in Florida. Buried in Arlington National Cemetery, Washington D.C.

Vida [Nerlin] Sweeny. Navy yeoman [F], WWI. Returned to Montana and worked for Northern Pacific Railroad. Married Chester Sweeney in Seattle. Died Nov 1975 in Seattle and is buried in Lakewood, WA.

Harriet [O'Day] Nielsen. ANC, WWI. Returned to Billings, Montana, and became head nurse and nursing instructor at Billings Polytechnic Institute [present Rocky Mountain College]. Married late in life to Jens Nielsen in Hardin, Montana. They had no children. She died Jan 1976, in Miles City, MT, and is buried next to Jens in Laurel City Cemetery, Laurel, MT. In 2014 the author submitted a proposal to the Montana congressional delegation to name the new U.S. Dept of Veterans Affairs, Billings, MT, medical clinic in honor of Harriet O'Day Nielsen. The Montana three-person naming committee (the author was not on the committee) rejected the recommendation.

Nellie [Ouldhouse] Shelton. ANC, WWI. Returned to Montana. Married George Shelton. Their son, Frederick, was killed-in-action in World War II. She died Dec 1979 and is buried next to her husband and son in Custer National Cemetery, Crow Agency, MT.

Marie [Paul] Adams. Army Signal Corps, WWI. Returned to Montana. May have died Dec 1965 in Butte. Possibly buried in St. Ignatius, MT.

Clara Peterson. ANC, WWI. After the war moved to Sheridan, Wyoming, and lived with her sister. Never married. Clara died Feb 1966 in Nebraska. Buried in Dannebrog, NE.

Alice Hough Ralston. ANC, WWI. Returned to Montana but moved many times. Never married. Died Oct 1967 in Bozeman, MT. Buried in New Hill Cemetery, Anaconda, MT.

Clara Ruff. ANC, WWI. Did not return to Montana. Never married. Nursed in Minneapolis, MN. Died Aug 1959 in St. Louis, Missouri. Buried in Jefferson Barracks National Cemetery, St. Louis.

Elizabeth [Sandelius] Benbow. ANC, WWI. Returned to Montana with her husband, Cebron Benbow. They moved to Los Angeles, California, and started a family. She died May 1983 in Harbor City, California. She is memorialized in Los Angeles National Cemetery, Los Angeles, CA. She may have received the French Croix de Guerre medal for her actions at FH 112. This is not yet confirmed.

Helen Sherry. Navy yeoman [F], WWI. Did not return to Montana. Lived and worked in Honolulu, HI. Never married. Retired to San Francisco, where she died June 1959. Buried in Golden Gate National Cemetery, San Bruno, CA.

Gertrude [Sloan] McDermott. ANC, WWI. Returned to Montana and married Frank McDermott, president of the Bon Marche department stores. She died Aug 1957 and is buried in Missoula, MT.

Violet Smith. Navy, yeoman [F], WWI. Lost to history.

Elizabeth Sterling. ANC, WWI. Moved to Portland, OR. Apparently never married. Died June 1969, Portland. Burial location unknown.

Margaret [Thompson] Dibb. ANC, WWI. Returned to Montana and married Harold J. Dibb. She died 1988 and is buried with Harold in Toledo, WA.

Henrietta Vineyard. ANC, WWI. Returned to Montana but continued in Red Cross nursing service. Never married. Died Jan 1972 in Silver Spring, MD. Burial location unknown.

Lucy Walters. ANC, WWI. Returned to Montana and owned and operated the Malta Clinic/hospital, Malta, MT. Never married. Moved to New Mexico for a time, then to Ohio. Relocated to Los Angeles. Died there Jan 1961. Buried in Forest Lawn Memorial Park, Los Angeles, CA.

Susie [Welborn] McCrumb. ANC, WWI. Returned to Montana. Married briefly but divorced. Had no children. Nursed throughout Montana until her retirement. Died Aug 1996 in Billings. At her death at age 103, she is thought the last surviving member of the Army Nurse Corps of World War I. Buried in Sunset Gardens, Billings, MT.

Irma Myrtle [Wright] Smith. Navy, yeoman [F], WWI. Served as telephone operator at Puget Sound Naval Yard, WA. Honorably discharged from naval service on May 11, 1918, due to physical disability. She moved to San Diego, CA. Wright married in 1932 to Clyde B. Smith of Waukegan, IL. She died Nov 28, 1954, in Los Angeles, CA, and is presumed buried there.

Mary [Vannier] Anderson. Army Signal Corps, WWI. Married Otto E. Anderson. She died Aug 1976 in Wenatchee, WA. Buried in Wenatchee cemetery.

APPENDIX B

Montana Towns Where Women Entered Military Service in WWI

Alton
Melott	Alta	Army Nurse Corps

Anaconda
Cosgrove	Mary	Army Nurse Corps
Jordan	Katherine	Army Nurse Corps
Morrow	Hazel	Army Nurse Corps

Baker
Hodgson	Violet	Army Nurse Corps

Belmont
Lynch	Elizabeth	Navy Yeoman (F)

Billings
Ames	Florence	Army Nurse Corps
Barrow	Minnie	Army Nurse Corps
Covert	Emily	Army Nurse Corps
Darcy	Agatha	Army Nurse Corps
Flynn	Catherine	Army Nurse Corps
Lifbom	Emma	Army Nurse Corps
Link	Clara	Army Nurse Corps
Mecklenburg	Dora	Army Nurse Corps
O'Day	Harriet	Army Nurse Corps
Osborne	Maude	Army Nurse Corps
Petersen	Clara	Army Nurse Corps
Rasmussen	Agnes	Army Nurse Corps

Box Elder
Vineyard	Henrietta	Army Nurse Corps

Bozeman
Anderson	Lena	Army Signal Corps
Benedict	Georgia	Navy Yeoman (F)
Bohart	Ruby	Navy Nurse Corps
Brown	Maude	Army Nurse Corps
Butler	Beatrice	Army Nurse Corps
Coffey	Thea	Army Nurse Corps
McGinn	Mary	Army Nurse Corps
Redle	Josephine	Navy Yeoman (F)
Rust	Mary	Army Nurse Corps

Buffalo
Shouse	Frances	Army Nurse Corps

Appendix B   249

Butte

Alexander	Sara	Army Nurse Corps
Callaghan	Cassie	Army Nurse Corps
Cariher	Margaretha	Army Nurse Corps
Collins	Eunice	Army Nurse Corps
Connor	Sally	Army Nurse Corps
Dolan	Josephine	Army Nurse Corps
Dowling	Amy	Army Nurse Corps
Duval	Mary	Army Nurse Corps
Evster	Myra	Army Nurse Corps
Frey	Annabelle	Army Nurse Corps
Grimmeke	Celia	Army Signal Corps
Hart	Diana	Army Nurse Corps
Hornke	Ella	Army Nurse Corps
Howard	Lois	Army Nurse Corps
Jackson	Emily	Army Nurse Corps
Kelly	Elizabeth	Navy Yeoman (F)
Laughran	Katherine	Army Nurse Corps
McGregor	Agnes	Army Nurse Corps
Melia	Catherine	Army Nurse Corps
Noeth	Lillian	Army Nurse Corps
Ouldhouse	Nellie	Army Nurse Corps
Paul	Marie	Army Signal Corps
Pinchin	Anna	Army Nurse Corps
Purcell	Mary	Army Nurse Corps
Ralston	Alice	Army Nurse Corps
Regan	Helen	Army Nurse Corps
Rowe	Ethleen	Army Nurse Corps
Seymour	Mary	Army Nurse Corps
Small	Katherine	Army Nurse Corps
Smythe	Mary	Army Nurse Corps
Snyder	Mrs Cecilia	Army Nurse Corps
Stephens	Mary	Army Nurse Corps
Strutzel	Mary	Army Nurse Corps
Thompson	Bertha	Army Nurse Corps
Tippett	Minnie	Army Nurse Corps
Vannier	Mary Jane	Army Signal Corps
Wellcome	Charlotte	Army Nurse Corps

Casady

Miller	Florence	Army Nurse Corps

Clyde Park

Parsons	Jessie	Army Nurse Corps

Columbus

Sandelius	Elizabeth	Army Nurse Corps

Conrad

O'Brien	Mrs Irene	Army Nurse Corps

Culbertson

Larson	Julia	Army Nurse Corps

Deer Lodge
Herman	Josephine	Red Cross Nurse
Judy	Stella	Army Nurse Corps

Denton
Wright	Irma	Navy Yeoman (F)

Dillon
Lyons	Irene	Red Cross Nurse
Stahl	Esther	Red Cross Nurse

Drummond
Wells	Edna	Army Nurse Corps

East Kalispell
Rustad	Glenda	Army Nurse Corps

Florence
O'Hare	Mary	Army Nurse Corps

Forsyth
Newton	Lucinda	Army Nurse Corps

Ft. Benton
Patterson	Elizabeth	Navy Yeoman (F)
Sherry	Helen	Navy Yeoman (F)

Gardiner
Jones	Luella	Navy Nurse Corps

Gilman
McManus	Florence	Army Nurse Corps

Glasgow
Becker	Bertha	Army Nurse Corps
Dobias	Ann	Army Nurse Corps
Ford	Mrs. Florence	Army Nurse Corps
Lezie	Ethel	Navy Yeoman (F)
Walters	Lucy	Army Nurse Corps

Glendive
Slater	Margaret	Army Nurse Corps

Grace
Elder	Vera	Navy Yeoman (F)

Great Falls
Aasen	Mina	Army Nurse Corps
Aronson	Harriet	Army Nurse Corps
Baughman	Ida	Army Nurse Corps
Craig	Cora	Army Nurse Corps
Curran	Anna	Army Nurse Corps
Denny	Mary	Army Nurse Corps
Flanagan	Virginia	Army Nurse Corps
Fousek	Lydia	Army Nurse Corps
Fowler	Effie	Army Nurse Corps
Gibson	Grace	Army Nurse Corps
Gonczy	Emeline	Army Nurse Corps
Gregory	Mary	Army Nurse Corps
Held	Della	Army Nurse Corps
Hervin	Esther	Navy Yeoman (F)

Appendix B

	Hume	Wilhelmina	Army Nurse Corps
	Hutton	Mary	Army Nurse Corps
	Jefferson	Sophia	Army Nurse Corps
	Larson	Amanda	Army Nurse Corps
	McQuown	Fleda Mary	Army Nurse Corps
	Menzies	Bell	Army Nurse Corps
	Parslow	Alice	Navy Nurse Corps
	Peters	Cloe	Army Nurse Corps
	Reed	Elta	Army Nurse Corps
	Rollings	Sarah	Army Nurse Corps
	Ruff	Clara	Army Nurse Corps
	Shortreed	Elizabeth	Army Nurse Corps
	Thomson	Mary	Army Nurse Corps
Hamilton			
	Harrington	Lulu	Army Nurse Corps
Harlowton			
	Muncie	Maude	Army Nurse Corps
Havre			
	Boyle	Alice	Army Nurse Corps
	Coad	Nelle	Army Nurse Corps
	La Fournaise	Louise	Army Nurse Corps
	Lange	Marcia	Army Nurse Corps
	Mariette	Mabel	Army Nurse Corps
	Susag	G.	Army Nurse Corps
Helena			
	Blankvoort	Margaretha	Army Nurse Corps
	Daigle	Mary	Army Nurse Corps
	Dittus	W	Army Nurse Corps
	Egan	Merle	Army Signal Corps
	Forman	Mrs. Effie	Navy Nurse Corps
	Griffith	Jean	Army Nurse Corps
	Kennedy	Florence	Army Nurse Corps
	Larson	Fannie	Army Nurse Corps
	Larson	Genevieve	Army Nurse Corps
	Laws	Mary	Army Nurse Corps
	Martin	Ella	Navy Nurse Corps
	Martin	Julia	Army Nurse Corps
	Martin	Margaret	Army Nurse Corps
	O'Donnell	Katherine	Army Nurse Corps
	Opp	Mae	Army Nurse Corps
	Peterson	Rose	Army Nurse Corps
	Ryer	Gertrude	Army Nurse Corps
	Sands	Elizabeth	Army Nurse Corps
	Sandstrom	Nina	Army Nurse Corps
	Stabler	Erma	Army Nurse Corps
	Vollmer	Frances	Army Nurse Corps
	Walsh	Norah	Army Nurse Corps
	Zogarts	Mary	Army Nurse Corps

Joliet
Nerlin	Vida	Navy Yeoman (F)

Judith Gap
Vincent	Gertrude	Navy Nurse Corps

Kalispell
McIntyre	Regina	Army Nurse Corps

Lakeview
Zerr	Gertrude	Navy Yeoman (F)

Laurel
Docksteader	Maude	Army Nurse Corps

Lewistown
Baxter	Rue	Red Cross Nurse
Canon	Alice	Navy Nurse Corps
Shannon	Evelyn	Navy Yeoman (F)
Thorpe	Frances	Army Nurse Corps
Toland	Mary	Navy Nurse Corps
Witchen	Elsie	Army Nurse Corps
Wood	Eva	Army Nurse Corps

Livingston
Christensen	Anna	Army Nurse Corps
Dyer	Emma	Navy Nurse Corps
Kelly	Mary	Army Nurse Corps

Lothair
Fredrickson	Mary	Army Nurse Corps
Myhre	Rena	Army Nurse Corps

Malta
Sims	Jean	Army Nurse Corps

Miles City
Cantwell	Bridie	Army Nurse Corps
Clayton	Gladys	Army Nurse Corps
Hageman	Martha	Army Nurse Corps
Kell	Johnsie	Army Nurse Corps
Kemmer	Mrs. Ethel	Army Nurse Corps
Lee	Hannah	Army Nurse Corps
Lindeberg	Louise	Army Nurse Corps
Welborn	Susie	Army Nurse Corps

Missoula
Boles	Kate	Army Nurse Corps
Brunelle	Clara	Army Nurse Corps
Bryan	Frances	Army Nurse Corps
Burke	Honore	Army Nurse Corps
Butzerin	Eula	Army Nurse Corps
Clark	Zola	Army Nurse Corps
Cullop	Artie	Navy Yeoman (F)
Glasscock	Lillian	Army Nurse Corps
Hall	Mary	Army Nurse Corps
Hanson	Minnie	Army Nurse Corps

Appendix B

	Hassett	May	Army Nurse Corps
	Hollenbeck	Elizabeth	Army Nurse Corps
	Johnson	Alice	Navy Yeoman (F)
	Marshall	Lucy	Army Nurse Corps
	McClenahan	Harriet	Army Nurse Corps
	McVey	Ethel	Navy Nurse Corps
	Miller	Dorothy	Army Nurse Corps
	O'Brien	Madge	Army Nurse Corps
	Sloane	Gertrude	Army Nurse Corps
	Sterling	Elizabeth	Army Nurse Corps
Moore			
	Messner	Elizabeth	Army Nurse Corps
	Nicholson	Joan	Army Nurse Corps
Ollie			
	McManigal	Margaret	Navy Nurse Corps
Red Lodge			
	Becklen	Alice	Army Nurse Corps
	MacCauley	Margaretha	Army Nurse Corps
Roundup			
	Knudsen	Clara	Army Nurse Corps
Sand Springs			
	Clark	Etta	Navy Nurse Corps
Shelby			
	Smith	Violet	Navy Yeoman (F)
Stevensville			
	Hightower	Nancy	Army Nurse Corps
Sweetgrass			
	Martin	Nora	Army Nurse Corps
Three Forks			
	Joslin	Lucy	Army Nurse Corps
Toston			
	Connor	Charlotte	Army Nurse Corps
Townsend			
	Dean	Myrtle	Army Nurse Corps
	Vaughn	Myrtle	Army Nurse Corps
Unknown			
	Biddles	Florence	Army Nurse Corps
Whitefish			
	Kennedy	Ruth	Army Nurse Corps
Whitetail			
	Doerr	Aimee	Army Nurse Corps
Wickes			
	Dailey	June	Army Nurse Corps

APPENDIX C

Women Entering WWI Military Service in Montana

Aasen Mina
Army Nurse Corps

Alexander Sara
Army Nurse Corps

Ames Florence
Army Nurse Corps

Anderson Lena
Army Signal Corps

Aronson Harriet
Army Nurse Corps

Barrow Minnie
Army Nurse Corps

Baughman Ida
Army Nurse Corps

Baxter Rue
Red Cross Nurse

Becker Bertha
Army Nurse Corps

Becklen Alice
Army Nurse Corps

Benedict Georgia
Navy Yeoman (F)

Biddles Florence
Army Nurse Corps

Blankvoort Margaretha
Army Nurse Corps

Bohart Ruby
Navy Nurse Corps

Boles Kate
Army Nurse Corps

Boyle Alice
Army Nurse Corps

Brown Maude
Army Nurse Corps

Brunelle Clara
Army Nurse Corps

Bryan Frances
Army Nurse Corps

Burke Honore
Army Nurse Corps

Butler Beatrice
Army Nurse Corps

Butzerin Eula
Army Nurse Corps

Callaghan Cassie
Army Nurse Corps

Canon Alice
Navy Nurse Corps

Cantwell Bridie
Army Nurse Corps

Cariher Margaretha
Army Nurse Corps

Christensen Anna
Army Nurse Corps

Clark Zola
Army Nurse Corps

Clark Etta
Navy Nurse Corps

Clayton Gladys
Army Nurse Corps

Coad Nelle
Army Nurse Corps

Coffey Thea
Army Nurse Corps

Collins Eunice
Army Nurse Corps

Connor Sally
Army Nurse Corps

Appendix C

Connor	Charlotte	Egan	Merle
Army Nurse Corps		Army Signal Corps	
Cosgrove	Mary	Elder	Vera
Army Nurse Corps		Navy Yeoman (F)	
Covert	Emily	Evster	Myra
Army Nurse Corps		Army Nurse Corps	
Craig	Cora	Flanagan	Virginia
Army Nurse Corps		Army Nurse Corps	
Cullop	Artie	Flynn	Catherine
Navy Yeoman (F)		Army Nurse Corps	
Curran	Anna	Ford	Mrs. Florence
Army Nurse Corps		Army Nurse Corp	
Daigle	Mary	Forman	Mrs. Effie
Army Nurse Corps		Navy Nurse Corps	
Dailey	June	Fousek	Lydia
Army Nurse Corps		Army Nurse Corps	
Darcy	Agatha	Fowler	Effie
Army Nurse Corps		Army Nurse Corps	
Dean	Myrtle	Fredrickson	Mary
Army Nurse Corps		Army Nurse Corps	
Denny	Mary	Frey	Annabelle
Army Nurse Corps		Army Nurse Corps	
Dittus	W	Gibson	Grace
Army Nurse Corps		Army Nurse Corps	
Dobias	Ann	Glasscock	Lillian
Army Nurse Corps		Army Nurse Corps	
Docksteader	Maude	Gonczy	Emeline
Army Nurse Corps		Army Nurse Corps	
Doerr	Aimee	Gregory	Mary
Army Nurse Corps		Army Nurse Corps	
Dolan	Josephine	Griffith	Jean
Army Nurse Corps		Army Nurse Corps	
Dowling	Amy	Grimmeke	Celia
Army Nurse Corps		Army Signal Corps	
Duval	Mary	Hageman	Martha
Army Nurse Corps		Army Nurse Corps	
Dyer	Emma	Hall	Mary
Navy Nurse Corps		Army Nurse Corps	

Hanson Army Nurse Corps	Minnie	Jordan Army Nurse Corps	Katherine
Harrington Army Nurse Corps	Lulu	Joslin Army Nurse Corps	Lucy
Hart Army Nurse Corps	Diana	Judy Army Nurse Corps	Stella
Hassett Army Nurse Corps	May	Kell Army Nurse Corps	Johnsie
Held Army Nurse Corps	Della	Kelly Army Nurse Corps	Mary
Herman Red Cross Nurse	Josephine	Kelly Navy Yeoman (F)	Elizabeth
Hervin Navy (Yeoman)	Esther	Kemmer Army Nurse Corps	Mrs. Ethel
Hightower Army Nurse Corps	Nancy	Kennedy Army Nurse Corps	Ruth
Hodgson Army Nurse Corps	Violet	Kennedy Army Nurse Corps	Florence
Hollenbeck Army Nurse Corps	Elizabeth	Knudsen Army Nurse Corps	Clara
Hornke Army Nurse Corps	Ella	La Fournaise Army Nurse Corps	Louise
Howard Army Nurse Corps	Lois	Lange Army Nurse Corps	Marcia
Hume Army Nurse Corps	Wilhelmina	Larson Army Nurse Corps	Fannie
Hutton Army Nurse Corps	Mary	Larson Army Nurse Corps	Amanda
Jackson Army Nurse Corps	Emily	Larson Army Nurse Corps	Julia
Jefferson Army Nurse Corps	Sophia	Larson Army Nurse Corps	Genevieve
Jennings Red Cross Nurse	Alta	Laughran Army Nurse Corps	Katherine
Johnson Navy Yeoman (F)	Alice	Laws Army Nurse Corps	Mary
Jones Navy Nurse Corps	Luella	Lee Army Nurse Corps	Hannah

Lezie	Ethel	McQuown	Fleda Mary
Navy Yeoman (F)		Army Nurse Corps	
Lifbom	Emma	McVey	Ethel
Army Nurse Corps		Navy Nurse Corps	
Lindeberg	Louise	Mecklenburg	Dora
Army Nurse Corps		Army Nurse Corps	
Link	Clara	Melia	Catherine
Army Nurse Corps		Army Nurse Corps	
Lynch	Elizabeth	Melott	Alta
Navy Yeoman (F)		Army Nurse Corps	
Lyons	Irene	Menzies	Bell
Red Cross Nurse		Army Nurse Corps	
MacCauley	Margaretha	Messner	Elizabeth
Army Nurse Corps		Army Nurse Corps	
Mariette	Mabel	Miler	Florence
Army Nurse Corps		Army Nurse Corps	
Marshall	Lucy	Miller	Dorothy
Army Nurse Corps		Army Nurse Corps	
Martin	Julia	Morrow	Hazel
Army Nurse Corps		Army Nurse Corps	
Martin	Nora	Muncie	Maude
Army Nurse Corps		Army Nurse Corps	
Martin	Margaret	Myhre	Rena
Army Nurse Corps		Army Nurse Corps	
Martin	Ella	Nerlin	Vida
Navy Nurse Corps		Navy Yeoman (F)	
McClenahan	Harriet	Newton	Lucinda
Army Nurse Corps		Army Nurse Corps	
McGinn	Mary	Nicholson	Joan
Army Nurse Corps		Army Nurse Corps	
McGregor	Agnes	Noeth	Lillian
Army Nurse Corps		Army Nurse Corps	
McIntyre	Regina	O'Brien	Mrs Irene
Army Nurse Corps		Army Nurse Corps	
McManigal	Margaret	O'Brien	Madge
Navy Nurse Corps		Army Nurse Corps	
McManus	Florence	O'Day	Harriet
Army Nurse Corps		Army Nurse Corps	

O'Donnell Army Nurse Corps	Katherine	Rollings Army Nurse Corps	Sarah
O'Hare Army Nurse Corps	Mary	Rowe Army Nurse Corps	Ethleen
Opp Army Nurse Corps	Mae	Ruff Army Nurse Corps	Clara
Osborne Army Nurse Corps	Maude	Rust Army Nurse Corps	Mary
Ouldhouse Army Nurse Corps	Nellie	Rustad Army Nurse Corps	Glenda
Parslow Navy Nurse Corps	Alice	Ryer Army Nurse Corps	Gertrude
Parsons Army Nurse Corps	Jessie	Sandelius Army Nurse Corps	Elizabeth
Patterson Navy Yeoman (F)	Elizabeth	Sands Army Nurse Corps	Elizabeth
Paul Army Signal	Marie	Sandstrom Army Nurse Corps	Nina
Peters Army Nurse Corps	Cloe	Seymour Army Nurse Corps	Mary
Petersen Army Nurse Corps	Clara	Shannon Navy Yeoman (F)	Evelyn
Peterson Army Nurse Corps	Rose	Sherry Navy Yeoman (F)	Helen
Pinchin Army Nurse Corps	Anna	Shortreed Army Nurse Corps	Elizabeth
Purcell Army Nurse Corps	Mary	Shouse Army Nurse Corps	Frances
Ralston Army Nurse Corps	Alice	Sims Army Nurse Corps	Jean
Rasmussen Army Nurse Corps	Agnes	Slater Army Nurse Corps	Margaret
Redle Navy Yeoman (F)	Josephine	Sloane Army Nurse Corps	Gertrude
Reed Army Nurse Corps	Elta	Small Army Nurse Corps	Katherine
Regan Army Nurse Corps	Helen	Smith Navy Yeoman (F)	Violet

Appendix C

Smythe Mary
Army Nurse Corps

Snyder Mrs Cecilia
Army Nurse Corps

Stabler Erma
Army Nurse Corps

Stahl Esther
Red Cross Nurse

Stephens Mary
Army Nurse Corps

Sterling Elizabeth
Army Nurse Corps

Strutzel Mary
Army Nurse Corps

Susag G.
Army Nurse Corps

Thompson Bertha
Army Nurse Corps

Thomson Mary
Army Nurse Corps

Thorpe Frances
Army Nurse Corps

Tippett Minnie
Army Nurse Corps

Toland Mary
Navy Nurse Corps

Vannier Mary Jane
Army Signal Corps

Vaughn Myrtle
Army Nurse Corps

Vincent Gertrude
Navy Nurse Corps

Vineyard Henrietta
Army Nurse Corps

Vollmer Frances
Army Nurse Corps

Walsh Norah
Army Nurse Corps

Walters Lucy
Army Nurse Corps

Welborn Susie
Army Nurse Corps

Wellcome Charlotte
Army Nurse Corps

Wells Edna
Army Nurse Corps

Witchen Elsie
Army Nurse Corps

Wood Eva
Army Nurse Corps

Wright Irma
Navy Yeoman (F)

Zerr Gertrude
Navy Yeoman (F)

Zogarts Mary
Army Nurse Corps

NOTES

Introduction

1 Montana Memory Project.
2 38 CFR Ch.1, §3.7 (d).
3 Montana Memory Project
4 Ibid.
5 Cumming, Irene M. "Montana Homestead Girl Who Helped to Win the War." Biographical file of Cora V. Craig. Montana state library, Helena, MT.
6 Valley County, (Montana) Museum records for Louise C. LaFournaise (Schneider)
7 "Montana Nurse Is Cited for Bravery." *Helena Independent Record*, December 11, 1919.
8 Gail, 17.
9 Ibid., 16.
10 Billings Polytechnic School, Billings, Montana. School annual for year 1927.
11 Kemmick, Ed. "Women Veterans of WWI-so many stories yet to tell." *Last Best News*, March 23, 2017. Internet at: www.lastbestnews.com/site/2017/03woeman-of-wwi-so-many-stories-yet-to-tell/
12 Walters, Lucy. "*My Biggest Moment.*" American Legion Monthly, as told in the *Franklin Evening Star*. December 3, 1935.
13 "Nurses Awaiting Orders to Leave for War Zone." *Great Falls Tribune*, July 7, 1918.
14 The other two career officers, Lieutenant Colonel Alice Becklin, and Lieutenant Colonel Elizabeth V. Messner. Both were nurses and officers in the U.S. Army Nurse Corps. Becklin is buried in Red Lodge, Montana; Messner is buried in Arlington National Cemetery.
15 Bruhn.
16 Montana Memory Project.
17 Marcia Lucille Lange obituary. *Fennimore Times*, May 25, 1932.
18 "Slacker Nurses a Two-edged Menace." *New York Tribune*, June 9, 1918.
19 Montana Memory Project.
20 Saunders, Edward E. "Biographical Sketch of Eula Bernice Butzerin." Laurel, Montana, 2017.
21 "Memorial Observance Will Be a Fitting One." *Great Falls Tribune*, May 30, 1919.
22 Ethel McVey Hittinger, Elizabeth V. Messner, and Jean Griffith. All three nurses.
23 Benoit, Zach. "No Longer Forgotten: WWI nurse honored after nearly a century in unmarked Billings grave." *Billings Gazette*, May 6, 2015.
24 Pickett, Mary. "The Last of the World War I Veterans." *Billings Gazette* (date unknown.)

Notes   261

Chapter 1. A Train Came to Glasgow

25   "Valley County Quota Leaves," *Great Falls Tribune*, November 5, 1917.
26   Glasgow and Valley County, 98.
27   Records of the US Weather Service, Glasgow, Montana.
28   The original courthouse building was demolished in the 1970s and replaced with a far less ornate, but affordable building which still exists on the site of the original courthouse.
29   "Jail Breaking by a Murder." *Great Falls Tribune*, April 12, 1903.
30   "Hardee Shot to Death, Not Born to Be Hanged." *Kalispell Bee*, June 19, 1903.
31   "Murder in Great Falls." *Great Falls Tribune*, December 20, 1903.
32   Valley County Museum records, Glasgow, Montana.
33   Hidy, 17.
34   Present Billings, Montana, is named after the Northern Pacific president, Frederick Billings, who served as president from 1879 to 1881.
35   Malone, 114.
36   Lass, 108.
37   Ibid., 19.
38   Ibid., 108.
39   Ibid., 156.
40   Grand Union Hotel. Internet at www.grandunionhotel.com/about-frand-union-hotel.htm.
41   Ibid., 117.
42   Glasgow and Valley County, introduction.
43   For an extensive history of James J. Hill and his efforts building the Great Northern Railway, refer to Martin, Albro, *James J. Hill & The Opening of the Northwest*.
44   Malone, 120.
45   Ibid., 128.
46   Ibid., 132.
47   A statue of Stevens is at the summit of Marias Pass.
48   Glasgow and Valley County, 20.
49   Ibid., 16.
50   Ibid., 54.
51   Ibid.
52   Ibid.
53   Ibid., 125.
54   Public Law 57-1616.
55   Malone, 252.
56   Ibid., 261.
57   Glasgow and Valley County, 16.
58   "The Northern Pacific Railroad and the Country it Traverses." Brochure in collection, Montana State Library, Helena, Montana.
59   Ibid.
60   Ibid.

61	American Journal of Nursing, Vol XVIII, December 1917, No. 3, 232.
62	Glasgow and Valley County. Introduction.
63	"Paris Gibson's Views on Dixon's Homestead Bill." *Great Falls Tribune*, Feb 26, 1908.
64	Public Law 245. Sixtieth Congress, Session II, Chapters 150,160. 1909.
65	"Substitute Bill Reported For Two Homestead Bills." *Anaconda Standard*, March 7, 1908.
66	Rand McNally Corporation, *New Commercial Atlas, Map of Montana*. New York: Rand McNally, 1913.
67	"Fort Peck Lands Are Opened To Settlers." *Butte Daily Post*, May 4, 1917.
68	"8,406 Virgin Farms." *Harlem Enterprise*, August 21, 1913.
69	"Stream Of Applicants At The Glasgow Office." *Anaconda Standard*, September 2, 1913.
70	"More than 14,000 Registered Here." *Great Falls Tribune*, September 19, 1913.
71	"Registration Is Not Small." *Great Falls Tribune*, September 6, 1913.
72	"More Than 14,000 Registered Here." *Great Falls Tribune*, September 19, 1913.
73	"Hoosier Wins First Prize." *Montana Standard*, September 24, 1913.
74	"Miss Hazel Richardson, First Girl To Draw Claim." *Great Falls Tribune*, September 28, 1913.

Chapter 2. Lucy's Ticket

75	National Weather Service. Glasgow, Montana. Historical records.
76	Notification letters and War Department forms courtesy Bernice Welborn Hash.
77	"Montana Draft," *Great Falls Tribune*, July 13, 1917.
78	"Glasgow Nurse Reports for Duty at the Front," *Glasgow Courier*, November 2, 1917.
79	On the prairie daily meals were, and still are, called "breakfast, dinner, and supper." The meal at noon being "dinner time."
80	"Glasgow Bids Boys Farewell." *Great Falls Tribune*, October 5, 1917.
81	"Board Will Start Action on Monday." *Great Falls Tribune*, August 18, 1917.
82	"First Contingent of National Army Leaves Today." *Great Falls Tribune*, September 6, 1917.
83	"6000 Miles City Citizens Do Honor." *Miles City Daily Star*, September 6, 1917.
84	"Great Sendoff For The Boys." *Anaconda Standard*, October 23, 1917.
85	For beating the sheepherder, "Phillips Sheriff Arrested," *Great Falls Tribune*, June 26, 1918.
86	"Had No Liquor on Their Train," *Great Falls Tribune*, October 13, 1917.
87	"Ministers on Drink Matters," *Montana Standard*, October 2, 1917.
88	"Will Search Troop Trains for Booze," *Daily Missoulian*, September 26, 1917.

Notes

89   "Official Notice." *Daily Missoulian*, October 7, 1917.
90   "Troop Train to Be Searched for Liquor." *Montana Standard*, October 3, 1917.
91   "Last Contingent of Draft Men Leaves." *Glasgow Courier*, November 2, 1917.
92   "Valley County Quota Leaves," *Great Falls Tribune*, November 5, 1917.
93   "Funeral of Glasgow Young Man Takes Place in Helena," *Glasgow Courier*, October 25, 1918.
94   Pronounced "HAVE-er."
95   "North Montana Soldiers Leave," *Great Falls Tribune*, November 3, 1917.
96   Dyer, 14.
97   "See the elephant," a phrase Civil War veterans used to mean be in combat.
98   World War One Draft Registration Card A, June 5, 1917 version.
99   Ibid.
100   "558 Valley County Men Will Be Called," *Glasgow Courier*, July 27, 1917.
101   "Twenty-Nine Men Rejected at Camp Lewis," *Glasgow Courier*, December 7, 1917.
102   "Funeral of Glasgow Young Man Takes Place in Helena," *Glasgow Courier*, October 25, 1918.
103   "For Miss Walters." *Glasgow Courier*, October 12, 1917.
104   *Park City Record*, January 18, 1918.
105   Welsh, 63-64.
106   "Fast Train Schedules." *Yellowstone Monitor*, May 13, 1909.
107   Whyte system of locomotive classification developed by Frederick Whyte in the early 20th century.
108   Great Northern Railroad Steam Locomotives.
109   "The 4-4-2 Atlantic Type." American Rails, Internet at www.american-rails.com.
110   "Only 14 Times Late in a Year." *Leavenworth Echo*, April 30, 1915.
111   "A Wonderful Record." *King City Times*, March 5, 1915.
112   "G.N. Train in Smashup." *Tacoma Times*, June 3, 1916.
113   "Oriental Limited Train Directory." Original pamphlet in Montana state library, Helena, Montana.
114   Great Northern Railway Historical Society. 1924 Oriental Limited, Reference Sheet No. 217, June 1944. Internet at www.gnflyer.com.
115   "Fast Through Service to Minneapolis-St Paul," *Great Falls Tribune*, June 23, 1916.
116   "Summer Excursion Fares via Great Northern Railway." *Oregon Daily Journal*, July 17, 1917.
117   "Snow Blockade Continuing." *Great Falls Tribune*, December 29, 1917.
118   Montana Memory Project. Military Enlistments (Montana) World War I. Records of the Montana Adjutant General's Office. RS 223. Montana State Library, Helena, MT.
119   Goins, Karen. "The Parents of Lucy Walters." Unpublished manuscript.
120   Montana Memory Project. Lucy Walters.

121   "Lucy Walters Saves Women From Drowning." *Santa Fe New Mexican*, October 11, 1906.
122   "125 Years of Pioneering Healthcare." Research Medical Center. Internet at www.researchmedicalcenter.com.
123   "Denounce Vaterland *(sic)* and Change Name of Hospital." *Topeka State Journal*, March 16, 1918.
124   "Two Saved from the Blue By Lucy Walters, a Nurse." *Roswell Daily Record*, October 6, 1906.
125   "Glasgow and Valley County, 83.
126   Ibid., 8.
127   "History of Nursing in Montana." Montana state library, 28.
128   Ibid., 82.
129   Butzerin went with Base Hospital 28, Kansas City, Missouri; Ralston went with Base Hospital 10, Philadelphia, Pennsylvania. Base Hospital 10 was one of the first six base hospitals to deploy to France.

Chapter 3. The Draft

130   The grave of Edgar S. Merritt, Eastern Montana State Veterans Cemetery, Miles City, Montana; Section A, row 2, grave 1.
131   McPherson, 600.
132   American Bar Association Journal. "A Judicial Revisitation Finds Kneeder v. Lane Not So Amazing." December 1967, Vol. 53, 1133.
133   McPherson, 601.
134   Nevins, 465.
135   Chambers, John W. "Selective Service," in *The United States in the First World War, An Encyclopedia* (New York: Garland Publishing,1995), 540.
136   McPherson, 606-611.
137   Kneeder v. Lane, 45 Pa.St.238.
138   Annual Report of the Secretary of the Navy, 1920, p3.
139   Simpson, 1.
140   Tuchman, *Zimmerman Telegram*.
141   "Conscription Bill to Pass by Saturday." *New York Tribune*, April 27, 1917.
142   "House Passes War Resolution." *Anaconda Standard*, April 6, 1917.
143   "President Signs War Declaration." *Buffalo Commercial*, April 6, 1917.
144   Clements, Kendrick A. "Woodrow Wilson," in *The United States in the First World War, An Encyclopedia* (New York: Garland Publishing,1995), 793.
145   Congressional Medal of Honor Society, Mount Pleasant, SC. Internet at www.cmohs.org.
146   The Twenty-Second amendment to the U.S. Constitution limiting presidents to two four-year terms would be ratified by the states in 1952.
147   General Orders, No. 30. Headquarters Dept of the Army, Washington, April 30, 1898.
148   Trickey, Erick. "Why Teddy Roosevelt Tried to Bully His Way." Smithsonian Institute. Internet at www.smithsonianmag.com/history/why-teddy-roosevelt-tried-bully-way-onto-wwi-battlefield-180962840/Smithsonian.com.

149   Clements, "Woodrow Wilson."
150   "Wilson at Capitol to Push Army Bill." *New York Evening World*, April 18, 1917.
151   "Universal Draft." *Brooklyn Life*, April 14, 1917.
152   "Congress Shows a Leaning to Volunteers." *New York Times*, April 10,1917.
153   "Volunteers First, Roosevelt's Idea." *New York Times*, April 16, 1917.
154   "Conscription Bill In Danger." *Brooklyn Daily Eagle*, April 9, 1917.
155   "Divided Over Army Bill." *Wall Street Journal*, April 14,1917.
156   "Back Up Wilson Missoula's Reply to John Evans." *Missoulian*, April 15, 1917.
157   "Stand Firmly by the President." *New York Times*, April 28, 1917.
158   "Miss Rankin Couldn't Vote". *New York Times*, May 17, 1917.
159   "Wilson at Capitol Hill to Push Army Bill." *New York Evening World*, April 18, 1917.
160   "Roosevelt Wins Army Point." *New York Times*, May 16, 1917.
161   Trickey.
162   "Senate Passes Draft Bill." *New York Times*, May 18, 1917.
163   Ibid.
164   American Bar Association Journal. "A Judicial Revisitation."
165   Cox v. Wood, 247 U.S. 3, as stated in "A Judicial Revisitation Finds Kneeder v. Lane Not So Amazing." Later in United States V. Henderson, 180 F. 2d 711 (7th Cir. 1950) cert denied, the Supreme Court wrote, "Congress was expressly given the power, "To raise and support armies ..." U.S. Constitution Article I, Section 8, Clause 12. This is an unqualified power given to Congress in order that it may protect the very existent of government. There is neither express nor implied limitation in the Constitution to the power."
166   "Order For Draft Made Public." *Great Falls Tribune*, July 14, 1917,1.
167   Chambers, John W. "Selective Service," in *The United States in the First World War, An Encyclopedia* (New York: Garland Publishing,1995), 540.
168   "Dissatisfied with Quota." *Great Falls Tribune*, July 20, 1917.
169   "New Draft Plans to Go into Effect Soon." *Glasgow Courier*, November 16, 1917.
170   "The Conscientious Objector." *Great Falls Tribune*, July 10, 1917.
171   "Cannot Evade Military Duty." *Great Falls Tribune*, April 20, 1917.
172   "558 Valley County Men Will Be Called." *Glasgow Courier*, July 27, 1917.
173   "Must File Affidavits to Claim Exemptions." *Glasgow Courier*, July 27, 1917.
174   "Overworked Babes to Dodge Army." *Ronan Pioneer*, August 31, 1917.
175   "Initial Selection for America's Great Army." *Montana Standard*, July 21, 1917.

Chapter 4. Nursing in Montana

176   Gail, 17.
177   U.S. federal census, year 1880.

178   "William Ransom Ames." *Nebraska City Tribune*, March 21, 1903.
179   Schryver, 2.
180   Ibid., 30.
181   Ibid., 15.
182   Ibid., 31.
183   Ibid., 214.
184   "Florence Ames Leaves to Take Up Red Cross Work." *Billings Gazette*, May 3, 1918.
185   McPherson, 478.
186   Ibid., 480-483.
187   Ibid.
188   "Fair Nurses at War." *Billings Gazette*, March 12, 1907.
189   "Strong Backing For Nurses' Bill." *Rochester Democrat*, February 21, 1903.
190   "Bills Killed." *Daily Missoulian*, February 5, 1909.
191   "History of Nursing in Montana." Montana state library, 4.
192   Ibid., 3-4. This Catherine Flynn of Missoula is not to be confused with another Catherine M. Flynn, R.N, Billings, Montana, who entered the U.S. Army Nurse Corps from Billings in July 1917.
193   "Graduate Nurses Want Legislation." *Anaconda Standard*, January 19, 1913.
194   Montana Nurses Association Records. Montana Historical Society, MC 273.
195   "To License Nurses." *Butte Daily Post*, January 18, 1911.
196   St. Vincent's, Billings; Murray hospital, Butte; St. James hospital, Butte; Deaconess hospital, Bozeman; Frances Mahon hospital, Glasgow; Columbus hospital, Great Falls; Deaconess hospital, Great Falls; St. John's hospital, Helena; St. Peter's hospital, Helena; St. Patrick's, Missoula
197   Montana's biennial legislature meets in the odd year.
198   "Nurses Meet to Organize." *Great Falls Tribune*, July 4, 1913.
199   "Registration Of Nurses Is Desired." *Montana Standard*, January 18, 1913.
200   "History of Nursing in Montana." Montana state library, 51.
201   "Test For Nurses Will Begin Today." *Daily Missoulian*, January 6, 1914.
202   "Sisters Of Charity Under Nurses' Law." *Anaconda Standard*, November 16, 1913.
203   Pickett, Mary. "*The Last of the World War I Veterans.*" *Billings Gazette*, [undated].
204   The phrase "when and how bad," is a staple among rodeo riders.
205   "Eastern Montana Cowboy Dies of Hemorrhage." *Great Falls Tribune*, April 23, 1927.
206   Montana Memory Project.
207   Internet at FindaGrave.com.
208   "Death of Dr. S. A. Kell." *Yorkville* [SC] *Enquirer*, April 15, 1904.
209   "Johnsie Kell Visits Family." *Fort Mills* [SC] *Times*, June 22, 1922.
210   Certificate of the Registrar of the Land Office at Miles City, Montana, for Johnsie White Kell.

Notes   267

211   Montana Memory Project.
212   "Sisters Of Charity Under Nurses' Law." *Anaconda Standard*, November 16, 1913.
213   "Professional Nurses In Session At Helena." *Daily Missoulian*, May 28, 1913.
214   Montana Memory Project."

Chapter 5. The Profession of Care

215   The World Atlas, Internet at www.worldatlas.com.
216   Jones, 21-25.
217   Dock, 19.
218   Ibid., 18.
219   Ibid., 21.
220   Ibid., 26-35.
221   Ibid., 75.
222   Ibid., 40-60.
223   Ibid., 22.
224   Ibid., 90-91.
225   Dock, 75.
226   Ibid., 78.
227   Hutchinson, 230-233.
228   Jones, 139.
229   Ibid., 159-160.
230   Dock, 83.
231   Ibid., 79.
232   Ibid., 83.
233   Ibid., 78.
234   Ibid., 86-95.
235   Dock, 37.
236   Commission, War with Spain, 65-66.
237   Ibid., 76-77.
238   Ibid., 84.
239   Dock, 44.
240   Ibid., 46.
241   Ibid., 70.
242   Naval Reserve Regulations, Section 2, para 409.(3).
243   Dock, 687-88.
244   Ibid., 98-102.
245   Ibid., 111.

Chapter 6. The Yeomanettes

246   Register of Commissioned and Warrant Officers.
247   "Navy Reserve To Wind Up Today." *Anaconda Standard*, April 28, 1918.
248   The majority of planes flown by American pilots in World War I Europe

were French and English designed and built.
249 "E. J. Friedlander Dies in Seattle." *Minneapolis Star*, April 15, 1955.
250 Gavin, 3.
251 Ebbert, 59-60.
252 "Women in the News." *Asheville Citizen-Times*, April 9, 1917.
253 "Navy Reserves Plan to Return." *Montana Standard*, May 25, 1918.
254 "Annual Recital of College of Music." *Anaconda Standard*, June 30, 1917.
255 "Fort Benton." *Havre Herald*, June 3, 1908.
256 The commissioning of the USS Billings, (LCS-15) in 2017, makes the number thirty-two.
257 Commencement at Fort Benton." *Great Falls Tribune*, June 1, 1908.
258 "Fort Benton." *Great Falls Tribune*, February 23, 1909.
259 "Brother of Butte Woman Dies Suddenly." *Montana Standard*, July 26, 1917.
260 "Lost In The Storm." *Fort Benton River Press*, February 16, 1887.
261 "Patterson Has Sold A Carload." *Great Falls Tribune*, October 24, 1910.
262 "The House." *Great Falls Tribune*, January 3, 1901.
263 "Suppressing Scab." *Great Falls Tribune*, November 18, 1898.
264 "John F. Patterson Dead." The *Missoulian*, March 9, 1905.
265 "Elizabeth Patterson Dixon Obituary." *Great Falls Tribune*, June 29, 1985.
266 "Meaderville News." *Montana Standard*, July 21, 1918.
267 Ibid.
268 Montana Memory Project.
269 Ibid.
270 "The Haskin Letter." *Montana Standard*, July 23, 1918.
271 Craig. Preface.
272 Ibid., 109.
273 Ibid., 111-12.
274 Ibid., 221-22.
275 Ibid., 228-29.
276 Naval Reserve Regulations. Section 2., para 404. (1).
277 Ebbert, 5.
278 "Loretta Perfectus Walsh." The United States Navy Memorial. Internet at: www.navylog.navymemorial.org/walsg-loretta
279 Ebbert, 10.
280 Montana Memory Project.
281 Craig, 148-49.
282 U.S. Navy. Chief of Bureau Letter, N60-WAH-HEB, 2158-1140, February 5, 1919, Subject: Unofficial titles 'yeoman' and 'yeomanette.'
283 "The Haskin Letter." *Montana Standard*, July 23, 1918.
284 Ibid.
285 The records of the adjutant general of Montana do not have a service record card for Alice Johnson. How long she served and where/when she was eventually discharged is not known.
286 "Recruit of One Girl." *Anaconda Standard*, May 22, 1918.
287 Ebbert, 51-52.

288 Haskin Letter, "Marines Still Busy." *Great Falls Tribune*, December 25, 1918.
289 Gavin, 25-26.
290 Montana Memory Project.
291 Gavin, 27.
292 "Uniforms Specified for Yeomanettes." *Oregon Daily Journal*, March 27, 1918.
293 "Better Values for Yeomanettes." *Newport News Daily Press*, January 19, 1919.
294 Ebbert, 31-35.
295 "University Scholarships." *Daily Missoulian*, June 5, 1914.
296 "On the Square." *St. Louis Star and Times*, May 30, 1917.

Chapter 7. The Call

297 Montana State Historical Society. Naturalization Records of Mary Margaret Hughes, 1906-1929. Petition and Records, 1905-1913.
298 "Has Fought Death in Wilds." *Conrad Independent*, October 30, 1919.
299 Montana State Historical Society. Naturalization Records of Mary Margaret Hughes.
300 Ibid., Montana county naturalization records.
301 Ibid., MC170, Box 1, Folder 7.
302 Farwell, 26.
303 Ibid., 36.
304 Miller, 263.
305 Farwell, 38.
306 Miller, 230-238.
307 Farwell, 69-71.
308 "Merritte Weber Ireland." Internet at: www.arlingtoncemetery.net/mwireland.htm.
309 Ibid.
310 History of the American Red Cross, 314.
311 "Army Nurse Corps." The United States World War One Centennial Commission. Internet at: www.worldwar1centennial.org.
312 Medical Department of the United States Army in the World War, Vol VIII, Field Operations. Washington D.C.: Gvn't Printing Office, 1925.
313 Addington, Larry. "National Defense Act of 1916," in *The United States in the First World War, An Encyclopedia* (New York: Garland Publishing,1995), 399.
314 Ibid. 93.
315 Blair, 6.
316 Ibid., 22.
317 Ibid., 9-11.
318 Ibid., 107.
319 Ibid., 19.
320 National League of Nursing Education, 250-256.
321 History of the American Red Cross, 327.

322 Ibid., 316-340.
323 Medical Dept of the U.S. Army in the World War, Vol II, 20.
324 Ibid., 316.
325 History of the American Red Cross, 459.
326 "Hundreds Of Friends At Funeral Services." *Anaconda Standard*, June 22, 1914.
327 "Alice Ralston Funeral Slated." *Montana Standard*, October 31, 1967.
328 "Alice Ralston To Coeur d'Alene." *Montana Standard*, May 7, 1911.
329 "Hundreds Of Friends At Funeral Services." *Anaconda Standard*, June 22, 1914.
330 Montana Memory Project.
331 History of American Red Cross Nursing, 300-306.
332 "Registered Nurses in State Now Number 687" [*sic*]. *Ronan Pioneer*, December 7, 1917.
333 "Editorial Comment." The American Journal of Nursing, Vol. XVIII, Nov 1917, No. 2.
334 "Member of Early Day Benton Family, Dies." *The* [Ft Benton] *River Press*, May 31, 1961.
335 "Miss Flanigan [*sic*] Off For Front. *Great Falls Tribune*, July 1, 1917.
336 Extracts from Virginia Flanagan's World War No. 1 Diary. Montana State Library.
337 American Journal of Nursing, Vol XVIII, No. 5, Feb 1918, 366.
338 Montana Memory Project.
339 Montana State Board of Health, Bureau of Vital Statistics, Certificate of Death for Virginia E. Flanagan. No. 61 070263.

340 "Missoula Woman Goes To France As Nurse." *Daily Missoulian*, June 23, 1917.
341 American Journal of Nursing, Vol XVII, October 1916, No.1.

Chapter 8. A Telegram from Margaret

342 Western Union, 32.
343 Dept. of the Interior, 544.
344 Western Union.
345 Activation papers of Susie Lee Welborn. Courtesy Bernice Welborn Hash.
346 History of the Red Cross, 322-323.
347 Ibid., 388.
348 Medical Dept of the U.S. Army in the World War, Vol 5, 713.
349 The author took his Army basic training with the 9th Infantry Division at Fort Lewis.
350 Medical Dept of the U.S. Army in the World War, Vol 5, 713.
351 Montana Memory Project.
352 Private Lawrence Keegan, Co. L, 362nd Infantry Regiment, Butte, Montana, would be severely wounded in action in France, Oct 1, 1918. He would

Notes

be honorably discharged, May 3, 1919.
353   "Lucy Walters Writes From Training Camp." *Glasgow Courier*, February 22, 1918.
354   "Physical Exemptions For Various Reasons." *Anaconda Standard*, January 21, 1918.
355   "Lucy Walters Writes From Training Camp." *Glasgow Courier*, February 22, 1918.
356   Montana Memory Project.
357   "Thousands of Nurses Needed In Army." *Glasgow Courier*, January 4, 1918.
358   History of the Red Cross, 305.
359   Ibid., 956.
360   Ibid., 955.
361   "Red Cross Parade Cheered By 300,000." *New York Times*, October 5, 1917.
362   Montana granted women the vote in 1915.
363   "Nurses Needed For Army." *New York Times*, December 30, 1917.
364   Welborn, Alex. "*Lieutenant William T. Fitzsimons, MD: Good and Faithful Servant.*" University of Kansas School of Medicine. Internet at: www.kumc.edu.
365   "Campaign for Nurses Begins. *Anaconda Standard*, August 5, 1918.
366   "Montana First State to Secure Student Nurses." *Helena Independent Record*, September 1, 1918.
367   History of the Red Cross, 293-296.
368   Conrad hospital, Conrad; Columbus hospital, Great Falls; Frances Mahon Deaconess hospital, Glasgow; Kalispell General hospital, Kalispell; and Montana Deaconess hospital, Great Falls.
369   "Campaign for Nurses Reserve Begins." *Anaconda Standard*, August 5, 1918.
370   "25,000 Women to Enroll in Student Nurse Reserve." *Dillion Examiner*, July 24, 1918.
371   "Billings Dedicates Enduring Structure." *Billings Gazette*, May 31, 1924.
372   History of the Red Cross, 967.
373   Ibid., 293.
374   "Want Montana Nurses For Service In France." *Ronan Pioneer*, December 21, 1917.
375   Montana Memory Project.
376   Medical Dept of the U.S. Army in the World War, Vol V, 736-741.
377   "Nurses Going to France." *Great Falls Tribune*. November 10, 1917.
378   American Journal of Nursing, Vol XVIII, October 1917, No. 1. 695.
379   Ibid.
380   "Butte Girl Tells of Life Of Nurse. *Montana Standard*, April 23, 1918.
381   Ibid.
382   "Alice Becklin." *Great Falls Tribune*, July 17, 1945.
383   "Alice A. Becklin." *Carbon County* [MT] *News*, obituary. October 1984.
384   Medical Dept of the U.S. Army in the World War, Vol V, 490-493.
385   Ibid., 665

272   Notes

386   Extracts from Virginia Flanagan's World War No. 1 Diary. Montana State Library.
387   "English Is Taught Encamped Soldiers." *Anaconda Standard*, November 24, 1917.
388   "It's Great Life at Camp Dodge." *Anaconda Standard*, August 3, 1918.
389   Montana Memory Project.
390   Medical Dept of the U.S. Army in the World War, Vol V, 651-655.
391   Ibid., 651-656.
392   "Dr. Campbell Tells of Dodge Hospital." *Anaconda Standard*, June 19, 1918.
Montana Memory Project.

Chapter 9. The Great Falls Six

393   Bruhn, 13.
394   Ibid.,9.
395   "Utica Montana." Internet at www.russellcountry.com.
396   "Martin Messner Dead." *Great Falls Tribune*, November 8, 1907.
397   "Col. Messner Is Retired From Army Nurse Corps." *Battle Creek* (MI) *Enquirer*, June 14, 1946.
398   "Chas. Ray And Joan Nicholson Married." *The Inland Empire* (Moore, MT) November 20, 1913.
399   Montana Memory Project.
400   "Decree of Divorce." *Great Falls Tribune*, January 19, 1917.
401   "Former Treasurer Is Convicted On Charge." *Montana Standard*, December 6, 1929.
402   Montana Memory Project.
403   Ibid.
404   Ibid.
405   The author's father, Ross Saunders, U.S. Army, WWII, would land at Lingayen Gulf, January 1945, to complete the allied invasion of the Philippines.
406   Elizabeth Norman's book, "We Angels of Bataan," is a comprehensive account of the American Army and Navy nurses' ordeal as prisoners-of-war.
407   Bruhn, 1.
408   Ibid., 5-6.
409   Bridgewater, 26.
410   "Columbus Hospital Nurses' Training School Sends." *Great Falls Tribune*, May 27, 1917.
411   Montana Memory Project.
412   History of the Red Cross, 342.
413   Ibid., 344.
414   Ibid., 1446.
415   Montana Memory Project.
416   "Red Cross Nurses Entertained." *Great Falls Tribune*, July 7, 1918.
417   Bruhn, 6.
418   "Miss Fousek Is Anxious To Cross." *Great Falls Tribune*, October 13,

	1918.	
419	Medical Department of the U.S. Army in the World War, Vol I, 264.	
420	Ibid.,Vol VI., 352	
421	Byerly	
422	Medical Dept of the U.S. Army in the World War, Vol VI., 280.	
423	Ibid., 360.	
424	Ibid., 363.	
425	Medical Dept of the U.S. Army in the World War, Vol V, 656.	
426	"Miss Fousek Is Anxious to Cross." *Great Falls Tribune*, October 13, 1918.	
427	"One Thousand Die in Montana." *Great Falls Tribune*, December 18, 1918.	
428	"Fight Spread of Dread Influenza." *Conrad Independent*, October 11, 1918.	
429	Report of the Surgeon General, U.S. Army. 1919, Vol 2, 1044.	
430	"Limit Funeral Attendance." *Great Falls Tribune*, October 20, 1918.	
431	"Peace Will Lift Ban On Butte Bars." *Great Falls Tribune*, November 8, 1918.	
432	"Butte High School Becomes Hospital." *Anaconda Standard*. October 1918.	
433	Ibid.	
434	"Butte Methodists And Miners Immune." *Great Falls Tribune*, October 30, 1918.	
435	"Five Doctors Are Brot [*sic*] From Oregon." *Great Falls Tribune*, October 15, 1918.	
436	"Local Nurse Tells of 'Flu' Battle. *Glasgow Courier*, November 1, 1918.	
437	Venson, 741.	
438	Medical Dept of the U.S. Army in the World War, Vol VI, 362.	
439	History of the Red Cross, 290.	
440	Flanagan, 7.	
441	History of the Red Cross, 255-256.	
442	"To Train Nurses." *Butte Daily Post*, August 30, 1917.	
443	"To Train Nurses At Summer School." *Great Falls Tribune*, June 21, 1918.	
444	Ibid.	
445	"Slacker Like Custard Pie." *Montana Standard*, May 10, 1918.	
446	"Slacker Nurses A Two-Edged Sword." *New York Tribune*, June 9, 1918.	
447	"The Work of a Nurse." *Indianapolis Star*, June 15, 1918.	
448	History of the Red Cross, 405.	
449	"Slacker Nurses A Two-Edged Sword." *New York Tribune*, June 9, 1918.	
450	Bellafaire, Judith. *Native American Women Veterans*. The Women's Memorial, Internet at www.womensmemorial.org.	
451	In 2015 detailed and persistent research by the author in Montana military records and tribal census records of the Confederated Salish-Kootenai, headquartered in Pablo, Montana, identified and proved the World War I service of the only known, thus far, American Indian female from Montana. Regina McIntyre-Early.	
452	"Regina McIntire Early Dies in New York." Flathead [MT] Courier,	

February 15, 1923.
453   "A New Rate of Pay for the Army Men." *Anaconda Standard*, May 23, 1917.
454   "Laborers Employed in the Health Department." *Montana Standard*, June 25, 1917.
455   "Fix Fee Standard For Influenza Nurses." *Great Falls Tribune*, October 18, 1918.
456   Farwell, 69.

Chapter 10. Going Across

457   FY 1917 Annual Report of the Secretary of the Navy. GPO, Wash. D.C., 762.
458   Massie, Introduction.
459   Tuchman, 325.
460   Massie, 909-911.
461   Showell, 36.
462   Simpson, 140.
463   Ibid., 137.
464   Ibid., 74.
465   Farewell, 72.
466   Tuchman, 333.
467   Miller, 141.
468   "10 Ships Sunk; 8 Lives Lost." *New York Times*, February 2, 1917.
469   Annual Report of the U.S. Shipping Board, 1918, 8-10.
470   Ibid., 23.
471   American Journal of Nursing, Vol XVIII, 1917, 217.
472   Farwell, 81.
473   Washington Historical Quarterly, January 1923, 14.
474   Annual Report of the Surgeon-General, U.S. Navy, 1918. Washington D.C.: Government Printing Office, 59.
475   Farwell., 72.
476   Annual Report of the Navy Department, FY 1919, 25.
477   Ibid.
478   Farwell, 76.
479   Miller, 170.
480   "Coasting Frolic Ends with Broken Bones." *Daily Missoulian*, January 18, 1917.
481   "Judge J. L. Sloane Failed to Rally." *Daily Missoulian*, September 6, 1914.
482   "Miss Gertrude Sloane The Nurses' President. *Daily Missoulian*, July 24, 1913.
483   "Begins Journey to France." *Daily Missoulian*, September 27, 1917.
484   Internet at https://en.wikipedia.org/wiki/RMS_Baltic_(1903)
485   "Miss Sloane Reaches Europe With Nurses Unit." *Daily Missoulian*, November 15, 1917.
486   Ibid.

Notes 275

487   Port of Hoboken, NJ. Ships manifests, *Missanabie* and *Megantic* for June 11/12, 1918.
488   Flanagan, 12.
489   Miller, 116.
490   Venzon, 493.
491   Flanagan, 7.
492   Venzon, 489.
493   Ibid.
494   "Millions of Acres Given to Railroads." *Ronan* (MT) *Pioneer*, October 19, 1917.
495   "War Time Economy on Railways Near." *Daily Missoulian*, (Missoula, MT) July 8, 1917.
496   Venzon, 493.
497   American Journal of Nursing, 213.
498   American Red Cross Services. 1945 annual questionnaire for Butzerin, Eula B.
499   Eula's 1978 Washington State death certificate erroneously reads she was born in Montana.
500   "Train Wreck Fatal Near St. Regis." *Mineral Independent* (Superior, MT), Jan 31, 1918.
501   "Albert Butzerin for State Senate." *Daily Missoulian*, Sep 20, 1914.
502   "Society News." *Daily Missoulian*, May 18, 1913.
503   "Train Wreck Fatal Near St. Regis." *Mineral Independent*.
504   "Graduating Class Best Yet." *Daily Missoulian*, Jun 6, 1909.
505   American Red Cross Services.
506   "Miss Butzerin Honored." *Daily Missoulian*, Feb 14, 1918.
507   Young, James E., ed., *Teachers College Record* (New York: Columbia University Press, 1922, Vol XXIII, No. 1), 283.
508   "Few at the Institute." *Ottawa* (KS) *Herald*, Dec 22, 1917.
509   "Miss Butzerin Honored." *Daily Missoulian*, Feb 14, 1918.
510   "Medicine in the First World War, Forming Base Hospital 28." University of Kansas Medical Center. http://www.kumc.edu/wwi/base-hospital-28.html
511   "She Goes to France as Nurse." *Topeka* (KS) *Daily State Journal*. May 28, 1918.
512   Montana Memory Project.
513   U.S. Army Transportation Service, passenger manifest for *Mauretania*, June 30, 1918.
514   History of the Red Cross, 416-418.
515   American Journal of Nursing, 416.
516   Papers of Elizabeth Sandelius Benbow. Her grandson has Benbow's original dog tags.
517   War Risk Insurance Report, 5.
518   Ibid.,8.
519   American Journal of Nursing, 243.
520   History of the Red Cross, 420.
521   Ibid.

522 "Knott Hotels for Nurses." *New York Herald*, April 20, 1918.
523 "Lyons Opens Headquarters." *New York Sun*, October 10, 1917.
524 History of the Red Cross, 421.
525 Ibid. 422.
526 Flanagan, 8-9.
527 American Journal of Nursing, 620.
528 Bigelow had no ties to Montana.
529 Stimson, 8.
530 Ibid., July 30, 1917.
531 Flanagan, 10.
532 American Journal of Nursing, 1918, 336.
533 Flanagan, 10.
534 Stimson, 1.
535 Flanagan, 10.
536 Internet at https://en.wikipedia.org/wiki/SS_Megantic
537 Flanagan, 12.
538 Ibid.,11.
539 "Nurses Killed by Rebounding Shell." *United Press International*, May 22, 1917.
540 The author was an ordnance ammunition officer while on active duty in the Army.
541 "Two Nurses Killed During Ship Practice." *Butte* [MT] *Standard*, May 21, 1917.
542 "Deer Lodge Nurse on Armed Merchantman." *Butte Daily Post*, May 23, 1917.
543 "Blame Gun Cup For Mongolia Accident." *Daily Missoulian*, May 30, 1917.
544 History of the American Red Cross, 365.
545 Annual Report of the Secretary of the Navy, 1918, 1405.
546 Annual Report of the Surgeon-General of the Navy, 1918; 60.
547 Another Montana nurse, Mary Hall, may have been on board one of the ships, but this is not confirmed.
548 History of the American Red Cross, 423.
549 Flanagan, 12.
550 Walters, Lucy. *Just in Time*. American Legion magazine, December 3, 1935.
551 Ibid.
552 Flanagan, 12.
553 *Missanbie*. Internet at https://uboat.net
554 Ibid., *Carpathia*.
555 Steel, Jeanette. "What Sank the USS San Diego?" *San Diego Union-Tribune*, September 15, 2017.

Chapter 11. Over There

556 Clay, 154.

557 Flanagan, 13.
558 Wigle, 43.
559 Tuchman, 259.
560 Horne, 13.
561 Ibid.
562 Frum, David. *"The Lessons of the Somme."* Atlantic Monthly, July 1, 2016.
563 Ibid.
564 Ibid.
565 Farwell, 91.
566 Griess, 8.
567 Farwell, 93.
568 "The Fighting First, History of the First Division." Internet at: www.fdmuseum.org.
569 "Second to None." History of the 2nd Infantry Division. Internet at: www.2id.korea.mil.
570 History of the American Red Cross, 415.
571 Ibid., 414.
572 Hoeber, 34-38.
573 State Department Passport Records, London, England.
574 Fairchild, Stambaugh, and McCelland had no ties to Montana.
575 Rote.
576 Hober, 83.
577 History of the American Red Cross, 460.
578 Horne, 45-49.
579 Hoeber, 87.
580 Farwell, 88.
581 Ibid.
582 Ibid., 90.
583 Ibid.
584 Griess, 202.
585 Farwell, 101.
586 Ibid.
587 Bradley, 18.
588 Annual Report of the Chief Signal Officer, 1919.
589 Ibid., 540.
590 Cobbs, 72.
591 "The American Women's Telephone Unit Abroad." *Baltimore Sun*, June 30, 1918.
592 Ibid.
593 Ibid.
594 "American 'Hello Girls' Do Important War Work in France." *Greenville [SC] News*, May 19, 1918.
595 Ibid.
596 "Line Busy." *Daily Missoulian*, September 29, 1917.
597 Cobbs, 45.
598 Ibid., 46.

599   Gaines, E. L. *"Principles of Telephone Traffic."* Telephony, The American Telephone Journal, Chicago: Telephony Pub Corp., July 2 to December 31, 1921. 18.
600   "Hello Girls Strike For Higher Salaries." *Montana Standard*, July 4, 1917.
601   "Compromise Ends Missoula's Phone Strike." *Daily Missoulian*, July 8, 1917.
602   "Hello Girls, Leaders in West Coast 'Phone Strike." *Daily Missoulian*, November 3, 1917.
603   "Montana Federation of Labor Opens Annual Sessions." *Butte* [MT] *Miner*, August 17, 1909.
604   Annual Report of the Chief Signal Officer, 1919, 539.
605   "Miss Vannier Wins." *Anaconda Standard*, March 1, 1918.
606   James, 28.
607   U.S. Immigration Service. Passenger manifest for the SS *Lapland*, from New York City to Liverpool, June 28, 1918.
608   Cobbs, 67.
609   Annual Report of the Army Surgeon General, 1919, Vol 2. Washington D.C.: Government Printing Office, 1047.
610   "French-Speaking Girls Wanted." *Harrisburg* [PA] *Telegraph*, February 16, 1019.
611   "Montana Lassie One of the 150 Volunteer Hello Girls." *Fallon County* [MT] *Times*, May 9, 1918.
612   "American 'Hello Girls' Do Important War Work in France." *Greenville* [SC] *News*, May 19, 1918.
613   "Telephone Company In Its New Building." *Fergus County* [MT] *Democrat*, April 8, 1913.
614   "Butte Girl To Help Transform Phone Bells into Liberty Bells." *Montana Standard*, August 24, 1918.
615   Annual Report of the Chief Signal Officer, 1919, 195.
616   Ibid., 539.
617   Ibid., 94.
618   "Phone Chief To Go 'Over There.'" *Montana Standard*, August 18, 1918.
619   Ibid.
620   "Butte Women Who Served Overseas." *Anaconda Standard*, October 26, 1919.
621   "Miss Celia Grimmeke Sails Today For France." *Montana Standard*, September 11, 1918.
622   "Louis Paul Dies at 85." *Daily Missoulian*, May 23, 1957.
623   Banker had no ties to Montana.
624   Annual Report of the Chief Signal Officer, 1919, 540.
625   "American Girls in the War Zone." *Glasgow* [MT] *Courier*, October 18, 1918.
626   Ibid.
627   Annual Report of the Surgeon-General, U.S. Navy, 1918. Washington D.C.: Government Printing Office, 11.
628   Annual Report of the Navy, FY 1919, 2070.

629 "Alice Canon Goes to Los Angeles." *Great Falls Tribune*, September 9, 1911.
630 Montana Memory Project.
631 Annual Report of the Surgeon-General, U.S. Navy, 1918. 194.
632 Ibid.
633 Ibid.
634 Hoeber.

Chapter 12. Under Fire

635 Fussell.
636 Griess, 107.
637 Ibid., 118-120.
638 Hart, 341.
639 Griess, 124.
640 The author spent two tours-of-duty in Europe with the U.S. Army Europe.
641 Hoeber, 49.
642 Ibid., 57.
643 Hoeber, 85.
644 Ibid.
645 The author fought in the Persian Gulf War. During the war, the initial aerial, ground, and sea bombardment on Iraq lasted over a month. When the bombardment stopped, it seemed the quietest day of the war. We couldn't sleep in the desert as the evenings were too quiet.
646 Hart, 356.
647 Terraine, introduction.
648 Medical Dept of the U.S. Army in the World War, Vol VII,
649 "Marvelous Achievements in Medicine Due to War". *Anaconda Standard*, August 4, 1918.
650 History of the Red Cross, 447.
651 These women had no ties to Montana.
652 Hoeber, 86.
653 History of the Red Cross, 467.
654 Stimson, June 30, 1917.
655 Ibid.
656 Dent, 25.
657 Ibid., 13.
658 Medical Dept of the U.S. Army Report, Vol VIII,15-18.
659 Hart, 425-426.
660 Budreau, 231.
661 History of the Red Cross, 466.
662 Ibid., 468.
663 Miller, 378.
664 Bradley, 445.
665 Venzon, 295.

666	Farwell, 163.
667	History of the Red Cross, 503.
668	Medical Dept of the U.S. Army in the World War, Vol II, 91.
669	Ibid., 669.
670	Farwell, 211-212.
671	Ibid., 169-170.
672	Ibid.
673	History of the American Red Cross, 515.
674	"Missoula Nurse Will Go To Camp." *Missoulian*, February 1, 1918.
675	Report of the Army Surgeon General, 1919, 1695.
676	History of the American Red Cross, 645.
677	Report of the Army Surgeon General, 1919, 1696.
678	"Missoula Nurse Will Go To Camp." *Missoulian*, February 1, 1918.
679	Hall left no known record of her war experiences.
680	Biographical Sketch of Ann E. Dobias. Internet undated.
681	Montana Memory Project.
682	Ibid.
683	Medical Report of the U.S. Army, Vol VIII, 1919, 175.
684	History of the American Red Cross, 1685.
685	"Nurse Dobias Writes of Her Army Life." *Glasgow Courier*, December 20, 1918
686	"Ann Dobias Letter Home." *Glasgow Courier*, undated.
687	Montana Memory Project.
688	History of the American Red Cross, 534.
689	Medical Dept of the U.S. Army in the World War, Vol VII, 1075.
690	History of the American Red Cross, 619.
691	Montana Memory Project
692	Report of the Surgeon General of the U.S. Army, 1919, 2058.
693	Ibid., 1753,
694	Miller, 373.
695	Montana Memory Project.
696	Base Hospital 57 in time became the American Hospital in Paris. The American Hospital is still open.
697	"Nurse in Glasgow Is Decorated By The King of Siam For Services." *Great Falls Tribune*, June 18, 1919.
698	Diary of Virginia Flanagan. Montana Historical Society.
699	Montana State Board of Examiners for Nurses, Certificate of Registration for Elizabeth D. Sandelius.
700	"T.C. Benbow at World's Fair." *Great Falls Tribune*, Nov 23, 1941.
701	U.S. War Dept Certificate of Identification for Elizabeth D. Sandelius.
702	The post cards and her dog tags survive in the possession of her grandson, James Benbow, Los Angeles, California.
703	History of the Army Medical Dept in World War I, Vol VIII, 437.
704	Both nurses had no ties to Montana.
705	History of the American Red Cross, 752-753.
706	Bowling had no ties to Montana.

707 History of the American Red Cross, 662-663.
708 History of the Twenty-Eighth Division, 176-178.
709 Headquarters, 28th Division, Camp Dix, NJ. General Orders No. 1, 1919.
710 Farwell, 209.
711 "Butte Girl Is Cited by Pershing for Valor." *Great Falls Tribune*, November 16, 1919.
712 "Switchboard Soldier Dances with Pershing." *Anaconda Standard*, April 25, 1919.
713 No known record reads of Vinnier's and Adam's wartime experiences,
714 Griess, 161-162.
715 Farwell, 224-225.
716 *Billings Gazette*, June 2, 1908.
717 Ibid., August 23, 1907.
718 Montana Memory Project.
719 History of the American Red Cross, 653-654.
720 Ibid.
721 Report of the Surgeon General of the U.S. Army, 1919, 1691-1694.
722 National Archives and Records Administration, Records of the American National Red Cross, 1917-1934, Record Group 200, Box 850, 942.11/102.
723 Ibid.
724 Ibid.
725 Ibid.
726 "Billings Nurse with Army of Occupation." *Billings Gazette*, February 13, 1919.
727 In the official dispatch, O'Day's name is misspelled as "Helen M. Day."
728 History of the American Red Cross, 1476.
729 "History of Base Hospital No. 53." Internet at www.ourstory.info/library/2-ww1/BH53/hosp53.htm.
730 Ibid.
731 National Archives and Records Administration, Records of the American National Red Cross, 1917-1934, Record Group 200, Box 850, 942.11/102.

Chapter 13. Going Home

732 Montana Memory Project.
733 American Battle Monuments Commission.
734 "Nurse Finds Grave of Soldier Brother." *Great Falls Tribune*, March 14, 1919.
735 Internet at https://thelandpatents.com.
736 Montana Memory Project.
737 Annual Report of the Surgeon General of the U.S. Navy, 1918, 109-110.
738 Ibid., 111.
739 American Battle Monuments Commission. Internet at www.abmc.gov.
740 The Trained Nurse and Hospital Review. NY: Lakeside Pub. Co., 1913. 177.

741   Report of the Surgeon General of the U.S. Army, 1919, 1122.
742   Ibid., 1362.
743   History of the American Red Cross, 1011.
744   "New York Society Girls Commit Suicide." *Great Falls Tribune*, January 25, 1919.
745   Obituary of Marcia Lange. *Fennimore* [CA] *Times*, May 25, 1932.
746   Memoirs of Bill Schira. Internet at net.lib.byu.edu.
747   Annual Report of the Surgeon-General of the Navy, 1918; 69.
748   Ibid., 81.
749   "Billings Nurse with Army of Occupation." *Billings Gazette*, February 13, 1919.
750   "Former Warren Nurse Writes from France." Warren Michigan, undated newspaper article.
751   "What the Chevron Means." *Iola* [KS] *Register*, undated.
752   History of the American Red Cross. 1066-1075.
753   Army-Navy Nurse Act of 1947, and Public Law 36, 80th Congress
754   "Miss Mary Vannier Home From Three Years War Work." *Helena Independent Record*, January 18, 1920.
755   "Helena Hello Girl Holds Key Position in Peace Maneuvers." *Great Falls Tribune*, January 4, 1919.
756   Gavin, 92.
757   Ibid., 289.
758   "Siberian Rail Forces Get Veteran Status." *New York Times*, Apr 29, 1973.
759   Ibid., 299-300.
760   History of the American Red Cross, 1018.
761   Ibid., 1019.
762   Ibid., 1129.
763   Diary of Virginia Flanagan. Montana state library.
764   Saunders, Edward E. "John E. Moran, Medal of Honor Biographical Sketch." Unpublished.
765   "Presentation of Medals." *Great Falls Tribune*, July 4, 1919.
766   History and Roster, Cascade County Soldier and Sailors, 1919.
767   "War Conditions Affect Homesteads." *Miles City* [MT] *Star*, undated.

Epilogue

768   The veteran was Jimmy Kerr, U.S. Navy, Vietnam War, from Billings, Montana.
769   Joint veterans' color guard, Billings, Montana.
770   Saunders, Edward E. Commemorative remarks at dedication ceremony, Women's World War I memorial, Billings, Montana, April 6, 2017.
771   The bugler was Mr. Randy Grow, Billings, Montana. Story of the bugle as told by him. Used with his permission.

SELECTED BIBLIOGRAPHY

Books

Bradley, Omar N. *A Soldier's Story*. New York: Holt, 1951.

Bruhn, Gladys. *Memories of Mina. Bruhn*:1982.

Clay, Catrine. *King, Kaiser, Tsar: Three Royal Cousins Who Led the World to War*, London: John Murray, 2006.

Cobbs, Elizabeth. *The Hello Girls: America's First Women Soldiers*. Cambridge: Harvard University Press, 2017.

Craig, Lee A. *Josephus Daniels, His Life and Times*. Chapel Hill: University of North Carolina Press, 2013.

Davison, Henry P. *The American Red Cross in the Great War*. New York: MacMillan, 1919.

Dent, Olive. *A Volunteer Nurse on the Western Front*. London: Random House, 2014.

Dock, Lavina, R.N., Sarah E. Pickett, Clara Noyes, R.N., Fannie Clement, R.N., Elizabeth Fox, R.N., Anna Van Meter. *History of American Red Cross Nursing*, New York: MacMillian, 1922.

Dyer, Gwynne. *War*. New York: Crown Publishers, 1985.

Dumenil, Lynn. *The Second Line of Defense: American Women and World War I*. Chapel Hill: University of North Carolina Press, 2017.

Ebbert, Jean, and Marie-Beth Hall. *The First, The Few, The Forgotten, Navy and Marine Corps Women in World War I*. Annapolis: Naval Institute Press. 2002.

Farwell, Byron. *Over There: The United States in the Great War, 1917-1918*. New York: W. W. Norton, 1999.

Fussell, Paul. *The Great War and Modern Memory*. New York: Stirling Pub. Co. 2009.

Griess, Thomas E. *The Great War: The West Point Military History Series*. Wayne, New Jersey: Avery Pub. Co., 1986.

Hart, Peter. *The Great War*. London: Oxford University Press. 2013.

James, Reginald W (editor). *The Marine Engineer and Naval Architect*. London:1909, 28.

Miller, James Martin, and H.S. Canfield. *The People's War Book*. Cleveland: R. C. Barnum Co. 1920.

Gail, William W. *Yellowstone County, Montana, in the World War, 1917 to 1918*. Billings: War Publishing Co., 1919.

Gavin, Lettie. *They Also Served: American Women in World War I.* Boulder: University of Colorado Press, 1997.

Glasgow and Valley Historical Society. *Glasgow and Valley County.* Charleston, SC: Arcadia Publishing C0, 2010.

Hallett, Christine E. *Veiled Warriors: Allied Nurses of the First World War.* Oxford: Oxford University Press, 2014.

Hart, Peter. *The Great War, A Combat History of the First World War.* Oxford: Oxford University Press, 2013.

Hidy, Ralph W., Muriel E. Hidy, Roy V. Scott, and Don L. Hofsommer. *The Great Northern Railroad, A History.* Minneapolis: University of Minnesota Press, 1988.

Hoeber, Paul. *History of the Pennsylvania Hospital Unit, (Base Hospital No, 10, U.S.A.) In the Great War.* New York, 1921.

Horne, Alistair. *The Price of Glory, Verdun 1916.* New York: Penguin Books, 1964

Hutchinson, John F. *Champions of Charity, War and the Rise of the Red Cross.* Boulder: Westview Press, 1996.

Jensen, Kimberly. *Mobilizing Minerva: American Women in the First World War.* Urbana: University of Illinois Press, 2008.

Jones, Marion M. *The American Red Cross, from Clara Barton to the New Deal.* Baltimore: The John's Hopkins Press, 2013.

Lass, William E. *A History of Steamboating on the Upper Missouri River.* Lincoln: University of Nebraska Press, 1962.

Malone, Michael P. *James J. Hill: Empire Builder of the Northwest.* Norman: University of Oklahoma Press, 1996.

Martin, Albro. *James J. Hill & The Opening of the Northwest.* St. Paul: Minnesota Historical Society Press, 1976.

Massie, Robert K. *Dreadnought: Britain, Germany, and the Coming of the Great War.* New York: Random House, 1991.

McPherson, James. *Battle Cry of Freedom.* New York: Oxford University Press, 1988.

National League of Nursing Education. *Proceedings of the Twenty-Fourth Annual Convention.* Baltimore: Williams and Wilkins, 1919.

Nevins, Allan. *The War for the Union, War Becomes Revolution, 1862-1863.* New York: Schribner's, 1960.

Norman, Elizabeth M. *We Band of Angels: The Untold Story of American Nurses Trapped on Bataan by the Japanese.* New York: Pocket Books, 1999.

Schryver, Grace F. *A History of the Illinois Training School for Nurses.* Chicago: Illinois Training School for Nurses, 1930.

Showell, Jak Mallman. *Battle Beneath the Waves; U-boats at War.* Arms and Armor/Sterling Publishing.

Simpson, Colin. *The Lusitania.* New York: Ballantine Books, 1972.

Stimson, Julia Katherine. *Finding Themselves; the Letters of an American Army Chief Nurse in a British Hospital in France.* New York: MacMillian and Co., 1918.

Terraine, J. *The Road to Passchendaele: The Flanders Offensive, 1917.* London: Leo Cooper, 1997.

Tuchman, Barbara W. *The Guns of August.* New York: Ballantine Books, [1962] 1994.

---------- *The Zimmerman Telegram.* New York: Ballantine Books, [1958] 1994.

Venzon, Anne Cipriano, ed. *The United States in the First World War: An Encyclopedia.* New York: Garland, 1999.

Welsh, Joe, Bill Howes, and Kevin J. Holland. *The Cars of Pullman.* Minneapolis: Voyageur Press, 2010.

Western Union Telegraph Co. *The Western Union Telegraph Directory.* New York: 1874.

Wigle, Shari Lynn. *Pride of America, We're With You: The Letters of Grace Anderson U.S. Army Nurse Corps, WWI.* Rockville, MD: Seaboard Press, 2007.

Zeiger, Susan. *In Uncle Sam's Service: Women Workers with the American Expeditionary Force, 1917-1919.* Philadelphia: University of Pennsylvania Press, 2004.

Government Documents

Blair, Emily N. *The Women's Committee of the United States Council of National Defense.* Washington D.C.: Government Printing Office, 1920.

Budreau, Lisa M. and Lt. Col. Richard M. Prior, eds. *Answering the Call: The U.S. Army Nurse Corps, 1917-1919, A Commemorative Tribute to Military Nursing in World War I.*, Washington D.C.: Government Printing Office, Office of the Surgeon General, Department of the Army, 2008.

Commission Appointed By The President To Investigate The Conduct Of The War Department In The War With Spain, Vol 1. Washington D.C.: Gov'n't Printing Office, 1899.

Department of the Navy. Annual Report of the Surgeon-General for Fiscal Year 1918. Washington D.C. Gvnt Printing Office: 1918.

Department of the Interior. *Annual Report for Fiscal Year 1897, Vol 3.* Washington D.C.: Gvnt Printing Office: 1897.

Director of the Bureau of War Risk Insurance. Annual Report for 1920. Washington D.C., Gvnt Printing office: 1920.

Feller, Carolyn M. Lt.Col., and Constance J. Moore, Major, eds. *Highlights in the History of the Army Nurse Corps.* Washington D.C.: U.S. Army Center of Military History, 1995.

Griess, Thomas E. ed. *Atlas for the Great War: The West Point Military History Series.* Wayne, NJ: Avery Publishing, 1986.

Regulations Governing the Organization and Administration of the Naval Reserve Force. Washington D.C.: Gov'n't Printing Office, 1918.

Sarnecky, Mary T., Col, USA (ret). *A Contemporary History of the U.S. Army Nurse Corps.* Washington D.C.: Government Printing Office, Office of the Surgeon General, Department of the Army, 2010.

United States Shipping Board, Second Annual Report. Wash D.C., Gvn't Printing Office. 1918.

Manuscript Collections

Montana Historical Society, Helena, Montana.

Montana Memory Project.

Goins, Kathy. Unpublished papers of Lucy Walters, U.S. Army Nurse Corps.

Bridgewater, Octavia, Anna Sherrick, Henrietta Crocket, Catherine Flynn, Lily Morris, Hazel Uppington. *Nursing in Montana.* Montana Nurses Association. Undated.

Walters, William D. and Vernon Beck. *An Illinois Nurse in Europe, The Letters of Zella Maude Judy, 1917-1920.*

Newspapers and News Periodicals

Asheville (NC) Citizen-Times

Baltimore Sun

Billings (MT) Gazette

Brooklyn (NY) Life

Selected Bibliography

Brooklyn (NY) Daily Eagle
Buffalo (NY) Commerical
Butte (MT) Daily Post
Butte (MT) Independent
Conrad (MT) Independent
Daily Missoulian, Missoula, MT
Fallon County (MT) Times
Fennimore (CA) Times
Fergus County [MT] Democrat
Flathead (MT) Beacon
Fort Mills [SC] Times
Franklin (IN) Evening Star
Glasgow (MT) Courier
Greenville [SC] News
Harlem (MT) Enterprise
Harrisburg (PA) Telegraph
Havre (MT) Herald
Helena (MT) Independent Record
Inland Empire. Moore, MT
Kalispell (MT) Bee
Last Best News. Billings, Montana. (Internet news).
Leavenworth (WA) Echo
Miles City (MT) Daily Star
Miles City (MT) Independent
Montana Standard
Newport News (VA) Daily Press
New York Times
New York Tribune

Oregon Daily Journal
Park City (UT) Record
Rochester (NY) Democrat
Ronan (MT) Pioneer
Roswell (NM) Daily Record
Santa Fe New Mexican
Tacoma (WA) Times
Topeka (KS) State Journal
Yellowstone (Glendive, MT) Monitor
Yorkville [York, SC] Enquirer

Magazines and Periodicals

Rote, Nelle Fairchild. "Nurse Helen Fairchild, My Aunt, My Hero." Daughters of the American Revolution Magazine, November 1997, Vol 131, N0. 9

American Journal of Nursing. Baltimore: American Journal of Nursing Company.

American Red Cross. *The Red Cross Bulletin.*

————*Red Cross Magazine*

Collier's Magazine

Saturday Evening Post

Internet

Great Northern Railway-Steam Locomotives. Internet at www.gngoat.org/gn_steam_locomotives.htm.

Grand Union Hotel. Internet at www.visitmt.com/listings/general/hotel-motel/frand-union-hotel.html.

Montana Memory Project. Military Enlistments (Montana) World War I. Records of the Montana Adjutant General's Office. RS 223. Montana State Library, Helena, MT. Internet at www.mtmemory.org.

Washington Historical Quarterly.

Unpublished papers.

Saunders, Edward E. Biographical Sketch of Eula Bernice Butzerin. Laurel, MT, 2017.

Index

A

Aasen, Mina Andy xviii, 121
Adams, Marie Paul 182, 208
AEF. *See* American Expeditionary Force
Alice Hough Ralston xiv
American Battle Monuments Commission 224, 281
American Battle Monuments Commisson 224
American Civil War. *See* Civil War
American Expeditionary Force 90, 91, 92, 133, 134, 147, 157, 173, 174, 181, 182, 184, 189, 192, 193, 194, 195, 196, 197, 198, 201, 202, 203, 204, 207, 208, 209, 210, 212, 213, 214, 224, 225, 229
American Federation of Nurses 62, 63
American Journal of Nursing 60, 62, 112, 136, 262, 270, 271, 274, 275, 276
American Legion 230, 260, 276
American National Red Cross Society. *See* American Red Cross
American Nurses Association 63, 230
American Red Cross xvii, xx, 17, 57, 58, 59, 60, 61, 62, 63, 67, 68, 69, 89, 95, 96, 97, 98, 99, 103, 104, 107, 108, 109, 112, 126, 127, 134, 135, 137, 138, 145, 148, 153, 154, 157, 162, 166, 169, 194, 198, 201, 202, 209, 213, 230, 232, 243
American Telephone and Telegraph Company 178, 181

Ames, Florence 41, 42, 43, 54, 55, 120, 239, 240
Amiens, France 192
ANC. *See* Army Nurse Corps
Anderson-Roy, Lena 179, 180, 183
ARC. *See* American Red Cross
Arlee, Montana 182
Arlington National Cemetery xix, 92, 224, 245, 260
Army Appropriations Act 151
Army Nurse Corps xiv, xviii, xix, xx, 12, 25, 26, 54, 62, 64, 66, 67, 68, 69, 92, 97, 103, 109, 116, 117, 121, 122, 123, 126, 131, 137, 138, 145, 147, 149, 157, 158, 190, 192, 195, 198, 200, 201, 202, 204, 206, 207, 209, 214, 224, 225, 228, 229, 240, 241, 242, 243, 244, 245, 246, 247
Army Nursing Reserve 68
Army Reorganization Bill 66, 229
Army Signal Corps xiv, 173, 174, 178, 179, 180, 182, 183, 208, 229, 240, 243, 246, 247, 248, 249, 251, 254, 255
   Hello Girls xiv
Army War College 179
Arras, France 186, 192
Arthur, Chester A. 58

B

Baker, Newton, Sec of War 34, 93, 101, 117, 172, 194, 195, 248
Banker, Grace 182, 229
Barrow, Minnie 104
Barton, Clara 13, 45, 57, 58, 59, 60, 62
Base Hospital 2 96
Base Hospital 3, Navy 184
Base Hospital 4 96
Base Hospital 5 96, 97
Base Hospital 10 96

Base Hospital 12 96
Base Hospital 15 200, 201, 204, 207, 208, 209
Base Hospital 18 198
Base Hospital 21 96
Base Hospital 28 153, 154, 221
Base Hospital 43 196, 209
Base Hospital 53 212, 213, 214, 222, 225
Base Hospital 57 202
Base Hospital 88 212, 213
Base Hospitals 95, 96, 107, 112, 127, 138, 153, 169, 189, 190, 192, 195, 198, 212, 225, 227, 264
Bataan, Philippine Islands xviii, 120, 123, 124, 240, 272
Becker, Bertha 26, 240
Bell, Bessie S. 127, 175, 195, 251, 257
Belleau Wood, Battle of 169, 197
Benbow, Cebron 204, 246
Benbow, Thomas 204
Bennett, Mrs. Lester 55
Biddles, Florence 213, 214, 241, 253, 254
Billings, Montana xii, xiii, xviii, xx, 2, 41, 43, 45, 54, 55, 68, 70, 104, 111, 120, 147, 196, 209, 213, 226, 237, 240, 241, 242, 245, 247, 248, 260, 261, 266, 268, 271, 281, 282
Blackwell, Elizabeth MD 44
Black women in US Navy 78
Blaine County, Montana 18
Blois, France 195, 196, 202
Boardman, Mable Thorp 61, 62, 68
Bohart, Ruby 55, 240
Boles, Kate 119
Bowles, Charles S. 56
Bowling, Gertrude 206
British General Hospital 16 171
British Women's Voluntary Aid Detachment 170
Brown, Ethel Lezie 26
Brunelle, Clara 146
Buckles, Frank xiv
Bureau of Information, Nurses 230
Bureau of Navigation, US Navy 78, 79
Bureau of War Risk Insurance 154
Burlingame, James M. 48, 144
Butte, Montana xii, xiv, xvi, xviii, 4, 5, 6, 15, 16, 26, 36, 40, 45, 49, 54, 55, 70, 71, 72, 73, 75, 84, 96, 97, 106, 113, 119, 127, 132, 133, 135, 147, 175, 177, 181, 182, 184, 196, 213, 222, 243, 246, 249, 262, 266, 268, 270, 271, 273, 276, 278, 281, 287
Butzerin, Arthur 222
Butzerin, Eula xix, 153, 154, 221, 241, 260
Butzerin, Roy 222

C

Camp Custer, Michigan 127
Camp Devens, Massachusetts 130
Camp Dodge, Iowa 105, 118, 119, 120, 128, 131, 132, 137, 151, 222, 272
Camp Funston, Kansas 113, 114, 116, 131, 151
Camp Kearney, California 134, 149, 151
Camp Lewis 12, 20, 21, 26, 54, 103, 105, 106, 107, 131, 135, 148, 151, 263
Canon, Alice 183, 279
Cariher, Margaret 127
Cascade County, Montana 16, 17, 110, 231, 232, 282
Casualty Clearing Stations 189, 190, 192
Central Pacific Railroad 3, 6

Champagne, France 209
Chateau-Thierry, France 197, 200, 202, 203, 204, 205, 209, 210, 222, 223
Chaumont, France 173, 182, 198, 201, 204, 212, 213
Children's Bureau, Dept of the Interior 9
Chinook, Montana 18
Choteau County, Montana 18, 74, 99
Christensen, Anna 113, 114
Civil War 13, 18, 23, 28, 29, 30, 31, 33, 34, 38, 44, 45, 52, 56, 57, 63, 79, 116, 124, 145, 263
Clayton, Gladys R. 53
Cleveland, Grover 76, 77
Cokedale, Montana xvi, xviii, 147, 196, 203, 204
Columbus, Montana 203, 204
Committee on Nursing 89, 94, 95
Connor, Sally 184
Conscription. *See* Draft
Corregidor 124
Council of National Defense 93, 94, 95, 108, 109
Crab, Rolla 15
Craig, Cora V. xvii, 26, 202, 241
Croix de Guerre 212
Crowder, BG Enoch 38
Cullop, Artie 82
Curran, Anna 126

D

Daigle, Martha 184
Daniels, Josephus 2, 3, 4, 5, 6, 7, 8, 9, 10, 17, 18, 25, 33, 37, 143, 229
Daughters of the American Revolution 64
Davison, Maude C. 123
Deer Lodge, Montana 45, 102, 123, 161, 177, 242, 243, 250, 276

DeFao, Joseph 17
Delano, Jane A. 68, 69, 97, 98, 107, 126, 134, 137
Dent, Olive 191
Dewey, Admiral Thomas 140
Dix, Dorothea 45
Dobias, Ann 26, 227, 233, 280
Doerr, Aimee 127
Dolan, Josephine 127
Draft xiii, 4, 13, 15, 19, 25, 28, 29, 30, 31, 33, 34, 35, 36, 37, 38, 39, 40, 66, 71, 72, 105, 107, 118, 130
Dunlop, Margaret A. 171, 187
Duval, Mary 127

E

Ecury-sur-Coole, France 209
Egan, Merle 180, 181, 220, 229
Elderkins, Mary US Navy 205
Elder, Vera May
   Yeomanette 72
Ellis Island 152, 153, 154, 155, 162
Evacuation Hospital 4 208, 209, 210, 212, 214
Evacuation Hospital 5 200, 201
Evacuation Hospital 6 198, 199, 202
Evacuation Hospitals xviii, 198
Evans, John Morgan 35
Evashenko, Billy 17

F

Fairchild, Helen 96, 170, 189, 190
Fergus County, Montana 209
Field Hospital 109 205
Field Hospital 110 205
Field Hospital 111 205
Field Hospital 112 205, 206, 207
Field Hospitals 124, 200, 205, 212
Fitzsimons, William T. 109, 271
Flanagan, Virginia 99, 100, 117, 134, 147, 149, 196, 202, 231,

233, 242, 270, 272, 280, 282
Flynn, Catherine 47, 266
Ford, Florence 26
Fort Benton, Montana 4, 5, 6, 18, 45, 72, 73, 74, 75, 99, 102, 231, 268
Fort Riley 105, 113, 114, 115, 116, 131, 138, 150, 151, 202, 204, 209, 218
Fort Shaw, Montana 102
Fourth Marine Brigade 197
Fousek, Albert J. 126
Fousek, Lydia 120, 126, 128, 131, 132
Fowler, Effie 196
French Army 167
Frey, Annabelle 113
Friedlander, Ensign Eugene J. 70, 71, 72, 268
Friend, Bernice 126
Fromerville, France 210, 211, 212
Frontiers, Battle of the 167

G

Geneva Convention of 1864 56, 58
George, David Lloyd 185
Germany 32, 35, 40, 61, 90, 141, 142, 167, 185, 192, 202, 226, 227
Gibson, Grace 105, 147, 148, 196
Gibson, Paris 4, 10, 262
Gibson, Paris, Montana senator 4, 10, 262
Glasgow, Montana
  Founding of 1
  Glasgow women in WWI 26
  Land lottery office at 10
  Layout of 8
  Lucy Walters departs from 12, 20
  Lucy Walters writes home 106
  Mark Hoyt, mayor of 5
  Nurses arriving at BH43 196
  Oriental Limited stops at 148
  Preparations for land lottery 11
  Quota of draftees depart 17
  Siding 45 7
  Vigilantes at 2
Goethals, General George W. 194, 195
Gonczy, Emeline 113
Great Falls, Montana xii, xviii, xix, 4, 5, 6, 10, 11, 13, 14, 15, 17, 36, 39, 46, 48, 49, 70, 72, 74, 75, 76, 81, 83, 99, 100, 105, 110, 113, 117, 120, 121, 125, 126, 127, 128, 129, 131, 132, 133, 144, 147, 196, 213, 225, 231, 232, 233
Great Northern Railway 3, 6, 7, 8, 10, 11, 12, 14, 15, 21, 22, 25, 70, 143, 148, 162, 261, 263
Gregory, Mary 120, 126, 243
Grimmeke, Celia 181, 220

H

Haig, Field Marshal Douglas 186
Hall, Mary 196, 276
Hamilton, Montana 36, 88
Hardee, William, convicted killer 1
Harding, Warren G. 37, 115
Harrison, Benjamin 77
Havre, Montana xviii, 6, 8, 10, 18, 73, 125, 148, 171, 225, 244, 251, 268
Helena, Montana xii, 4, 5, 6, 14, 20, 45, 54, 55, 69, 70, 73, 87, 88, 89, 94, 102, 103, 127, 144, 177, 180, 181, 203, 229, 243, 251, 260, 261, 263, 266, 267, 271, 282
Hello Girls 174, 182, 277, 278. *See* Army Signal Corps
Higbee, Lenah S. 67
Hill, Charles, posse member killed 2
Hill County, Montana 18

Index

Hill, James J. 2, 3, 4, 5, 6, 7, 8, 9, 10, 18, 25, 33, 37, 143
Hodgson, Violet 101
Hornkey, Ella 119
Hovland, John 17
Hoyt, Mark MD 5, 25
Hughes, Margaret 55, 69, 87, 88, 89, 98, 103, 104, 105, 112, 133, 138, 243, 269
Hume, Minnie 120, 126
Hutton, Alma 120, 126

I

ICRC 57, 58, 59, 61
Influenza Epidemic xv, xix, 131, 133, 134, 136, 137, 179
International Committee of the Red Cross. *See* ICRC
Ireland, MGen Merritte W. MD 91

J

Jellicoe, Admiral Sir John 142
Johnson, Alice 81, 83, 244, 268
Johnson, Maj Hugh 38, 81, 82, 83, 244, 253, 256, 268
Johnson, Opha May 82
Jorgensen, Sigrid M. 156, 209, 210, 211, 214
Jutland, Battle of 141

K

Kell, Johnsie 53, 54, 266
Kingdom of Siam 202
King George V 166
Kinney, Dita H. 67
Kyte, Sylvia 126

L

LaFournaise, Louise xvii
Lange, Marcia xviii, 225, 244, 251, 256, 260, 282
Lange, Marsha xviii, 244, 282

Langres, France 212, 213, 214
Larson, Fannie 127
Larson, Genevieve 184
Laurel, Montana xiii, 213, 245, 260
Letterman Army General Hospital 127
Lewistown, Montana 122, 180, 183, 209, 243, 244, 252
Limoges, France 221, 222
Lindeberg, Louise 113
Liverpool, England 130, 146, 147, 154, 163, 164, 165, 169, 170, 172, 182, 278
Lusitania 32, 142

M

MacCauley, Margaret 196
Malta, Montana xii, 8, 15, 18, 27, 133, 148, 242, 247, 252
Manila, Philippine Islands 23, 121, 122, 124, 140
Marine Corps, US 82, 197, 205, 232, 269
Marne, Battle of the 167, 198, 199, 201, 202, 203, 204, 207, 208, 209, 222
Marshall, Geroge C. 208
Marshall, Lucy A. 55
Martin, Julia 127
Martin, Margaret 127
McCarthy, Katherine US Navy 205
McClelland, Helen G. 170, 190
McGee, Anita N. MD 64, 66, 67
McGinnis, Martin 4
McIntyre-Early, Regina xviii, 137, 273
McIsaac, Isabel 68
Mecklenberg, Dora 104
Melia, Catherine 127
Menzies, Bell 127
Messner, Elizabeth V. 122
Meuse-Argonne American Cemetery 222

Meuse-Argonne Offensive 199
Miles City, Montana xii, 14, 28, 52, 53, 54, 101, 113, 213, 244, 245, 252, 262, 264, 266, 282
   Eastern Montana Veterans Cemetery 28
   Miles City WWI nurses 53
Miller, Dorothy 127
Minot, North Dakota 6, 99, 121, 124, 125, 240, 244
Mobile Hospital 1 202
Mobile Hospitals 201
Montana Association of Graduate Nurses 46
Montana Central Railway 5
Montana Graduate Nurses Association 48, 89
Montana Naval Forces Monument 73
Moran, John E. Medal of Honor 232
Morse, Samuel F. B. 102

N

National Defense Act of 1916 33, 92, 269
National Guard 14, 34, 38, 39, 59, 90, 92, 105, 109, 114, 169
National Security League 32
Navy Cruiser and Transport Force 225
Navy Nurse Corps xiv, 67, 68, 83, 97, 184, 240, 248, 250, 251, 252, 253, 254, 255, 256, 257, 258, 259
Newlands Act of 1902 8
New Mexico 23, 24, 25, 107, 247
New York City xix, 23, 30, 58, 67, 68, 88, 96, 97, 101, 104, 108, 128, 137, 138, 145, 147, 148, 150, 151, 152, 154, 155, 156, 157, 158, 160, 162, 169, 178, 181, 182, 200, 231, 245, 278

New York City Draft Riot 30
Nightingale, Florence 42, 44, 57
Nivelle, Robert Georges 185
Northern Pacific Railroad 4, 5, 6, 9, 10, 14, 52, 54, 153
Noyes, Clara 103, 104, 126, 169, 230
Nye, Sylvene 212

O

O'Day, Harriett xviii, 147, 150, 196, 209, 212, 226, 245, 248, 257, 281
O'Donnell, Katherine 127
Oise-Aisne American Cemetery 223
Oise-Aisne Offensive 201, 223
Oldhouse, Nellie 119
Olson, Olaf 17
Opp, May 127
Oriental Limited 12, 13, 17, 21, 22, 23, 148, 152, 263
Orleans, France 195
Osborne, Maude 213, 248, 258

P

Paris, France 4, 10, 151, 167, 172, 173, 174, 175, 182, 183, 185, 186, 195, 197, 198, 200, 201, 202, 203, 207, 221, 222, 224, 229, 262, 280
Paris Peace Conference 229
Passchendaele, Battle of 168, 184, 187, 188
Patterson, Elizabeth 73, 268
Patton, George S. Jr. 208
Pershing, Gen John J. 91, 92, 134, 168, 172, 173, 174, 179, 180, 181, 182, 193, 194, 195, 197, 207, 208, 209, 212, 213, 224, 281
Peters, Cleo 127
Peterson, Elsie 126

Index

Phillips County, Montana xii, 15, 18
Post-Traumatic Stress Disorder 225

R

Rackham, Evelyn 126
Ralston, Alice xiv, 26, 96, 97, 147, 169, 170, 172, 184, 187, 188, 189, 192, 195, 227, 246, 249
Rankin, Jeanette 32, 36
Ray, Joan Nicholson 122
Reed, Elta 127
Relative Rank for Nurses 228, 229
Research Hospital, Kansas City 24
Richardson, Linna G. 69
Rickham, Susannah 126
Roosevelt, Theodore 32, 33, 34, 35, 37, 38, 59, 60, 64, 77, 264, 265
Rouen, France 190, 192, 193
Ruff, Clara 213, 225, 246, 251, 258

S

Samson, Anne xix
Sandelius, Elizabeth "Sandy" xviii, 147, 150, 196, 203, 204, 205, 207, 246, 249, 258, 275, 280
Santo Tomas Internment Camp 121
Savenay, France 196, 225, 226, 231
Selective Service. *See* Draft, the
Sherry, Helen
  Yeomanette 72, 73, 75, 246
Ship Convoys 130, 143, 144, 146, 147, 163, 164, 187, 190
Shira, Bill 225
Shortreed, Elizabeth 127
Silver Star Medal 192
Sisters of Charity of Leavenworth 45, 51
Sloane, Gertrude 144, 145, 184, 201, 274

Small, Katherine 127
Snearly, Charles, murder victim 2
Somme, Battle of the 35, 167, 168, 185, 277
Somme River 167
Soreng, Knute 17
Spanish-American War 34, 59, 63, 64, 66, 77, 91, 224, 233
SS Mongolia Deck Gun Tragedy 161
Stabler, Erma 127
Stars and Stripes newspaper 182
Sterling, Elizabeth 101, 213, 247
Sternberg, BG George M. 63, 64, 65, 66, 68, 121, 122, 123
Stevens, John F. 6, 7, 72
St. Ignatius, Montana 137, 182, 246
Stillwater County, Montana 203
St. Mihiel, France 207, 208
St. Paul, Minneapolis & Manitoba Railway 4, 5, 6
Strutzel, Mary 127
Student Nurse Reserve 109, 110, 111, 271

T

Taft, William H. 59, 61
Talcott, Agnes 111
Telegraph 9, 102, 103
Thirteenth Naval District, US Navy 70, 75
Thompson, Bertha 127
Thompson, Dora E. 158
Thompson, Margaret 120, 126
Tours, France 182, 183, 195, 229
Truman, Harry S. 208
Truscott, Fred 17

U

U-boats 141, 142, 144, 161, 162, 169
Union Pacific Railroad 3, 6, 102
United States Railroad Administra-

tion 152
United States Sanitary Commission 44, 45, 56, 57
United States Shipping Board 143, 274
U.S. First Infantry Division 168, 178
U.S. Second Infantry Division 168, 169

V

Valley County, Montana xii, 1, 2, 3, 13, 17, 18, 19, 21, 25, 26, 106, 133, 233, 244, 260, 261, 262, 263, 264, 265
Vannier, Mary 177, 178, 208, 229, 247, 278, 282
Vatne, John 17
Verdun xviii, 35, 167, 185, 199, 208, 209, 210, 211, 212
Verdun, Battle of 167
Veterans Administration 230
Vineyard, Henrietta 113, 115, 247
Virginia City, Montana 45, 99, 102
Vladivostok, Siberia 154, 222
Vollmer, Francis 127

W

Walsh, Loretta P. 78, 268
Walter Reed Army Hospital 128
Walters, Lucy xiv, xviii, 11, 12, 21, 23, 27, 103, 104, 105, 133, 140, 147, 148, 164, 196, 233, 242, 247, 263, 264, 271
War Risk Insurance 154, 275
WCAR 44
Welborn, Susie xix, xx, 46, 51, 52, 53, 213, 222, 223, 247, 252, 259, 270
Welborn, Ulysses 222
Welter, Katherine 126
Western Union Telegraph 102, 285
White, Cassie 212

Williams, Jack, Valley County deputy sheriff killed 2
Wilson, Woodrow xvii, 10, 31, 32, 33, 34, 36, 37, 38, 61, 77, 90, 92, 93, 135, 151, 172, 197, 229, 264, 265
Winters, Charlotte Berry xv
Women's Christian Temperance Union 15
Women's Telephone Unit of the American Signal Corps 174, 240
Worden, Montana 105
Wright, Irma Myrtle 76
WTU. *See* Women's Telephone Unit of the American Signal Corps

Y

Yeomanettes, US Navy 79, 80, 81, 82, 85, 268
Yeoman, US Navy xiv, xv, 19, 26, 68, 70, 71, 72, 75, 76, 77, 78, 79, 80, 81, 84, 85, 229, 241, 242, 243, 244, 245, 246, 247, 268
YMCA 179, 213
Ypres, Belgium 185, 186, 187, 188, 190, 201
YWCA 183

Z

Zerr, Gertrude Alice 19, 76, 84, 85, 252, 259

ABOUT THE AUTHOR

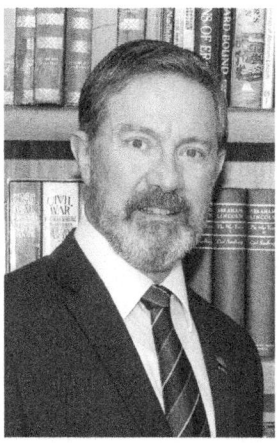

Edward E. "Ed" Saunders is a retired lieutenant colonel, U.S. Army. He served a career in the regular Army, and is a veteran of the Persian Gulf War. Saunders grew to manhood in the American West. He directed the effort to create the World War I Women's Memorial in Billings, Montana. Saunders previously wrote, "*Sentinels, The History of Yellowstone National Cemetery, From Prairie to Hallowed Ground.*" He and his wife live in Laurel, Montana.

Made in the USA
Coppell, TX
30 March 2024

30728686R10187